THE FUNDAMENTAL MECHANISMS OF SHOCK

Volume 1
THE RETICULOENDOTHELIAL SYSTEM AND ATHEROSCLEROSIS
Edited by N. R. Di Luzio and R. Paoletti • 1967

Volume 2
PHARMACOLOGY OF HORMONAL POLYPEPTIDES AND PROTEINS
Edited by N. Back, L. Martini, and R. Paoletti • 1968

Volume 3
GERM-FREE BIOLOGY: Experimental and Clinical Aspects
Edited by E. A. Mirand and N. Back • 1969

Volume 4
DRUGS AFFECTING LIPID METABOLISM
Edited by W. L. Holmes, L. A. Carlson, and R. Paoletti • 1969

Volume 5
LYMPHATIC TISSUE AND GERMINAL CENTERS IN IMMUNE RESPONSE
Edited by L. Fiore-Donati and M. G. Hanna, Jr. • 1969

Volume 6
RED CELL METABOLISM AND FUNCTION
Edited by George J. Brewer • 1970

Volume 7
SURFACE CHEMISTRY OF BIOLOGICAL SYSTEMS
Edited by Martin Blank • 1970

Volume 8
BRADYKININ AND RELATED KININS: Cardiovascular, Biochemical, and Neural Actions
Edited by F. Sicuteri, M. Rocha e Silva, and N. Back • 1970

Volume 9
SHOCK: Biochemical, Pharmacological, and Clinical Aspects
Edited by A. Bertelli and N. Back • 1970

Volume 10
THE HUMAN TESTIS
Edited by E. Rosemberg and C. A. Paulsen • 1970

Volume 11
MUSCLE METABOLISM DURING EXERCISE
Edited by B. Pernow and B. Saltin • 1971

Volume 12
MORPHOLOGICAL AND FUNCTIONAL ASPECTS OF IMMUNITY
Edited by K. Lindahl-Kiessling, G. Alm, and M. G. Hanna, Jr. • 1971

Volume 13
CHEMISTRY AND BRAIN DEVELOPMENT
Edited by R. Paoletti and A. N. Davison • 1971

Volume 14
MEMBRANE-BOUND ENZYMES
Edited by G. Porcellati and F. di Jeso • 1971

Volume 15
THE RETICULOENDOTHELIAL SYSTEM AND IMMUNE PHENOMENA
Edited by N. R. Di Luzio and K. Flemming • 1971

Volume 16A
THE ARTERY AND THE PROCESS OF ARTERIOSCLEROSIS: Pathogenesis
Edited by Stewart Wolf • 1971

Volume 16B
THE ARTERY AND THE PROCESS OF ARTERIOSCLEROSIS: Measurement and Modification
Edited by Stewart Wolf • 1972

Volume 17
CONTROL OF RENIN SECRETION
Edited by Tatiana A. Assaykeen • 1972

Volume 18
THE DYNAMICS OF MERISTEM CELL POPULATIONS
Edited by Morton W. Miller and Charles C. Kuehnert • 1972

Volume 19
SPHINGOLIPIDS, SPHINGOLIPIDOSES AND ALLIED DISORDERS
Edited by Bruno W. Volk and Stanley M. Aronson • 1972

Volume 20
DRUG ABUSE: Nonmedical Use of Dependence-Producing Drugs
Edited by Simon Btesh • 1972

Volume 21
VASOACTIVE POLYPEPTIDES
Edited by N. Back and F. Sicuteri • 1972

Volume 22
COMPARATIVE PATHOPHYSIOLOGY OF CIRCULATORY DISTURBANCES
Edited by Colin M. Bloor • 1972

Volume 23
THE FUNDAMENTAL MECHANISMS OF SHOCK
Edited by Lerner B. Hinshaw and Barbara G. Cox • 1972

THE FUNDAMENTAL MECHANISMS OF SHOCK

Proceedings of a Symposium Held in Oklahoma City, Oklahoma, October 1-2, 1971

Sponsored by
UNITED STATES NAVY PROJECT THEMIS

and THE UNIVERSITY OF OKLAHOMA
HEALTH SCIENCES CENTER
The University of Oklahoma Medical School
The Oklahoma Medical Research Foundation
The Veterans Administration Hospital

Edited by
Lerner B. Hinshaw
Veterans Administration Hospital
Departments of Physiology–Biophysics and Surgery
University of Oklahoma Health Sciences Center
Oklahoma City, Oklahoma

and

Barbara G. Cox
Editorial Consultant
Learning Resources Center
University of Oklahoma Health Sciences Center
Oklahoma City, Oklahoma

PLENUM PRESS • NEW YORK–LONDON • 1972

Library of Congress Catalog Card Number 72 - 77225
ISBN-13:978-1-4615-9016-3 e-ISBN-13: 978-1-4615-9014-9
DOI: 10.1007/978-1-4615-9014-9

Softcover reprint of the hardcover 1st edition 1972
A Division of Plenum Publishing Corporation
227 West 17th Street, New York, N. Y. 10011

United Kingdom edition published by Plenum Press, London
A Division of Plenum Publishing Company, Ltd.
Davis House (4th Floor), 8 Scrubs Lane, Harlesden, London,
NW10 6SE, England

UNITED STATES NAVY PROJECT THEMIS RESEARCH GROUP

Petar Alaupovic, Ph.D.
Cardiovascular Section
Oklahoma Medical Research Foundation
Oklahoma City, Oklahoma

Jacqueline J. Coalson, Ph.D.
Department of Pathology
University of Oklahoma Medical Center
Oklahoma City, Oklahoma

Ervin G. Erdös, M.D.
Department of Pharmacology
University of Oklahoma Medical Center
Oklahoma City, Oklahoma

Lazar J. Greenfield, M.D.
Department of Surgery
University of Oklahoma Medical Center
Oklahoma City, Oklahoma

Clarence A. Guenter, M.D.
Department of Medicine
University of Oklahoma Medical Center
Oklahoma City, Oklahoma

Chesterfield G. Gunn, M.D.
Department of Medicine
University of Oklahoma Medical Center
Oklahoma City, Oklahoma

Lerner B. Hinshaw, Ph.D.
Department of Physiology-Biophysics
University of Oklahoma Medical Center
Oklahoma City, Oklahoma

Donald D. Holmes, D.V.M.
Department of Pathology
University of Oklahoma Medical Center
Oklahoma City, Oklahoma

Eugene D. Jacobson, M.D.
Department of Physiology
University of Texas Medical School at Houston
Houston, Texas

This volume is dedicated to
The United States Navy Project THEMIS
whose resources and encouragement have
so greatly advanced our knowledge of
the mechanisms and therapy of shock

FOREWORD[1]

Research, to which so much discussion and thought will be devoted at this symposium, appears to have been downgraded in our society. Yet, learning and education *per se* rank high in our set of values, from the point of view of both lay people and professional workers. For some reason, we fail to detect the illogic inherent in this value system—for, what is research but the learning of *new* information? Apparently our society associates "learning" only with known, long-gathered information.

This symposium, I believe, will generate new information about shock through the integration of knowledge of many investigators, who have come to share a common meeting ground. Hopefully, the worth of this and similar endeavors will gain the recognition and, more important, the support of the public. In the next decade or so, I believe that shock research workers will be channeling their efforts more and more into investigating the repair of damaged cells. The individual cell and its products must be scrutinized just as carefully as we examine the whole organism or its collections of cells.

Shock is an exciting area of research, but it involves years of painstaking work. Moreover, the society which will reap its fruits must be persuaded to share the burden of its support.

John A. Schilling, M.D.

---

[1]Abstracted from Dr. John A. Schilling's *Opening Statement* at the symposium on October 1, 1971.

PREFACE

A concerned group of approximately forty investigators from the United States and Canada met in Oklahoma City in 1964 to carry out experiments on animals in endotoxin shock. Nearly all of the proposed and then-current forms of therapy to prevent irreversible shock and death were attempted (J. Okla. State Med. Assoc. 59:407-484, 1966). Unfortunately, no clearly demonstrable therapeutic benefits accrued from this massive effort. However, this meeting was without historic precedence, marking the first time in which reportedly successful therapies had been attempted on a large scale. The results left most investigators puzzled and disappointed, and a pall descended over many laboratories of shock research. It seemed clear that we had failed to penetrate the hidden barriers to our understanding of the mechanisms of endotoxin shock. Even as this postmortem is laid bare eight years later, we still have no unequivocal proof of the precise chain of events leading to irreversible shock and death.

Since the Shock Tour of 1964, the Oklahoma research group has regularly examined its position relative to an understanding of endotoxin shock. The critical need to clarify its mechanisms became apparent at that time, and we set to work conceiving experimental designs which might solve the problem. A great deal of research has been accomplished. Yet it appears that we are still skirting the core of the shock problem, endlessly wrestling with peripheral components, but never quite reaching the basic mechanisms. We have not advanced far enough in sequentially dissecting out those critical pathophysiological events early in shock which most assuredly lead to the irreversible state.

The Oklahoma-based U.S. Navy Project THEMIS research group, activated in 1968 and composed of surgeons, internists, physiologists, pathologists, pharmacologists, and biochemists, represents the faculties and staff of the University of Oklahoma Medical School, the Veterans Administration Hospital, and the Oklahoma Medical Research Foundation. This group has attacked experimental septic shock with a wide spectrum of approaches, ranging from molecular to clinical studies. At times, we have become discouraged.

The obstacles which block our understanding of the intimate mechanisms in shock have often seemed insurmountable.

Nevertheless, these interdisciplinary efforts have stimulated an underlying conviction that the shock problem will be most effectively solved by vigorous team research. Well-trained, highly motivated investigators from the basic and clinical sciences must join together in a concerted effort to sort out and define the fundamental mechanisms in shock. The results of such studies are most likely to yield clinically applicable therapeutic procedures.

In the spirit of this approach, we met with investigators from the United States, Canada, and Europe in Oklahoma City in October, 1971, to encourage an exchange of data and ideas, and hopefully to begin to unravel the fundamental mysteries of shock. These meetings were unique. A single, topically oriented conference provided a forum for an interdisciplinary group of research workers who might otherwise never have met in a single conference room for cross-pollination and challenge of one another's ideas. We hope that this symposium has proven its worth and that it establishes a pattern for future meetings.

The pages that follow represent a compilation of the latest findings, hypotheses, ideas, and suggestions of a dedicated group of investigators. The mosaic which emerges provides insight into many of the interlocking mechanisms which operate during shock. We hope that both our present and future colleagues, in all areas of research, will find this volume a useful tool.

Lerner B. Hinshaw, Ph.D.

ACKNOWLEDGMENTS

We wish to express our thanks to Dr. Arthur B. Callahan, Office of Naval Research, for his unfailing help in the many facets of important administrative matters. To Dr. Clifford M. Herman, Naval Medical Research Institute, goes our appreciation for his intellectual stimulation, as well as his active collaboration in evaluating and helping design research to clarify the mechanisms of shock. We are grateful, also, to Dr. Charles Brodine, National Naval Medical Center, for his early interest and wise counsel on the critical role of shock research, particularly as it relates to the pathologic events following trauma.

We also thank Jeanette Glasgow, whose skillful attention to the typing and assembly of the material in this volume helped make its publication possible. Finally, we appreciate the enthusiasm and assistance of Joy Provost in getting its production underway.

CONTENTS

THE FUNDAMENTAL MECHANISMS

OF SHOCK

INTRODUCTION: AN OVERVIEW OF THE SHOCK PROBLEM

Maurice B. Visscher, Ph.D., M.D.
Distinguished Service and Regents' Professor Emeritus

Department of Physiology, University of Minnesota,
Minneapolis, Minnesota

Shock is a problem that has interested surgeons and physiologists for a long time, but now internists, immunologists, and biochemists are becoming heavily involved. I note that the organizers of this symposium have invited eighteen surgeons, ten physiologists and eight internists, plus experts from several other fields to participate. I was interested in reviewing the questions which 23 of the participants said they would like to discuss, or hear discussed. The largest number dealt with endogenously released vasoactive agents, including catecholamine release. The "lung lesion" interested four participants. Effects upon cellular energy metabolism also stimulated interest, among other subjects relative to the shock state.

The range of partially or completely unanswered questions being dealt with in these sessions truly reflects the complexity of the problems characteristic of the various types of shock. Perhaps one of the greatest problems relates to the choice of suitable animal models for study. One of the earliest observations that my associates and I made in studying endotoxin shock was that species differences in the early responses to *E. coli* endotoxin were very great. No one species constitutes an adequate model. The shock literature also raises questions as to whether endotoxin shock is an adequate model for the study of clinical septic shock in general. No *a priori* reason exists why different bacterial toxins might not operate through differing intermediate target organs and chemical mechanisms. In fact, it would seem more than likely that they do.

In my opinion, investigators of shock should adopt an approach involving a number of different animal models. Thus, not only would different species be studied, the etiologic agents would be varied—as well as the mode of application of the shock-producing agents or procedures.

My main function here is to briefly discuss where we stand in relation to the problems of the physiology and experimental therapeutics of circulatory shock. The unsatisfactory nature of our present position may be gleaned from the introduction to one of the papers in the symposium on the physiological basis of circulatory shock presented at the 1970 meeting of the Federated Societies for Experimental Biology. The first sentence in Richard Lillehei's paper reads: "Mortality rate from septic and cardiogenic shock remains high in man, with death rates of 70-80% or more being the rule". The fact is that we know a great deal about specific elements in the shock picture. What clouds the main issue is that so much interplay occurs between various processes, and the correction of one defect may either exacerbate other defects or leave them free to progress to a completely irreversible state as far as the organism as a whole is concerned.

In preparing this brief presentation, I examined the abstracts of papers presented at the XXV International Congress of Physiological Sciences in Munich last July, and found thirteen papers on various aspects of shock, ranging from one on "Alterations in cation content of liver mitochondria" and "The relation of lysosomal hydrolases to irreversible experimental shock" to "The effect of administration of exogenous ATP in oligaemic shock". The interesting changes in the cation composition of mitochondria were a threefold increase in sodium, a large decrease in potassium, and a large increase in calcium. Other contributions dealt with myocardial function, transcapillary water movement, species differences, disturbances in capillary circulation, the effects of glucocorticoids, and the role of the reticuloendothelial system, to mention some of the topics.

Failure to solve the problem of the physiological mechanisms in circulatory shock is certainly not due to lack of interest and attention. But interest in isolated shock phenomena is not enough. A symposium like this one should encourage individual investigators to examine the problem of shock in broader ways than they may be inclined to do when their attention is focused on a specific element in the shock picture, or when they employ a single animal model in which the most prominent elements in the shock picture may differ from those in man. I suppose that all of us who have been interested in analyzing the pathophysiology of shock have been stimulated to do so primarily because of its importance in human medicine.

Underperfusion of some tissue beds in various parts of the body is, in my opinion, the common denominator in all forms of circulatory shock and in all species of animals. One other generalization can probably be made, namely, that the homeostatic mechanisms for regulating blood pressure probably contribute to the progression of the shock state through the route of underperfusion of organs, in which vasoconstriction follows a blood pressure fall. This in itself will aggravate cell damage.

It is by no means clear, however, what particular cells have to be damaged, and in what way, in order for hypotensive states to become progressive and irreversible. Yet, this is the crux of the shock problem. Ultimately, myocardial damage may be the final devastating blow causing death. In some circumstances, it may undoubtedly be true that if the myocardial-depressing substances liberated from damaged cells could be antagonized or their production inhibited, one might be able to effect recovery from what would otherwise be irreversible shock. Unfortunately, the attempts to increase survival rates by these means have been notably unsuccessful. Nevertheless, this does not mean that additional systematic work along these lines would not be profitable.

One point which I should like to stress most strongly is that undue emphasis upon restoration of arterial blood pressure rather than attention to factors which decrease resistance to blood flow in critical organs may have been an unfortunate element in much past research on shock. In the last analysis, one is not interested in the blood pressure. One is interested in perfusion rates, particularly of critical organs. Possibly, more useful therapeutic procedures would be generated by increased attention to possible ways to increase tissue perfusion in the kidney, intestines, pancreas, and liver (as well as the heart and brain, of course), when they are under the influence of the several vasoactive agents circulating in the blood stream in shock.

The application of computer techniques in multivariate analysis of the prognostic significance of various abnormalities in the evolution of clinical septic shock appears to be promising. However, I think we all realize that much work remains to be done before such procedures become useful in practice. Obviously, intact whole animals, and not cell or tissue cultures, must be used to study the various actions and interactions with which one has to deal in the analysis of the shock state.

Unfortunately, a movement is afoot not only in the United States, but in Europe, to discourage the use of living animals in biomedical research. In fact, the most vigorous campaign is being waged in the Council of Europe—an organization of Prime Ministers of all Western European countries, which recommends uniform, model laws for the member countries. One of its special commissions, The Commission on Science and Technology, took up a proposal by Professor S. T. Aygun, a veterinarian who runs a tissue culture laboratory in Ankara, Turkey, and who is Scientific Director of the International Association Against Painful Experiments on Animals. Basically, this proposal would severely limit the use of living animals for scientific purposes, the rationale being that not only is animal experimentation cruel, but medical science would progress faster using the more modern tools of cells and tissue cultures, computer technology, and statistics. Amazingly, the Commission on Science and Technology endorsed this proposal, despite the fact that the Commission on Health condemned it, along with other competent scientific experts. The matter now lies before the Prime Ministers themselves. Attempts to persuade them of the fallacies and hazards of this proposal are being made by the General Assembly of the International Union of Physiological Sciences, numerous leading European physiologists, and at least one International Surgical Society. In this country, the National Society for Medical Research (of which I am President) has taken a leading role in publicizing the falsity of the notion that computers, statistics, and tissue cultures can replace experimentation on intact animals.

For me to attempt an outline of the sorts of detailed investigations needed to elucidate the circulatory shock problem would be presumptuous. Let us consider some general principles, however. I have already alluded to some, but I should like to be a little more explicit. An examination of the literature soon makes it apparent that numerous contradictory conclusions seem to be drawn from studies in various laboratories. For example, the demonstration that the plasma concentration of one or more myocardial depressant substances rises during shock, and the demonstration that the isolated rat myocardial trabeculi respond by decreasing tension production to addition of endotoxin, seem to conflict directly with other data. For example, in perfused dog hearts, no deterioration in work capacity was apparent for long periods of time after endotoxin administration. One of the objectives of work on the shock problem should, I believe, be to attempt to account for apparently deviant conclusions. Simple experimental error is unlikely to account for differences in results of studies on the capacity of myocardium to develop tension and to do work. It seems much more likely that some factors are ignored in one or another set of experiments.

Another suggestion is that no single common path may lead to the state of practical irreversibility in shock. In other words, several types of damage may be possible, any one of which, if allowed to progress, can cause ultimate death. Investigative efforts should, I believe, be directed at elucidating all possible avenues of damage in the various types of shock, without the presupposition that the various pathways are of equal importance in all forms of the disorder.

A further thought is that hypoperfusion in any tissue may (and probably does, if severe enough) so extensively damage all oxygen-dependent metabolic processes that recovery after some critical point has been reached becomes impossible. The correction of some of the secondary alterations induced by such metabolic deficiencies may, then, offer little or nothing in the way of therapeutic benefit. I refer particularly to such phenomena as metabolic acidosis or ATP depletion.

In general, a warning seems appropriate against the temptation to think that correction of some of the epiphenomena of shock is likely to be rewarding. By epiphenomena, I mean secondary or tertiary effects of a primary disorder. The shock mechanisms are undoubtedly characterized by several orders of primacy, so to speak, in the pathogenesis of shock. Moreover, these undoubtedly differ in the various forms of shock.

As yet, we do not know exactly what specific effects of organ underperfusion or of toxic actions in shock are primary phenomena or epiphenomena and how many secondary processes need correction to bring about recovery. We do not yet know how far back in the chain of events occurring in bacterial toxin shock we need to go in order to forestall irreversibility.

It is the principle that I wish to emphasize. We do not yet have a satisfactory working analysis of the interrelationships between the various primary events, secondary events, and epiphenomena in shock of various etiologies. We are making progress, and this symposium will hopefully assist in the integrative process.

SESSION I

SHOCK AND THE CARDIOVASCULAR SYSTEM

Panel Moderator:

William C. Shoemaker, M.D.
Department of Surgery
Mount Sinai School of Medicine
The City University of New York
New York, New York

SESSION I: INTRODUCTORY REMARKS

William C. Shoemaker, M.D., *Panel Moderator*

Department of Surgery, Mount Sinai School of Medicine,
The City University of New York, New York, New York

The purpose of this program is to explore the conceptual basis of the mechanisms of shock. What precisely do we mean by mechanisms? It occurs to me that they fall into at least three large categories: those that may be pathogenic, those which are regulatory or controlling, and terminal mechanisms. Each of these three classes may relate to specific organs or specific controlling systems.

In a study of 180 patients at our institution, a sequential description of hemodynamic values according to six etiologic classifications of shock permitted separation of events into early, middle, and late stages. We believe that the events which precede the development of the hypotensive shock episode may have pathophysiologic significance. I should like to point out that the cardiac index is increased in all of these circumstances save two, *i.e.,* in patients with hemorrhage and in those with myocardial failure or tamponade. The heart rate is increased, presumably representing the neurogenic mechanism involved in regulation at the onset of shock. In patients with myocardial lesions, central venous pressure increases, which may improve filling pressure and effectiveness of the ventricle.

From derived calculations of hemodynamics, we see that only in the groups of patients with hemorrhage and myocardial failure are there transient increases in peripheral resistance. Thus, with respect to human shock, the low output/high resistance syndrome is really confined to patients with hemorrhage or those with myocardial problems, and it is transient and of limited scope. In most other shock patients, the resistance tends to fall progressively. The patients with hemorrhage and myocardial problems have a diminished central blood volume, but all of the other groups have an adequate blood volume with adequate ventricular filling. The patients with trauma have an increase in stroke index and stroke work. The other patients tend to have low values, presumably because of an increase in heart rate, but the ventricle does not fill.

If one looks at oxygen transport changes, one sees a decrease in arterial pO_2 only late in the course of the disease. Oxygen extraction drops markedly in the groups with hemorrhage and cardiac problems, but in most of the other patients there is a fall in oxygen content differences. If the increased cardiac output is generated by an increase in tissue needs, one would not expect these to fall. Therefore, we must conclude that other mechanisms are involved. It is our opinion that an increase in both cardiac drive and respiratory drive characterizes most of the patients in shock except those with hemorrhage or myocardial limitations. Also, in all patients in the early and middle periods, there is a time when oxygen consumption is limited, which reflects failure to deliver oxygen at some time in the early stages of shock.

In summary, we believe that the hemodynamic defect of shock is a tendency for the cardiac and respiratory drives to increase unless limited by either lack of blood volume to be pumped or inability of the heart to pump it.

PROPOSED RECLASSIFICATION OF SHOCK STATES WITH SPECIAL REFERENCE TO DISTRIBUTIVE DEFECTS[1]

Max Harry Weil, M.D., and Herbert Shubin, M.D.

The Shock Research Unit and the Department of Medicine, University of Southern California School of Medicine, the Los Angeles County/USC Medical Center, and the Center for the Critically Ill, Hollywood Presbyterian Hospital, Los Angeles, California

Some years ago, for lack of better knowledge, most of us were tempted to classify shock on an etiologic basis. We referred to: (a) shock due to blood loss (hypovolemic shock); (b) cardiogenic shock (pump failure); (c) bacterial shock (bacteremia, endotoxin); (d) acute hypersensitivity reactions (anaphylactic shock); (e) neurogenic shock (barbiturate and narcotic overdose, transection of the spinal cord; (f) shock associated with obstruction to blood flow, *e.g.*, pulmonary embolization; and (g) endocrine forms of shock (myxedema, pheochromocytoma, adrenocortical insufficiency, insulin excess).

Workers are now less attracted to classifications which stress a unitarian hypothesis. Little doubt exists that terminal mechanisms are similar, but these represent the end stages of the disease processes and do not necessarily pinpoint the options for therapeutic intervention. For practical purposes, a diagnostic classification serves mainly to identify primary mechanisms in relationship to priorities of treatment. To this extent, etiologic schemes of classification have been attractive. On the basis of additional

---

[1]This study was supported by USPHS Research Grants HE-00570 from the National Heart and Lung Institute, GM-16462 from the National Institute of General Medical Sciences, and HS-00238 from the National Center for Health Services Research and Development, HSMHA.

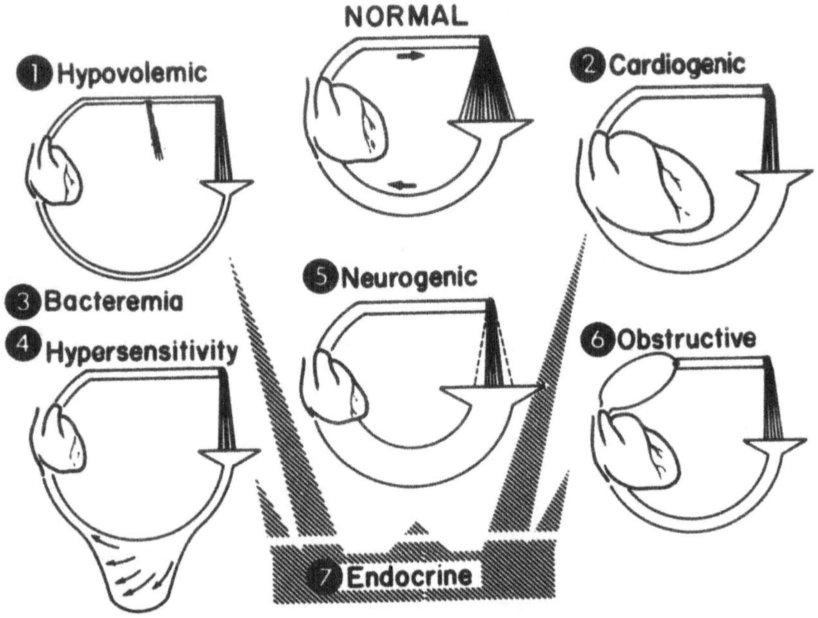

FIG. 1. Earlier classification of shock states. (From *Diagnosis and Treatment of Shock*, Baltimore: Williams & Wilkins, 1967, p. 10).

information, gathered principally from studies on patients, our group has recently proposed a modification of our earlier classification scheme.

MODIFICATIONS OF CLASSIFICATION

The earlier classification (4), which related etiology and mechanisms, is shown in Figure 1. Our revision (Fig. 2) is here presented for the first time. It reflects some advances in our understanding of hemodynamic mechanisms, particularly those which help to pinpoint the priorities of management of shock states due to causes other than hypovolemia and cardiac failure.

Let us briefly present the classification now used by our group. As previously, we refer to *hypovolemia* as the cause of shock states when the volume contained within the intravascular compartment is inadequate for purposes of perfusion. We refer to *cardiogenic* shock as a condition in which the cardiac pump is impaired to the extent that it cannot competently circulate available volume. *Obstruction* in the great veins, in the heart itself (pericardial tamponade, ball-valve thrombus), in the pulmonary

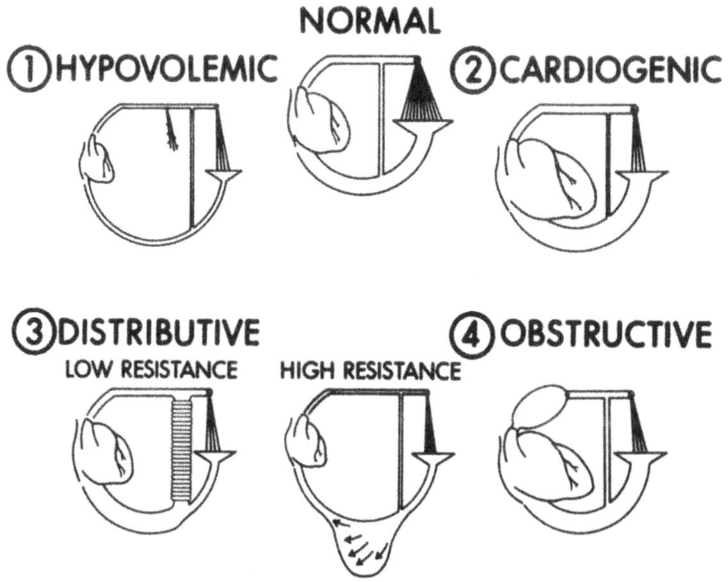

FIG. 2. Revised classification of shock states.

arteries (pulmonary embolism), or in the aorta (dissecting aneurysm) physically impedes the main stream of blood flow. These three categories are essentially the same as those included in our previous classification. In our new classification, we introduce a term which designates alterations in the distribution of blood volume. We have amalgamated bacteremia, hypersensitivity, and neurogenic types of shock into a single category which we have named *distributive* forms of shock. Each of these represents a distributive defect due to a major defect in arterial resistance, venous capacitance, or a combination of the two. In contrast to the three companion categories, the locus of the defect is primarily in the peripheral circuit, particularly in the small arteries and veins which make up the resistance and capacitance portions of the circuit.

We have not only combined three categories but also excluded one of the previous designations. Our experience during the past 10 years failed to justify the inclusion of *endocrine* shock as a discrete entity. Adrenocortical insufficiency, myxedematous coma, pheochromocytoma, and other endocrine crises which may be complicated by shock do, in fact, represent volume, cardiac, or distributive defects and, more often, a combination of defects.

TABLE 1

RECLASSIFICATION OF SHOCK STATES

Type of shock	Cause
I. Hypovolemic shock	
A. Exogenous	A. Blood loss due to hemorrhage Plasma loss due to burn, inflammation Electrolyte loss due to diarrhea, dehydration
B. Endogenous	B. Extravasation due to inflammation, trauma, application of a tourniquet, anaphylaxis, and pheochromocytoma
II. Cardiogenic shock	
	A. Myocardial infarction B. Cardiac failure C. Arrhythmia
III. Distributive shock	
A. High or normal resistance (increased venous capacitance; selective or general)	A. Bacillary shock Barbiturate intoxication CNS injury Ganglionic blockade
B. Low resistance (Arteriovenous shunt)	B. Inflammatory vasodilation due to pneumonia, peritonitis, abscess; reactive hyperemia
IV. Obstructive shock (by anatomic site)	
A. Vena cava	A. Compression
B. Pericardium	B. Tamponade
C. Cardiac chambers	C. Ball-valve thrombus
D. Pulmonary circuit	D. Embolism
E. Aorta	E. Dissecting aneurysm

DISTRIBUTIVE FORMS OF SHOCK

We have listed the clinical syndromes which we include among these distributive forms of shock and have further subdivided them as prototypes of high resistance and low resistance states (Table 1). In doing so, we must be cautious lest our scheme imply a level of understanding not yet attained. As with all other classifications, ours should be regarded as provisional and most assuredly subject to change if current hypotheses and extrapolations from animal experimentation are not corroborated.

We regard bacterial shock, *i.e.*, the shock state following intravascular injection or release of endotoxin or endotoxin-like materials, as a primary disorder of venous capacitance. We do not really know the locus of the alteration in the capacitance compartment, but blood appears to be selectively sequestered in the venous circuit. The defect does not appear to be reversed by infusion of large volumes of fluid, in contrast to the more generalized increase in venous capacitance which responds to "fluid distention" in shock states due to altered neuromotor controls, *e.g.*, barbiturate intoxication, ganglionic blockade, and transection of the spinal cord. Arterial resistance is usually increased or normal, and cardiac output is reduced. In addition, we recognize a low-resistance type of shock which is associated with inflammatory vasodilatation and arteriovenous shunting. It is more often observed in infection due to gram-positive organisms or a combination of gram-positive and gram-negative bacteria, as in cases of peritonitis and pneumonitis. Arterial resistance is decreased and cardiac output is usually increased. Nevertheless, a critical perfusion deficit exists, characterized by progressive increase in the lactate concentration and relatively low oxygen extraction. Oxygen content in mixed venous blood is characteristically increased. This high-output state with perfusion failure has been designated as a low-resistance type of capacitance defect.

ENDOTOXIN AND BACTERIAL SHOCK STATES AS DISTRIBUTIVE DEFECTS

After intravenous injection of endotoxin into the dog (3), there may be some question whether the peripheral resistance rises, but a decline in resistance *per se* does not explain the hypotensive state which follows injection of endotoxin. It is primarily the profound decline in cardiac output, as a consequence of a decline in venous return, which accounts for the hypotension (Fig. 3). We share concern with many other investigators lest the animal model be presumed to have direct applicability to human patients. Hence, we use the model only as a basis for approaching studies in patients under much less controlled conditions.

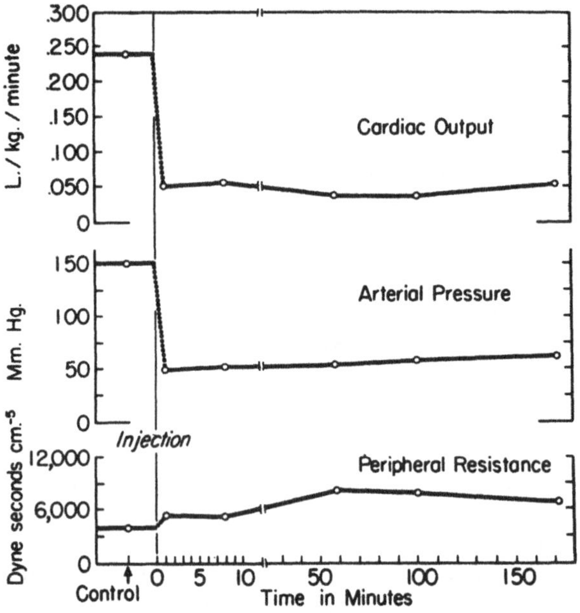

FIG. 3. Hemodynamic responses of the dog to endotoxin shock.

If we now turn our attention to the human patient, who has been our primary experimental model over the last decade, we recognize that the patient with bacterial shock due to bacteremia caused by gram-negative enteric organisms is likely to have a low arterial pressure associated with a low cardiac index and at least a numerically high peripheral arterial resistance. Mean circulation time is increased; hence the velocity of blood flow is decreased. These are the changes which are included in our new classification as characteristic of high or normal resistance distributive defects (Fig. 4). Infusion of large volumes of fluid usually fails to restore hemodynamic balance. We conceptualize ballooning of a selective portion of the venous capacitance bed with selective sequestration of volume.

The hemodynamic defect in patients with peritonitis is quite different. A decline in the blood pressure is associated with a relative increase in the cardiac index and a fall in peripheral arterial resistance. Despite the normal or increased cardiac index, perfusion is critically compromised, since the concentration of lactate is substantially elevated in the arterial blood. Mean circulation time, which is prolonged in shock states associated with bacteremia due to gram-negative organisms, is normal or low in

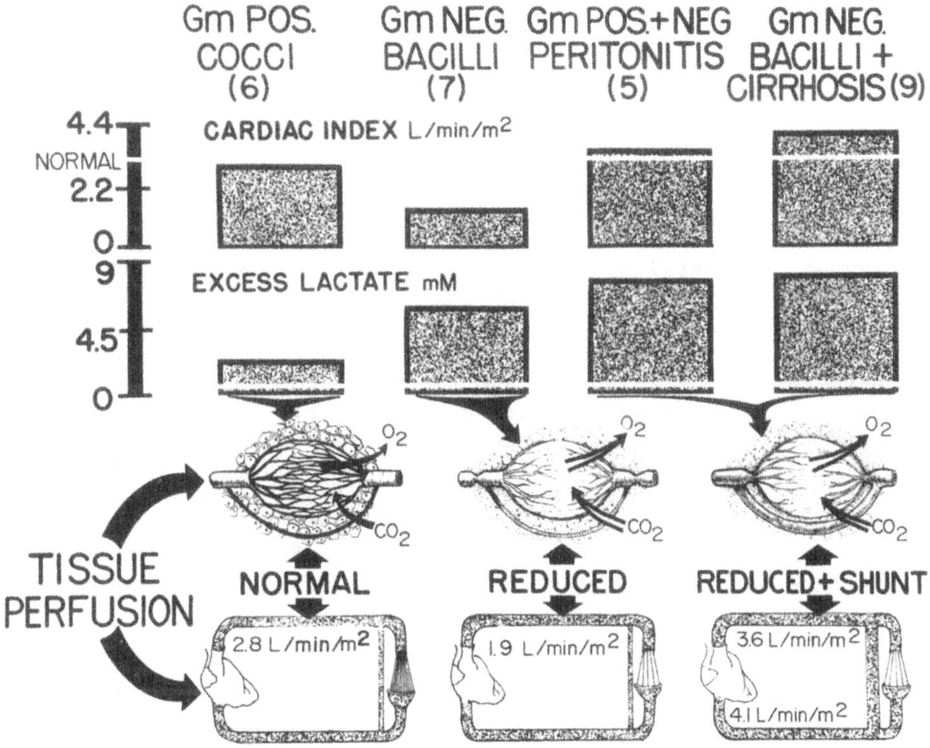

FIG. 4. Differences in cardiac index, excess lactate, and tissue perfusion in patients suffering from various forms of bacterial shock.

---

patients with peritonitis. Since the mean circulation time provides a reciprocal measure of the velocity of blood flow, not only the cardiac output but the velocity of flow tends to be high in patients with mixed gram-positive and gram-negative infections. These characteristics are best explained by arteriovenous shunting; in the context of the new classification, they are referred to as the low-resistance type of distributive shock.

The differences are graphically illustrated in Figure 4. When hypotension follows infections due to gram-positive cocci, the changes resemble those observed in peritonitis, although a severe perfusion defect with lactic acidosis is much less likely. Differentiations between the high-resistance defect characteristic of bacillary shock and the low-resistance distributive defect characteristic of peritonitis and other generalized mixed infections are shown. In both instances, marked deficits in perfusion are indicated by substantial increases in arterial lactate. Incidentally shown is the fact that patients with cirrhosis, who already have an underlying low-resistance distributive defect, are likely to give the false impression of having a low-resistance distributive defect, a subject discussed extensively in an earlier publication (2).

Related though somewhat different mechanisms operate in patients with barbiturate intoxication (1). Here, we find no reduction of peripheral arterial resistance (Fig. 5). On the contrary, in many such patients arterial resistance is increased, and clinical examination leaves no doubt that the arterial bed is constricted. We can load the intravascular compartment with fluid, increase the plasma volume to two to three times its normal value, and essentially reverse the hemodynamic defect. This is known as the "generalized distributive defect." These patients subsequently have diuresis and tend to establish normal hemodynamics. This understanding has been very useful clinically. Among our last 12 cases of barbiturate intoxication, we have not lost a single patient with potentially fatal blood levels of barbiturate, whereas we lost the first five out of eight in the early 1960's prior to treatment by volume expansion.

COMMENT

Our understanding of hemodynamic mechanisms depends not so much on the total volume of blood that flows past the aortic valve or the cardiac output as on the amount of blood delivered to the exchange sites. Even though cardiac output may be substantial, if that blood flow does not arrive at the exchange sites, the ultimate metabolic detriment is no different from low cardiac output without shunt flow.

The capacitance bed, which occupies nearly 80% of the volume-containing portion of the circulatory compartment, plays an important role. Those who are interested in the gross hemodynamic aspects of shock are likely to find significant insights as they examine it for an understanding of such shifts of volume. It is in this context that we improve understanding of those forms of acute circulatory failure that are not selectively related to volume or to the pump alone.

SUMMARY

We have presented a modification of our earlier classification of shock states. As in the earlier scheme, hypovolemia, cardiac

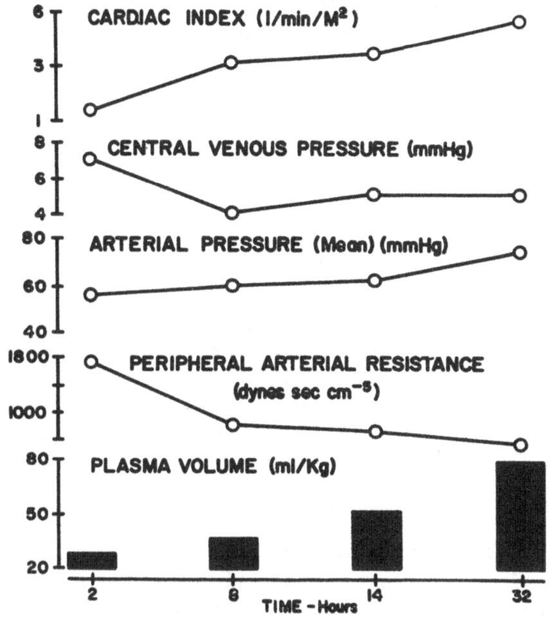

FIG. 5. Hemodynamic responses of a male patient in shock caused by barbiturate intoxication.

(pump) failure, and obstruction to the main stream of blood flow are still regarded as primary causes of shock. A new category designated as a distributive defect, which accounts for those types of shock due primarily to hemodynamic defects in the peripheral circuit, has been introduced. We have provided a differentiation between high- and low-resistance forms of shock, together with an indication of the importance of the venous capacitance bed in accounting for the changes. The applicability of these concepts to bacteremic shock and to shock associated with barbiturate intoxication has been discussed.

REFERENCES

1. Shubin, H., and M.H. Weil. The mechanism of shock following suicidal doses of barbiturates, narcotics, and tranquilizer drugs, with observations on the effects of treatment. Am. J. Med. 38:857, 1965.

2. Udhoji, V.N., and M.H. Weil. Hemodynamic and metabolic studies on shock associated with bacteremia: Observations on 16 patients. Ann. Intern. Med. 62:966-978, 1965.

3. Weil, M.H., L.D. MacLean, W.W. Spink, and M.B. Visscher. Studies on the circulatory changes in the dog produced by endotoxin from gram-negative microorganisms. J. Clin. Invest. 35:1194, 1956.

4. Weil, M.H., and H. Shubin. *Diagnosis and Treatment of Shock.* Baltimore: Williams & Wilkins, 1967, p. 10.

DISCUSSION

DR. W. C. SHOEMAKER, *Panel Moderator (New York, N.Y.):* If this venous capacitance system is central in circulatory failure, how do you regard the colloidal osmotic pressure and lactic acid concentrations? Are they adequate for diagnosis, and are they adequate as predictors of this? Are they useful as guides for therapy, and, when you reverse these changes, can you re-establish circulatory integrity?

DR. WEIL: Lactic acid concentrations have proven to be rather selective indicators of perfusion failure, in contrast to ventilatory failure, where lactate doesn't increase even in the most profound forms. Therefore, lactic acidosis is, I think, a selective indication of failure to deliver blood to the exchange sites at the capillary level. With regard to colloid osmotic pressure, we've now had an opportunity to measure this on about 150 patients, and it becomes helpful in understanding fluid shifts at the capillary level. These, then, would make the fluid shifts significant in regard to the total volume contained within the intravascular compartment, and it would make them somewhat separate, at least conceptually, of the size of the capacitance bed. Stated in another form, the colloid osmotic pressure appears to do just what you would expect it to do, as Dr. Landis pointed out many years ago (and Dr. Visscher's teacher long before him, Starling). That is, it controls to some extent the shift of fluid. Another important point is that when fluid shifts into one selective area (namely, the lung), it can do selectively a lot of harm. So, both lactic acidosis and colloid osmotic pressures might best be looked at as components of activities that go on at the exchange sites, in contrast to gross plumbing changes in the capacitance bed.

DR. SHOEMAKER: Are there questions from the audience?

DR. E. D. JACOBSON *(Houston, Texas):* I'd like to take issue with the notion that resistance rises in endotoxin shock on the precapillary side. It was shown, many years ago, by your colleague, Gilbert, with the pump-perfused heart, that the resistance falls in the dog. Where we have made direct measurements with flowmeters, in the same situation in the dog, we also find a fallen resistance in endotoxin shock. Using subhuman primates, which are presumably closer to man, Reynolds and Swan and our own group, studying the baboon and the monkey, respectively, have found that the splanchnic circulation actually vasodilates markedly in endotoxin shock.

DR. WEIL: Gene [Dr. Jacobson], I think I alluded to the fact that there may be some controversy with regard to changes in the numerical resistance values. Also, however, the quantitative changes in resistance, which have been reported by the workers you quoted, including yourself, seem on calculation not to account for the gross hemodynamic changes that are observed. Even if there were subtle changes or moderate decreases in peripheral arterial resistance, the decreases that are observed do not, of themselves, account for the volume that fails to be returned in the intact organism to the venous inflow into the heart. I think that the argument really hinges on the gross economy of blood returned. Also, harking back to measurements in human patients and taking into consideration the right atrial filling pressures, we're on fairly safe grounds when we say that a major component of the gross defect is a reduction in effective venous return.

PARTICIPATION OF ENDOGENOUS VASOACTIVE AGENTS IN THE PATHOGENESIS OF ENDOTOXIN SHOCK

Thomas E. Emerson, Jr., Ph.D.

Michigan State University, Department of Physiology, College of Human Medicine, East Lansing, Michigan

I would like to briefly present the views of a physiologist on the problem of shock. I will limit my comments primarily to endotoxin shock in the dog. Arterial pressure, as we all know, is controlled by cardiac output and total peripheral resistance. Dr. Weil has mentioned that there seems to be a primary defect in cardiac output, at least in early shock, which results secondarily from a reduced venous return. Figure 1 is an incomplete schema of some known events occurring in the dog during endotoxin shock. It also suggests, at least in my mind, some unknown areas. In the canine model, endotoxin shock is followed by a release of vasoactive agents. Many of these are known, but some are unknown—for example, histamine or histamine-like agents leading to hepatic venous constriction, pooling in the hepatosplanchnic vasculature, a decrease in venous return, and subsequent decreases in cardiac output and arterial pressure. Of course, other vasoactive agents are released (acetylcholines, serotonins, bradykinin-like polypeptides, *etc.*). More recently, a myocardial depressant factor has been identified which has also been shown to be vasoactive in the peripheral circulation. Moreover, various electrolyte and water abnormalities arise later in shock.

In summary, the arterial pressure drops due primarily to the decrease in venous return and problems in the circulatory system, mainly on the venous side. The fall in pressure activates the sympathicoadrenal system, with release of more vasoactive agents (in this case, constrictors such as epinephrine) and acceleration of sympathetic nerve activity. These phenomena, in turn, increase precapillary and postcapillary resistances in various organs. A decrease in the precapillary-to-postcapillary resistance ratio

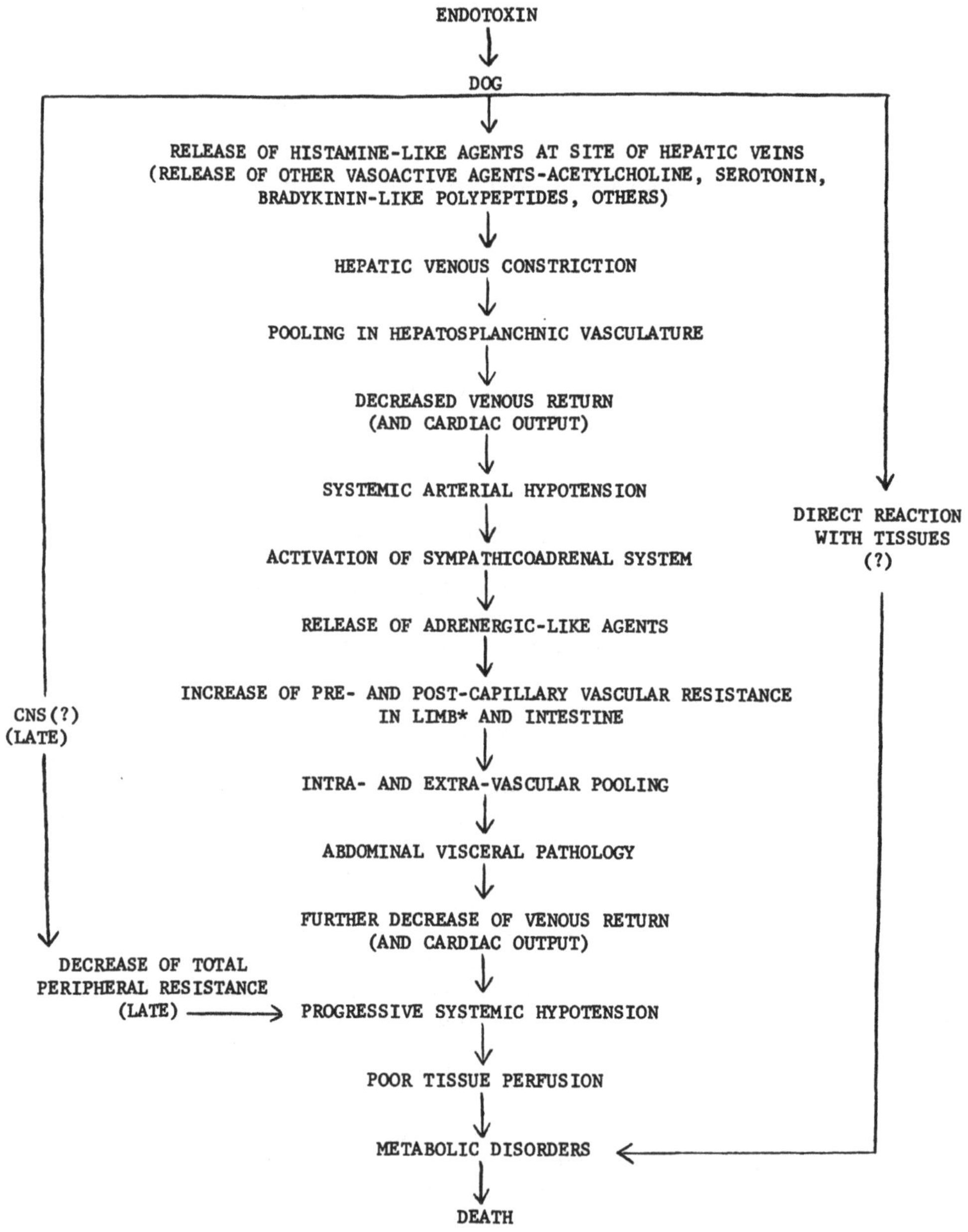

FIG. 1. Schema showing some known and some possible events during irreversible endotoxin shock in the dog; * = recently shown by L.B. Hinshaw and S.E. Owen (J. Appl. Physiol. 30:331, 1971) and G.J. Grega and F.J. Haddy (Am. J. Physiol. 220:1448, 1971) that no extravascular fluid loss occurs in forelimb.

favors intravascular and extravascular pooling, hemoconcentration, and further decreases in venous return and cardiac output. These changes are followed by a progressive systemic hypotension. As a result, poor tissue perfusion ensues. This is the primary defect in shock, ultimately leading to the death of the animal. In addition to starvation of the cells for oxygen, a release of other vasoactive agents occurs (*e.g.*, lysosomes, proteases), which is detrimental. These agents might well play a role later in the progression of shock, particularly in late shock, when there is a devastating effect on peripheral resistance. Some recent data have been reported by Hinshaw and Owen at the University of Oklahoma and Weidner, Grega, and Haddy at Michigan State University concerning capillary filtration as influenced by changes in precapillary and postcapillary resistance. Their findings indicate that a net reabsorption of fluid occurs in the canine forelimb during endotoxin shock. I might mention briefly that we can block most of the vasoactive agents (those that are released early) and alter the early hypotension, but we cannot prevent death. Thus, I doubt that we can call these agents the primary trigger mechanism or say that they are ultimately responsible for death. As far as a direct reaction of endotoxin with tissue goes, most evidence would not support this. Right now, I think the central nervous system might well be a main issue in shock. I, at least, am seriously inclined to think that the central nervous system may play an important role in shock, particularly during the late phase.

Figure 2 illustrates the effects of endotoxin in the monkey and the cat. Again, the central nervous system is implicated. Endotoxin causes venous pooling in the monkey, a decrease in venous return and cardiac output, and the other events that we see in the dog. The primary difference is that this decrease in venous return in the monkey occurs very slowly, over a long period of time, and we have been unable to identify the sites of pooling. We suspect the capacitance system but have been unable to pinpoint this. After the initial phase, the responses of the monkey are fairly similar to those of the dog, with very poor tissue perfusion and ultimate death.

A shock workshop was held in Oklahoma City in 1964 at the Civil Aeromedical Research Institute and the University of Oklahoma Medical Center. (For detailed data, see Table 1). Investigators from all over the country carried out their various therapeutic procedures using a group of standardized dogs and a standardized method for endotoxin shock. Most forms of therapy attempted were not successful on this particular occasion. For example, fibrinolysin treatment was associated with a survival rate of 20%, whereas 25% of the controls survived. Isoproterenol plus blood and low-molecular-weight dextran produced a survival of 10%, compared to

TABLE 1

SHOCK WORKSHOP DATA: ENDOTOXIN CANINE SURVIVAL STUDIES[a]

Investigators	Treatment	Percent survival at: 0-48 hr	49-96 hr	97-168 hr	Permanent survivors (No. and %)
Cavanagh	Fibrinolysin	20%	20%	20%	2/10 (20%)
	Control	25%	25%	25%	1/4 (25%)
Duff, Peretz	Isoproterenol + blood + LMW dextran	30%	20%	10%	1/10 (10%)
	Control	25%	25%	25%	1/4 (25%)
Emerson, Brake, Hinshaw	Splanchnic denervation	10%	10%	10%	1/10 (10%)
	Control	0%	—	—	0/5 (0%)
Fine, Palmerio, Minton, Nahor	Celiac blockade (xylocaine in alcohol)	0%	—	—	0/5 (0%)
	Celiac blockade (xylocaine in saline)	50%	50%	40%	4/10 (40%)
	Control	0%	—	—	0/1 (0%)
Hardaway, Elovitz, Kuida	Heparin + phenoxybenzamine	0%	—	—	0/3 (0%)
	Methyldopa + promethazine	14%	14%	14%	1/7 (14%)
	Control	50%	50%	50%	2/4 (50%)

Longerbeam, Lillehei, Block, Rosenberg	Hydrocortisone + dextran	20%	20%	20%	1/5 (20%)
	Phenoxybenzamine + plasma	50%	30%	10%	1/10 (10%)
	Control	25%	25%	0%	0/4 (0%)
Masucci, Hinshaw	Phenoxybenzamine + plasma	45%	33%	33%	3/9 (33%)
Spink, Reddin, Starzecki	Aldosterone + angiotensin	30%	30%	20%	2/10 (20%)
	Control	40%	40%	40%	2/5 (40%)
Sukhnandan, Wilson, Thal	Phenoxybenzamine + dextran + blood + norepinephrine	40%	0%	—	0/10 (0%)
	Control	0%	—	—	0/5 (0%)
Weil, Shubin, Bradley	Hydroxycortisone	0%	—	—	0/5 (0%)
	Dexamethasone	67%	67%	50%	3/6 (50%)
	Phentolamine	20%	20%	20%	1/5 (20%)
	Dexamethasone + metaraminol	60%	40%	20%	1/5 (20%)
	Control	50%	33%	17%	1/6 (17%)

Note: Total number of experimental and control dogs, 158. Endotoxin dose, LD_{82}. Final control group survival, 18%.

[a]Modified from J. Oklahoma State Med. J. 59:477, 1966.

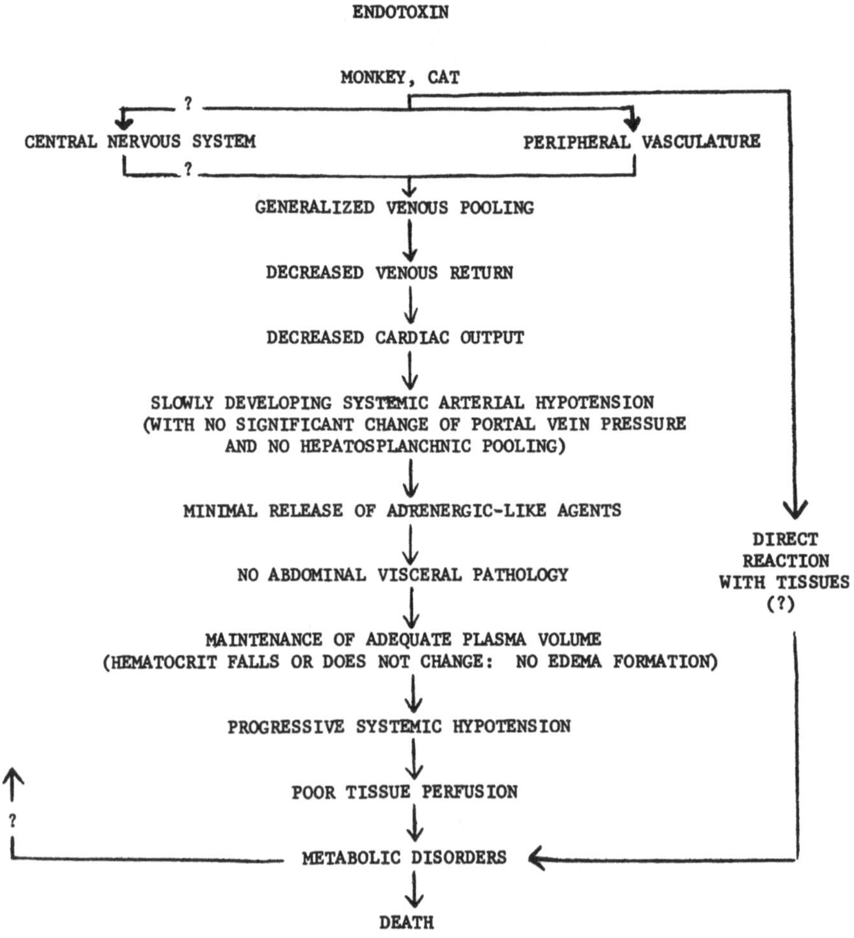

FIG. 2. Schema showing some known and some possible events during irreversible endotoxin shock in the monkey and cat.

25% for the untreated controls. With splanchnic denervation, 10% survived. With celiac blockade (again, splanchnic denervation), survival rates were zero and 40%. With heparin plus phenoxybenzamine, survival was zero, and so on. Unfortunately, Dr. Visscher's suggestion apropas of these data in 1964 still seems to apply, *i.e.,* that perhaps no therapeutic regimen at all is better than what is currently available to us.

I would now like to comment in more detail on some of the evidence concerning release of various vasoactive agents and their possible role in the pathogenesis of endotoxin shock. Since a comprehensive review of the literature on this subject is beyond the scope of this paper, only a few specific references will be cited to document important points.

HISTAMINE

One of the first humoral agents to be put on the firing line was histamine, a potent vasodepressor which can promote intravascular fluid loss under certain conditions (25). Hinshaw and colleagues (33,34,37), as well as others (40,41,59,60), have shown that histamine is released within seconds after intravenous injection of *Escherichia coli* endotoxin. In the dog, histamine release immediately precedes the marked fall in arterial blood pressure which is due to a decreased cardiac output after hepatic venous constriction, pooling of blood in the splanchnic viscera, and decreased venous return. The hepatic venous effect can be initiated by histamine (9) and can be ameliorated by histamine-blocking agents (1,31).

Several of our studies suggest that histamine may be intimately involved in the early hemodynamic response to endotoxin (29,31). Very recently, Vick and co-workers reinvestigated this problem (58). They concluded that histamine release must somehow be involved in the early cardiovascular changes and lethality in endotoxin shock. However, while our work and that of others clearly implicates histamine in the early cardiovascular changes in endotoxin shock, as well as some of the later vascular alterations, the fact remains that prevention or amelioration of the early vascular effects of histamine (1,31) does little to prevent mortality (29). Other indirect evidence exists which does not favor histamine, and the early hemodynamic changes associated with its release, as the major trigger mechanism in the pathogenesis of endotoxin shock (14,18). In one study, lethal amounts of endotoxin were slowly infused intravenously (14). Hemodynamic, metabolic, and survival data were compared to data from another group of dogs receiving the same dose of endotoxin as an intravenous bolus injection. In another study (18), live *E. coli* cells were administered and the results were compared to those obtained from dogs intravenously injected with lethal amounts of *E. coli* endotoxin. Bolus injections of endotoxin produced the characteristic early changes in pressure and other parameters, while purified *E. coli* endotoxin given as a slow infusion and live *E. coli* cells did not. When all three groups of dogs were compared, however, within a few hours there was little difference in arterial pressure or other parameters and no difference in mortality.

Histamine may have a long-term detrimental effect by promoting fluid efflux into skeletal muscle or skin. We performed some experiments on nonshocked dogs to evaluate this. Histamine infused intravenously at doses high enough to markedly lower systemic blood pressure had little effect on capillary filtration in the skin or muscle vascular beds of the dog forelimb (4). While histamine given in this manner decreased the precapillary-to-postcapillary resistance ratio, which alone would increase capillary filtration, it also lowered large artery (aorta) and large vein (central) pressure sufficiently to offset this one determinant of capillary pressure. If there is any direct effect on capillary permeability, this is also overridden (4).

While histamine release is no doubt harmful, the available evidence fails to support the hypothesis that this endogenous agent is responsible, either directly or indirectly, for the irreversibility of endotoxin shock.

CATECHOLAMINES

Perhaps the most controversial area concerning endotoxin shock, vasoactive hormones, and death involves the catecholamines and the sympathetic nervous system. Evidence has been gathered both for and against this hormonal system being responsible for the irreversibility of gram-negative endotoxin shock.

Plasma catecholamine levels are clearly elevated during endotoxin shock (27,40,44,54,55) as a result of increased sympathetic nerve activity and release from the adrenal glands (7,49). The studies of Hinshaw *et al.* (38) and others (40,63,65) show that the vascular responsiveness to catecholamines is altered during endotoxin shock. Hinshaw's data are particularly relevant, since they suggest a depressed arterial response and enhanced venous sensitivity to catecholamines, a situation which favors intravascular pooling and increased capillary filtration.

Other data show that adrenergic blocking agents ameliorate or prevent the intestinal pathology and improve survival rates in dogs given lethal amounts of endotoxin (44,47).

This impressive body of data strongly implicates the sympathicoadrenal system as a prominent contributor to the pathogenesis of endotoxin shock. However, conflicting data have also been reported. A number of earlier papers (13,29,38) suggest considerable fluid loss in muscle and perhaps skin during shock, based on experiments on the dog forelimb perfused with constant flow. The findings were thought to explain part of the decrease in effective circulating blood volume which accompanies the progression of shock. Studies have also shown that sympathetic nerve stimulation or catecholamine infusion in the forelimb perfused with constant flow can cause edema due to venous constriction and subsequent increase in capillary hydrostatic pressure (15). While these data are valid under constant-flow conditions, they do not necessarily reflect what happens in the natural situation in which flow is not constant. This is a critical consideration, since capillary hydrostatic pressure is directly determined by capillary blood volume and wall compliance. Capillary volume is determined by capillary inflow and outflow, which, in turn, depend upon aortic pressure and organ arterial resistance and central venous pressure and organ venous resistance, respectively. Thus, in the intact animal during shock all of these factors are changed, and not all in the direction to promote transcapillary fluid efflux. Two recent studies have been performed on the skeletal muscle and skin beds of the dog forelimb perfused by natural flow; they emphasize this point (36,61). The results are particularly significant since skeletal muscle comprises over half of the body mass and represents a large potential space for vascular volume loss. Both groups of workers simultaneously and independently found that fluid efflux from the vascular system did not occur in the dog forelimb perfused with natural flow, even after several hours of endotoxin shock. On the contrary, tissue fluid was actually reabsorbed during this period. While the precapillary-to-postcapillary resistance ratio was markedly reduced, which alone would elevate capillary hydrostatic pressure, other factors which influence capillary hydrostatic pressure (aortic pressure, central venous pressure, and limb flow) were altered sufficiently to completely offset the local resistance changes. These findings negate earlier conclusions, based on data from constant-flow experiments, that vascular fluid is lost to muscle tissue space during endotoxin shock.

One other recent study bears on this point. Grega and Haddy (24) investigated the involvement of skin and skeletal muscle vasculatures and transcapillary fluid flux in the dog forelimb perfused with natural flow during catecholamine shock. A 3-hour intravenous infusion of large amounts of epinephrine or norepinephrine regularly produced shock. However, fluid efflux was seen only shortly after catecholamine infusion was started, and the amount was small. Progression of shock was associated with net fluid reabsorption into the vasculature. These findings do not support the reported marked reduction in blood volume in catecholamine shock. The authors mentioned the evidence for whole-blood loss into the intestinal lumen and fluid loss into the small intestine and pericardial sac during catecholamine shock, but pointed out that these losses were apparently small. They concluded from their work and that of others that "sympathetic hyperactivity does not initiate the development of irreversibility by causing extensive fluid efflux into skin and skeletal muscle during severe hemorrhagic hypotension."

While these studies do not prove that an overactive sympathicoadrenal system is not prominently involved in the pathogenesis of endotoxin shock, they do suggest that: (a) the massive potential interstitial space of skeletal muscle and skin is not an area of fluid loss during endotoxin shock; and (b) prolonged, high plasma concentrations of catecholamines associated with hypotension do not promote vascular fluid loss in these areas. It is also of interest that fluid loss into the forelimb does not occur during endotoxin shock in the monkey or cat (13,32).

Other studies performed in Dr. Hinshaw's laboratories during my tenure at Oklahoma are relevant to the participation of the sympathicoadrenal system during endotoxin shock. We completed a number of studies designed specifically to answer this question, which I will briefly summarize. In one study, a "venous return" preparation was used to evaluate possible alteration of vascular responses to endotoxin by adrenergic blockade (1). Phenoxybenzamine (Dibenzyline), which also blocks or ameliorates the vascular effects of histamine, serotonin, and acetylcholine, was utilized to block the action of the catecholamines. Some of the animals were pretreated with phenoxybenzamine and others were not, thereby serving as controls. The dogs were then injected with a lethal dose of purified *E. coli* endotoxin and the measured parameters were followed for 100 minutes thereafter. Phenoxybenzamine caused no significant reversal of the trend towards acidosis, hemoconcentration, pooling of blood, reduction in venous return and cardiac output, or systemic hypotension during this period.

In another study (29), survival experiments were performed to evaluate the possible beneficial effects of adrenergic blockade, using appropriate levels of phenoxybenzamine as reported by others. The drug was given before or after shock and with or without supportive fluid therapy. Another group of dogs served as controls. Survival rates were essentially the same for treated and untreated dogs. We concluded that, although phenoxybenzamine had good blocking properties against the catecholamines and a number of other vasoactive agents, it failed to improve survival rate during endotoxin shock.

Clearly, we were unsuccessful in reversing the course of endotoxin shock by adrenergic blockade. We therefore approached the problem of an overactive sympathicoadrenal system by another route, *viz.*, by sympathetic denervation and adrenal ablation experiments (11,13,30). In the first of these studies, hemodynamic and metabolic evaluations were made in three groups of dogs receiving endotoxin. In one group, bilateral adrenalectomy was performed; in one, the splanchnic viscera were locally sympathectomized; and one group was sham-operated and served as a control. We found that hepatosplanchnic pooling in the dog during endotoxin shock does not depend upon an intact nerve supply to the abdominal viscera or upon the presence of adrenal glands. Neither sympathetic denervation of the splanchnic viscera nor adrenalectomy prevented portal hypertension, systemic hypotension, or intestinal hemorrhagic necrosis after endotoxin administration in the dog. Increases in vascular resistance and weight in the forelimb perfused by constant flow also occurred independent of intact adrenal glands. When the forelimb of the monkey and cat was similarly prepared (29), humorally induced vasoconstriction after endotoxin was minimal. Hemoconcentration was absent and net losses in limb weight occurred, indicating reabsorption of interstitial fluid. Therefore, this study provided no evidence to impugn the sympathicoadrenal system in the dog, cat, or monkey in endotoxin shock.

The contribution of the abdominal visceral sympathetic nervous system to the pathogenesis of endotoxin shock was further evaluated in dogs (11,13). Ten healthy dogs, subjected to splanchnic sympathectomy 2 1/2 - 8 weeks before the test, were injected intravenously with an LD_{80} of purified *E. coli* endotoxin. The animals were returned to their cages and observed until death, or for 7 days. Nine of the 10 dogs died within 5 1/2 to 19 hours after endotoxin injection; one survived permanently.

In summary, the role of the sympathicoadrenal system in the pathogenesis of endotoxin shock is uncertain. Certainly, the data are conflicting. Our research does not exclude the possibility that sympathetic nerve activity or circulating catecholamines have a negative effect in late endotoxin shock. However, our work does suggest that an overactive sympathicoadrenal system is not essential for hemodynamic or metabolic changes or death due to endotoxin shock.

SEROTONIN

Another vasoactive humoral agent thought to be involved in endotoxin shock is 5-hydroxytryptamine (serotonin). While numerous articles have stated that serotonin is released during endotoxin shock, a careful review of the literature makes it clear that this statement must be elaborated upon to indicate the full picture. *In vitro* and *in vivo* work of Kobold and co-workers (41) has demonstrated that serotonin is released from platelets in whole blood and from splanchnic visceral organs by endotoxin. The work of Davis *et al.* (5,6) has shown that, in the intact dog, plasma serotonin concentration rises slightly, peaking at about 30 seconds after intravenous injection of endotoxin and falling to control level within 5 minutes. Rosenberg and associates (54,55) and Jacobson *et al.* (40) have shown that plasma and serum serotonin levels drop markedly from 5 minutes after endotoxin administration onward. Apparently, then, if serotonin is released by endotoxin, the amount is small, the release occurs within a few seconds after the endotoxin challenge, and the elevation lasts only a few minutes.

The cardiovascular effects of serotonin are unimpressive, particularly at the doses under consideration. We have worked with this agent for a number of years in a variety of preparations, and using a wide range of doses. Serotonin always constricts skin vessels, whereas its effect on skeletal muscle vessels depends upon the initial level of resistance (4,19). If initial resistance is high, serotonin acts as a vasodilator in muscle and *vice versa* (19). In the *in vitro* vessel strip preparation, serotonin always increases smooth muscle tension in strips from skin and muscle vessels, regardless of the initial resistance (39). Serotonin has little effect on venous return or cardiac output in nonshocked dogs (9), and has negligible effects on capillary filtration (4). Animal experiments by Hinshaw performed on the blood or dextran-perfused lung suggest that serotonin can actively constrict the canine pulmonary vasculature (35). Therefore, serotonin may be involved in the transiently increased pulmonary vascular resistance which occurs in the dog immediately after intravenous endotoxin injection. This is not fatal to the dog, however, and in view of the available evidence I do not think we can assign a significant role to serotonin in the early or late events leading to irreversibility during endotoxin shock.

PROSTAGLANDINS

This family of naturally occurring, vasoactive substances has received considerable attention during the past few years. They are thought to play a role in circulatory regulation and perhaps possess other functions (17). The renal prostaglandin, PGA_1, is a potent vasodilator (50,51) which is released from the kidney during periods of ischemia (45), an established feature of endotoxin shock (21). We have recently noted that, in addition to causing active dilation of precapillary vessels of the skin and skeletal muscle beds in the dog forelimb (50), it also decreases total peripheral resistance and decreases cardiac output (51). This latter effect is secondary to peripheral pooling of blood and decreased venous return (51). Conceivably, then, PGA_1 could be a detrimental factor during endotoxin shock. However, further work is needed to determine this.

ANGIOTENSIN

The plasma concentration of angiotensin II rises early in endotoxin shock in the dog and cat, remaining elevated for at least

60-90 minutes after initiation of shock (27,64). Although angiotensin II is a potent vasoconstrictor in peripheral beds (4,15), this hormone seems unlikely to contribute significantly to the irreversibility of endotoxin shock. While venous return and cardiac output are decreased in the nonshocked dog during intravenous angiotensin II infusion (10), the renal vascular and systemic pressor responses to infused angiotensin II wane early during endotoxin shock and are essentially lost within 30-60 minutes (12).

VASOACTIVE PEPTIDES

Vasodilator polypeptides, of which bradykinin is often thought to be representative (25), have been identified during endotoxin shock in the rabbit (22), dog (41,58), and monkey (48). Thal's group (41,58) has pioneered this work, using a bioassay technique to identify release of bradykinin from dog whole blood and from splanchnic visceral organs.

Thal and Sardesai (58) have pointed out that the role of kinins in endotoxin shock is speculative but that they might be involved in some forms of septic shock in man associated with a low peripheral resistance and high cardiac output. While no doubt exists concerning the potent vasodilator properties of bradykinin (4,25) or its effect on venous return and cardiac output (8), little evidence is available to indicate that it has a detrimental effect in endotoxin shock. Additional research directed toward the vasoactive polypeptides might be in order.

More recently, Lefer (43) has identified a vasoactive peptide-like substance in the plasma of dogs during endotoxin shock. This substance has been shown to depress myocardial function in isolated cardiac tissue, as well as in the intact animal. Consequently, it was named myocardial depressant factor (MDF) (43). MDF also constricts superior mesenteric artery strips in the presence or absence of norepinephrine or angiotensin II (23). MDF, which is produced in the splanchnic viscera during shock, has been suggested to be responsible for a positive feedback system which would further constrict the superior mesenteric artery, thereby leading to the production of still more MDF (23). While this is an attractive hypothesis for the dog, it is difficult to extrapolate to other species such as the monkey, cat, or rabbit, which manifest little, if any, visceral pathology during irreversible endotoxin shock (29,32,33,42).

Some investigators doubt that MDF, as a cardiac depressant, contributes to irreversibility during endotoxin shock. Hinshaw *et al.* (28) have presented data showing no alteration of cardiac performance in the isolated, perfused dog heart for 3 hours after initiation of endotoxin shock. More recently, Hinshaw and colleagues (personal communication) found no evidence for a blood-borne myocardial depressant during a 6-hour period after injection of a lethal amount of endotoxin.

LYSOSOMES

As tissue ischemia and injury develop during endotoxin shock, lysosomal disruption may occur, with liberation of cytolytic enzymes, proteases, and certain phosphatases (3,43). This destructive process apparently occurs subsequent to the onset of shock and may well contribute to irreversibility. However, more data are needed to determine lysosomal contribution.

ELECTROLYTES

Certain electrolyte and water abnormalities occur during shock. For example, endotoxin shock in the dog is associated with hyperkalemia, hyperosmolarity, and acidosis (61). In addition to the well-known effects of these abnormalities on the heart, this combination causes vasodilation in isolated organs and depresses systemic arterial blood pressure in the intact dog (20,26,46), partly due to a decrease in total peripheral resistance (16). However, cationic abnormalities appear to cause minimal changes in the dog liver vasculature (2). Also, cationic abnormalities have little effect on veins. While there can be little doubt that these conditions are detrimental, the role of electrolyte and water abnormalities in the pathogenesis of shock is uncertain.

CENTRAL NERVOUS SYSTEM

Involvement of the central nervous system (CNS) in the pathogenesis of endotoxin shock is uncertain. In 1952, Penner and Klein (53) postulated that endotoxin acted directly on the CNS to produce the typical derangements of endotoxin shock. This conclusion was based on experiments in which the head and body circulations were isolated by a cross-perfusion technique. In paired dogs, the head of each animal was isolated from its own body circulation and perfused through one carotid artery with arterial blood from the other dog's body. Intravenously injected *Shigella* endotoxin produced shock only in the dog whose whole head was perfused with blood from the endotoxin-injected dog. Weil *et al.* (62) repeated and extended these experiments using *E. coli* endotoxin. Endotoxin injected intravenously into the trunk of the isolated, perfused head, or into decapitated dogs, or into spinal cats, caused early pathological changes resembling those seen in the intact animal. While it was concluded that the CNS was not essential for initiation of endotoxin shock, participation of the CNS in the subsequent course of shock was not ruled out. A problem in both of these studies (53,62) was an incomplete separation of the body and head circulations, which permitted endotoxin injected into one system to gain entrance into the other. Also, *Shigella* endotoxin apparently differs in certain ways from typical endotoxin obtained from gram-negative bacterial organisms (62).

Other approaches to this problem have been attempted. For example, shock has been induced by injection of small amounts of *Shigella* (52) or *E. coli* (56,57) endotoxin into the cerebral ventricular spaces. Simmons *et al.* (56,57) concluded that CNS effects of endotoxin may contribute to the development of shock, although several differences in response to endotoxin were noted between intraventricular or intracisternal *vs.* intravenous endotoxin injection. Possibly, then, the CNS may be involved in the pathogenesis of gram-negative endotoxin shock.

REFERENCES

1. Brake, C.M., T.E. Emerson, Jr., L.E. Wittmers, and L.B. Hinshaw. Alteration of vascular responses to endotoxin by adrenergic blockade. Am. J. Physiol. 207:149-151, 1964.

2. Chou, C.C., and T.E. Emerson, Jr. Local effects of Na^+, K^+, Mg^{++} and Ca^{++} on vascular resistances in the dog liver. Am. J. Physiol. 215:1102-1106, 1968.

3. Christy, J.H. Pathophysiology of gram-negative shock. Am. Heart J. 81:694-701, 1971.

4. Daugherty, R.M., Jr., J.B. Scott, T.E. Emerson, Jr., and F.J. Haddy. Comparison of intravenous and intra-arterial infusion of vasoactive agents on dog forelimb blood flow. Am. J. Physiol. 214:611-619, 1968.

5. Davis, R.B., W.R. Meeker, and W.L. Bailey. Serotonin release by bacterial endotoxin. Proc. Soc. Exptl. Biol. Med. 108: 774-776, 1961.

6. Davis, R.B., W.R. Meeker, and D.G. McQuarrie. Immediate effects of intravenous endotoxin on serotonin concentrations and blood platelets. Circ. Res. 8:234-239, 1960.

7. Egdahl, R.H. The differential response of the adrenal cortex and medulla to bacterial endotoxin. J. Clin. Invest. 38: 1120-1125, 1959.

8. Emerson, T.E., Jr. Changes of venous return and other hemodynamic parameters during bradykinin infusion. Am. J. Physiol. 212:1455-1460, 1967.

9. Emerson, T.E., Jr. Effects of acetylcholine, histamine, and serotonin infusion on venous return in dogs. Am. J. Physiol. 215:41-48, 1968.

10. Emerson, T.E., Jr. Effect of angiotensin, norepinephrine, epinephrine, and vasopressin on venous return. Am. J. Physiol. 210:933-942, 1966.

11. Emerson, T.E., Jr., C.M. Brake, and L.B. Hinshaw. Endotoxin shock in chronic splanchnic denervated dogs. J. Trauma 5: 737-740, 1965.

12. Emerson, T.E., Jr., C.M. Brake, and L.B. Hinshaw. Renal vascular response to angiotensin and other vasoactive agents in endotoxin shock. Am. J. Physiol. 207:1260-1264, 1964.

13. Emerson, T.E., Jr., C.M. Brake, and L.B. Hinshaw. Splanchnic sympathetic and adrenal participation in endotoxin shock. J. Oklahoma State Med. Assoc. 59:425-431, 1966.

14. Emerson, T.E., Jr., and C.C. Gill. Effect of slow intravenous infusion of endotoxin in dogs. J. Appl. Physiol. 22:874-878, 1967.

15. Emerson, T.E., Jr., L.B. Hinshaw, and C.M. Brake. Vascular effects of angiotensin and norepinephrine in the dog, cat, and monkey. Am. J. Physiol. 208:260-264, 1965.

16. Emerson, T.E., Jr., and G.W. Jelks. Effects of increased plasma cationic levels on venous return and other parameters in dogs. Fed. Proc. 29:526, 1970.

17. Emerson, T.E., Jr., G.W. Jelks, and R.M. Daugherty, Jr. Effects of prostaglandin E_1 and $F_{2\alpha}$ on venous return and other parameters in the dog. Am. J. Physiol. 220:243-249, 1971.

18. Emerson, T.E., Jr., and F.C. Kelly. Effect of living *E. coli* cells on hemodynamics and mortality in the dog. J. Appl. Physiol. 23:609-612, 1967.

19. Emerson, T.E., Jr., P.D. Meier, and R.M. Daugherty, Jr. Local vascular responses to serotonin in dog skeletal muscle at different levels of resistance. Fed. Proc. 30:212, 1971.

20. Emerson, T.E., Jr., J.B. Scott, and F.J. Haddy. Effects of acute multiple alterations in plasma electrolyte levels on dog blood pressure. Am. J. Physiol. 218:234-240, 1970.

21. Emerson, T.E., Jr., D.T. Wagner, and C.C. Gill. *In situ* kidney pressure-flow resistance relationship during endotoxin shock in dogs. Proc. Soc. Exptl. Biol. Med. 122:366-368, 1966.

22. Erods, E.G., and I. Miwa. Effect of endotoxin on the plasma kallikrein-kinin system of the rabbit. Fed. Proc. 27:92-95, 1968.

23. Glucksmann, E.E., and A.M. Lefer. Effects of a myocardial depressant factor on isolated vascular smooth muscle. Am. J. Physiol. 220:1581-1585, 1970.

24. Grega, G.J., and F.J. Haddy. Forelimb transcapillary fluid fluxes and vascular resistance in catecholamine shock. Am. J. Physiol. 220:1448-1462, 1971.

25. Haddy, F.J., T.E. Emerson, Jr., J.B. Scott, and R.M. Daugherty, Jr. The effect of kinins of the cardiovascular system. In: *Handbuch der Experimentellen Pharmakologie*. Berlin-Heidelberg: Springer-Verlag, 1970, vol. XXV, pp. 362-384.

26. Haddy, F.J., J.B. Scott, T.E. Emerson, Jr., H.W. Overbeck, and R.M. Daugherty, Jr. Effects of generalized changes in plasma electrolyte concentration and osmolarity on blood pressure in the anesthetized dog. Circ. Res. 24:159-173, 1969.

27. Hall, R.C., and R.L. Hodge. Vasoactive hormones in endotoxin shock: A comparative study in cats and dogs. J. Physiol. (London) 213:69-84, 1971.

28. Hinshaw, L.B., L.T. Archer, L.J. Greenfield, and C.A. Guenter. Effects of endotoxin on myocardial hemodynamics, performance and metabolism. Am. J. Physiol 221:504-510, 1971.

29. Hinshaw, L.B., C.M. Brake, and T.E. Emerson, Jr. Biochemical and pathological alterations in endotoxin shock. In: *Shock and Hypotension: Pathogenesis and Treatment*. New York: Grune & Stratton, 1965.

30. Hinshaw, L.B., C.M. Brake, T.E. Emerson, Jr., M.M. Jordan, and F.D. Masucci. Participation of the sympathoadrenal system in endotoxin shock. Am. J. Physiol. 207:925-930, 1964.

31. Hinshaw, L.B., T.E. Emerson, Jr., P.F. Iampietro, and C.M. Brake. A comparative study of the hemodynamic actions of histamine and endotoxin. Am. J. Physiol. 203:600-606, 1962.

32. Hinshaw, L.B., T.E. Emerson, Jr., and D.A. Reins. Cardiovascular responses of the primate in endotoxin shock: Mechanism of hypotension. Am. J. Physiol. 210:335-340, 1966.

33. Hinshaw, L.B., M.M. Jordan, and J.A. Vick. Histamine release and endotoxin shock in the primate. J. Clin. Invest. 40: 1631-1637, 1961.

34. Hinshaw, L.B., M.M. Jordan, and J.A. Vick. Mechanism of histamine release in endotoxin shock. Am. J. Physiol. 200:987-989, 1961.

35. Hinshaw, L.B., H. Kuida, R.P. Gilbert, and M.B. Visscher. Influence of perfusate characteristics on pulmonary vascular response to endotoxin. Am. J. Physiol. 191:293-295, 1957.

36. Hinshaw, L.B., and S.E. Owen. Correlation of pooling and resistance changes in the canine forelimb in septic shock. J. Appl. Physiol. 30:331-337, 1971.

37. Hinshaw, L.B., J.A. Vick, C.H. Carlson, and Y.L. Fan. Role of histamine in endotoxin shock. Proc. Soc. Exptl. Biol. Med. 104:379-381, 1960.

38. Hinshaw, L.B., J.A. Vick, M.M. Jordan, and L.E. Wittmers. Vascular changes associated with development of irreversible endotoxin shock. Am. J. Physiol. 202:103-110, 1962.

39. Iturri, S., and T.E. Emerson, Jr. Responses of arterial vessel strips from skin and muscle to serotonin. Proc. Soc. Exptl. Biol. Med. 137:416-420, 1971.

40. Jacobson, E.D., B. Mehlman, and J.P. Kalas. Vasoactive mediators as the "trigger mechanism" of endotoxin shock. J. Clin. Invest. 43:1000-1013, 1964.

41. Kobold, E.E., R. Lovell, W. Katz, and A.P. Thal. Chemical mediators released by endotoxin. Surg. Gynecol. Obstet. 118:807-813, 1964.

42. Kuida, H., R.P. Gilbert, L.B. Hinshaw, J.C. Brunson, and M.B. Visscher. Species difference of gram-negative endotoxin on circulation. Am. J. Physiol. 200:1197-1202, 1961.

43. Lefer, A.M. Role of a myocardial depressant factor in the pathogenesis of circulatory shock. Fed. Proc. 29:1836-1847, 1970.

44. Lillehei, R.C., J.K. Longerbeam, J.H. Block, and W.G. Manax. The nature of irreversible shock: Experimental and clinical observations. Ann. Surg. 160:682-708, 1964.

45. McGiff, J.C., K. Crawshaw, N.A. Terrangno, A.J. Lonigro, J.C. Strand, M.A. Williamson, J.B. Lee, and K.K.F. Ng. Prostaglandin-like substances appearing in canine renal venous blood during renal ischemia. Circ. Res. 27:765-782, 1970.

46. McKeag, D.B., T.E. Emerson, Jr., and F.J. Haddy. Effects of electrolyte abnormalities on blood pressure in spinally blocked dogs. Clin. Res. 17:514, 1969.

47. Motsay, G.J., A. Alho, T. Jaeger, R. Dietzman, and R.C. Lillehei. Effects of corticosteroids in shock: Experimental and clinical results. Fed. Proc. 29:1861-1873, 1970.

48. Nies, A.S., R.P. Forsyth, and H.E. Williams. Contribution of kinins to endotoxin shock in unanesthetized monkeys. Circ. Res. 22:155-164, 1968.

49. Nykeil, F., and V.V. Glaviano. Adrenal catecholamines in *E. coli* endotoxin shock. J. Appl. Physiol. 16:348-350, 1961.

50. Parker, J., T.E. Emerson, Jr., and R.M. Daugherty, Jr. Vascular responses in the canine forelimb during intra-arterial infusion of prostaglandin A_1. Physiologist 14: 206, 1971.

51. Parker, J., G. Jelks, and T. Emerson, Jr. Cardiovascular effects of prostaglandin A_1 in the dog. Fed. Proc., in press.

52. Penner, A., and A.I. Bernheim. Studies in the pathogenesis of experimental dysentery intoxication. J. Exptl. Med. 111:145-153, 1960.

53. Penner, A., and S.H. Klein. The pathogenesis of experimental dysentery intoxication. J. Exptl. Med. 96:59-69, 1952.

54. Rosenberg, J.C., R.C. Lillehei, J. Longerbeam, and B. Zimmerman. Studies on hemorrhagic and endotoxin shock in relation to vasomotor changes and endogenous circulating epinephrine, norepinephrine and serotonin. Ann. Surg. 154: 611-627, 1961.

55. Rosenberg, J.C., R.C. Lillehei, W.H. Moran, and B. Zimmerman. Effect of endotoxin on plasma catecholamines and serum serotonin. Proc. Soc. Exptl. Biol. Med. 102:335-337, 1959.

56. Simmons, R.L., R.W. Anderson, T.B. Ducker, H.K. Sleeman, J.A. Collins, and K.P. Boothman. The role of the central nervous system in septic shock. II. Hemodynamics, respiratory and metabolic effects of intracisternal or intraventricular endotoxin. Ann. Surg. 167:158-167, 1968.

57. Simmons, R.L., T.B. Ducker, A.M. Martin, R.W. Anderson, and H.E. Noyes. The role of the central nervous system in septic shock. I. Pathologic changes following intraventricular and intracisternal endotoxin in the dog. Ann. Surg. 167:145-157, 1968.

58. Thal, A.P., and V.M. Sardesai. Shock and circulating polypeptides. Am. J. Surg. 110:308-312, 1965.

59. Vick, J.A. Trigger mechanism of endotoxin shock. Am. J. Physiol. 206:944-946, 1964.

60. Vick, J.A., B. Mehlman, and H. Heiffer. Early histamine release and death due to endotoxin. Proc. Soc. Exptl. Biol. Med. 137:902-906, 1971.

61. Weidner, W.J., G.J. Grega, and F.J. Haddy. Changes in forelimb weight and vascular resistances during endotoxin shock. Am. J. Physiol. 221:1229-1237, 1971.

62. Weil, M.H., L.D. MacLean, W.W. Spink, and M.B. Visscher. Investigations on the role of the central nervous system in shock produced by endotoxin from gram-negative microorganisms. J. Lab. Clin. Med. 48:661-672, 1956.

63. Weiner, R., and B.W. Zweifach. Influence of *E. coli* endotoxin on serotonin contractions of the rabbit aortic strip. Proc. Soc. Exptl. Biol. Med. 123:937-939, 1966.

64. White, F.N., E.M. Gold, and D.L. Vaughn. Renin-aldosterone system in endotoxin shock in the dog. Am. J. Physiol. 212: 1195-1198, 1966.

65. Zweifach, B.W., A.L. Nagler, and L. Thomas. The role of epinephrine in the reactions produced by endotoxin of gram-negative bacteria. II. The changes produced by endotoxin in the vascular reactivity to epinephrine in the rat mesoappendix and the isolated, perfused rabbit ear. J. Exptl. Med. 104:881-896, 1956.

DISCUSSION

DR. W. C. SHOEMAKER, *Panel Moderator (New York, N.Y.):* I'm delighted with this skepticism of this therapeutic nihilism.

DR. M. H. WEIL *(Los Angeles, Calif.):* On the basis of experimental studies in the primate and other species besides the dog, do we have substantial evidence that changes in the resistance bed can be implicated as economically important, from the point of view of explaining the decrease in cardiac output and the subsequent damage that we attribute to perfusion failure in experimental shock states?

DR. EMERSON: In our experience in the monkeys, I agree with you. I think the primary defect, as we have seen it, is not on the arterial side or in the peripheral resistance. It seems to be on the capacitance side. There is a slowly progressive decrease in venous return, a pooling of blood, if you wish—where, I don't know. I think the primary defect lies in the capacitance system.

DR. SHOEMAKER: Dr. Emerson, my vision wasn't very good from up here. When the slides were shown, did you include, in this group of therapeutic fiascos, hydrocortisone per chance, or methylprednisolone?

DR. EMERSON: Yes, it was on that slide.

DR. G. MOTSAY *(Minneapolis, Minn.):* Could we ask what the dose was that was used there, please?

DR. EMERSON: It was Dr. Lillehei's procedure. I think it was 50 mg/kg, although I'm not sure. It was a high dose, in other words.

DR. MOTSAY: Was that hydrocortisone or methylprednisolone?

DR. EMERSON: I think it was hydrocortisone, but I'd have to check to be sure.

PULMONARY DYSFUNCTION IN SHOCK

Lazar J. Greenfield, M.D.

Department of Surgery, University of Oklahoma Medical Center, Oklahoma City, Oklahoma

Informal Presentation[1]

The pulmonary lesions associated with shock often seem to be the prime determinants of patient survival. These lesions are apparently manifested in two ways. The first is an early syndrome of acute hypoxia, most typically seen in the septic shock patient. We can duplicate this hypoxic state in the laboratory by insult with an endotoxin or live organism injection. In our animal experiments, the effects suggest some degree of pulmonary microembolic phenomena. Histologically, aggregates of leukocytes are evident which promote an increase in pulmonary vascular resistance and seem to produce shunting in the pulmonary vascular bed. We have corroborated this in different ways, primarily by using an isogravimetric lung perfusion model.

Perhaps more important, however, is the second or late syndrome. Progressive respiratory failure is seen, usually after more or less successful resuscitation of a patient. Here, a hemodynamically stable patient develops a form of respiratory dysfunction resistant to therapy, which proceeds to progressive respiratory failure and death. It is this late syndrome that has been the most refractory to treatment.

The mechanism which primarily interests us involves the pulmonary vascular bed and particularly the pulmonary capillaries. What

---

[1]This manuscript appears here as presented at the symposium, with minor editorial revisions.

occurs here may explain the interstitial pulmonary edema customarily found in the lungs of patients dying with the "shock lung" syndrome. These capillaries play a unique role in terms of the hydrostatic pressure gradient if we accept Guyton's premise that there is a large negative interstitial pressure. Alterations in these pressures must be involved in the sequence of edema formation in the lungs. We also must consider the role of osmotic pressures, which raises the question of the role of crystalloid therapy in shock and the genesis of the pulmonary lesion. The addition of large volumes of crystalloid, which are known to distribute themselves both without and within the vascular bed, presumably can facilitate the deposition of these fluids in the interstitial space. We suspect that interstitial edema is one of the common denominators in the lung during late progressive respiratory failure. However, after studying the sequence of edema formation in the isolated perfused lung, we found that the edema induced by hemodilution differs markedly from that induced by venous hypertension.

After infusion of the crystalloid, one can generate alveolar wall edema and confirm its presence by adding a dye to the perfusate which is seen throughout the alveolar interstitium on light and electron microscopy. In contrast to this, the edema that occurs with venous constriction is localized to the perivenular spaces and produces opposite effects on the pulmonary capillary pressures and on respiratory exchange. Although the pulmonary capillary pressures that we measure by the isogravimetric perfusion technique are just one portion of the Starling equation, all of the shock preparation animals show a paradoxical increase in pulmonary capillary pressures in contrast to systemic capillaries, where the decrease in pressures suggests an increase in capillary permeability. When we generate interstitial pulmonary edema by pulmonary venous constriction, the effects include an elevation in pulmonary capillary pressure similar to that observed in the shocked animals insulted either by endotoxin or live organisms. However, after inducing interstitial edema by dilution with Ringer's lactate solution, we observe a lower pulmonary capillary pressure and no interference with respiratory gas exchange at a comparable degree of added wet weight. The effects on the osmotic gradients may be entirely different in the two groups, depending on the protein concentration in the interstitial space. In addition, we see a decrease in pulmonary vascular resistance in both groups which begins to rise toward control values in the venous constriction group after accumulation of 30-40 g of edematous fluid. Also, at this level of edema we note beginning interference with gas exchange, perhaps on the basis of arteriovenous shunting.

SUMMARY

The edema induced by hemodilution and that induced by venous hypertension seem to have quite different effects on gas exchange and pulmonary capillary pressure, although they both impair lung mechanics. In animal experiments, effective compliance is altered to a similar extent in both groups, which show comparable increases in wet-to-dry weight ratios. One may speculate further on the validity of incriminating crystalloid infusion alone or whether it is necessary to explore the pressure relationships in the pulmonary venous capacitance bed. Certainly the minimal elevation of pulmonary venous pressure which is required to produce edema should ordinarily be well tolerated. The etiology of the "shock lung" then would seem to involve increased permeability of a capillary bed insulted by shock and the effectiveness of fluid clearance from the pulmonary interstitial space.

DISCUSSION

DR. W. C. SHOEMAKER, *Panel Moderator (New York, N.Y.):* Are you saying, then, Lazar [Dr. Greenfield], that when we treat a patient in shock, we have to fill him up with fluids and give him the appropriate volumes? If it's a burn, are we to follow the book formula? And now, you're telling us that, by so doing, we are prejudicing this patient and he is dying from respiratory failure. Is that correct?

DR. GREENFIELD: We may well be adding an insult, at least to his pulmonary vascular bed, if we recognize the fact that this is the first capillary bed that our infusion therapy encounters in terms of unloading. However, usually the increase in density and fluid in the lungs is handled pretty well by the patients who subsequently diurese the excess fluid. One can question whether or not we have added a significant degree of insult, since this may not be the sole factor, as we have already indicated.

DR. B. D. LOWERY *(Baltimore, Md.):* Dr. Shoemaker, may I ask Dr. Greenfield a question? The core to this issue is the site of the constriction in the pulmonary vascular bed, as you have indicated. Would you comment on the controversy that exists between the data of Dr. Webb and those of Dr. Vieth? One suggests that the site of constriction in shock due to hemorrhage in trauma is at the pulmonary venous level, the other that it's at the pulmonary arterial or arteriolar level.

DR. GREENFIELD: I think you have implied the question of whether we can accept a unified hypothesis of pulmonary arterial constriction, as Vieth has advocated. I, personally, am unwilling to accept this at the present time. We have approached this by using our pulmonary capillary pressures to separate pre- and post-capillary resistances. We find that there is, indeed, a change, but it is not the change we expect. When we induce the graded hydrostatic edema and progressively increase the perfusion of the lung, overcoming the usual inflation gradients in the lung, we find that vascular resistance on the precapillary side falls initially and then returns toward control. Therefore, there seems to be no significant change in vascular resistance until we reach a significant load on the vascular bed. This may become an intolerable load, with spillover into the alveolar spaces, which would be recognized as overt pulmonary edema.

DR. SHOEMAKER: Do you wish to comment? Are there further questions?

DR. M. H. WEIL *(Los Angeles, Calif.):* Dr. Stein in our group has just recently completed a study of four patients who had radiographically demonstrable pulmonary congestion and pulmonary edema clinically, of unequivocal sorts. They had normal wedge pressures and normal left ventricular end diastolic pressures. Their colloid osmotic pressure was reduced to an average of 16 mm Hg and their estimated left ventricular filling pressure was on the order of 11 mm Hg. This, I think, tends to corroborate exactly what Dr. Greenfield had reference to, namely, that there is a significant lowering of colloid osmotic pressure. These values are more than 2 SD units away from those of our normal patients. Yet, at the same time, there is something around a 5 mm gradient between what would theoretically be pulmonary edema and the pressure conditions existing within the pulmonary capillary bed. Whether this difference, Dr. Greenfield, is, as you suggest, partly explained by changes in the capillary permeability or whether it might be due to factors relating to tissue pressures in the lung is the sort of information that we'd like to have very soon.

THE LUNG LESION IN SHOCK

Irwin R. Berman, M.D.

Department of Surgery, New York University Medical Center, New York, New York

Informal Presentation[1]

In this discussion, I will describe some of the mechanisms which I feel are basic to the lung lesion in shock and will attempt to unify these features into a logical sequence of events. Emphasis will be placed upon one mechanism by which permeability of the pulmonary capillary membrane may be altered to permit transudation of fluid into the lung interstitium.

Overinfusion, transfusion of old blood, sepsis, hypoxemia, and numerous other mechanisms have been incriminated in the occurrence of pulmonary insufficiency after shock and trauma. Yet severe hemorrhage, major trauma, endotoxin shock, and massive transfusion have one very important element in common. This common denominator is the production of intravascular microaggregates which are composed, in part, of aggregated blood platelets. The occurrence of embolization of such blood aggregates has been recognized since the early 1940's (3) and is associated with shock, with limb ischemia, and with long-bone fracture. In addition, pulmonary microembolism has been implicated both in arterial hypoxemia following injury and in the elevation of pulmonary arterial pressure in shock experiments. Using the screen filtration pressure technique, we have studied the occurrence of intravascular microaggregation after hemorrhage, trauma, and burn injury. This technique involves passage of blood at a constant rate through a 20-micron micromesh filter. A side-arm proximal to the filter is connected

[1]This manuscript appears here as presented at the symposium, with minor editorial revisions.

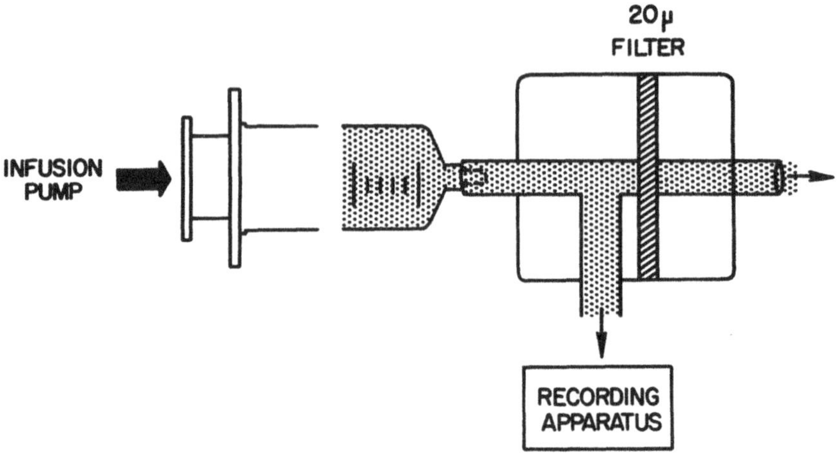

FIG. 1. Apparatus for determination of screen filtration pressure.

to a recording apparatus for measurement of screen filtration pressure (SFP) in millimeters of mercury (Fig. 1). The SFP of normal blood is less than 50 mm Hg.

A study of 89 moderately to severely injured young men was performed in the Republic of Vietnam (1). With rare exception, these patients were hospitalized within 2 hours after injury. At the time of admission, 59% of these men showed abnormal microaggregation by elevation of SFP. SFP was also elevated in 40-50% of the patients in the succeeding 4 days. During this period of study, 95% of patients with elevation of both arterial and venous SFP developed arterial hypoxemia, suggesting a relationship of hypoxemia to the occurrence of microaggregates in the systemic circulation. Since most patients with elevation of both arterial and venous SFP had sustained blast or fracture injury, it was tempting to postulate that suspension stability of blood elements was altered as the result of hemorrhage and transfusion superimposed upon a severe percussive injury.

To delineate more precisely the mechanisms operating in this series of seriously injured patients, we studied the occurrence of intravascular aggregation in the venous effluent of a very limited soft-tissue injury inflicted upon the hind limb of baboons (2). This injury was produced with a captive bolt pistol which produced a relatively uniform nonpenetrating wound. The fascinating finding in these studies was an almost immediate marked increase in SFP in

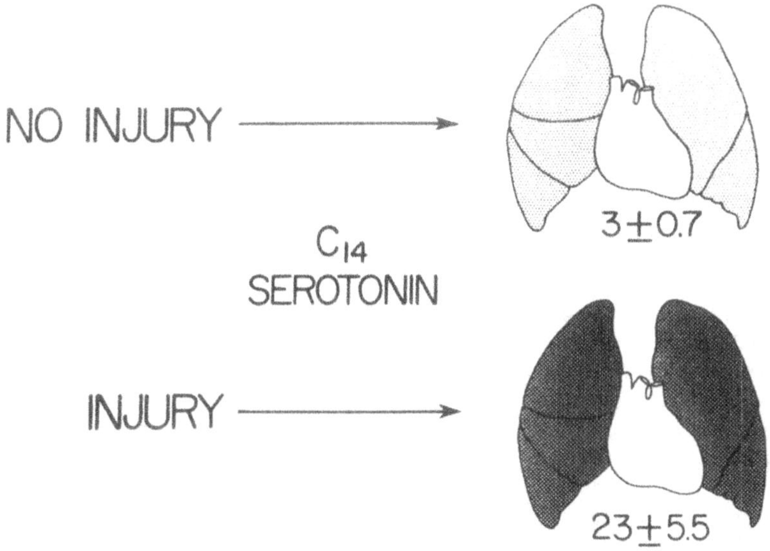

FIG. 2. Carbon-14 specific activity in lung tissue after limb injury in baboons. (Courtesy of Surgery 70:246, 1971.)

the venous effluent of injury. The extent of microaggregation was even greater if fracture was then produced, although femoral arterial ligation combined with injury produced SFP values comparable to those obtained with soft-tissue injury alone. Fall in platelet count in the venous effluent of injury suggested that intravascular aggregates detected by rising SFP were composed largely of blood platelets. In addition, the intravenous administration of a platelet label (^{14}C-labeled serotonin) to these animals showed a marked increase in ^{14}C specific activity in the lungs of injured baboons (23±5.5) compared to that of uninjured animals (3±0.7) (Fig. 2). More recently, these experiments have been repeated in baboons made thrombocytopenic before injury by the administration of platelet antiserum. These experiments further incriminated platelet aggregation in the sequelae of injury, since SFP failed to rise in the venous effluent of injury in these thrombocytopenic animals. Nevertheless, in animals made thrombocytopenic by this technique, pulmonary interstitial edema occurred with regularity. Although more work will be needed in this area, we believe that the occurrence of interstitial edema in these baboons is the result of massive intravascular aggregation of blood platelets induced by the antiserum. Presumably, this reaction establishes a matrix in the lung upon which pulmonary edema may occur.

As I have mentioned, altered blood aggregation, pulmonary

microembolism, and arterial hypoxemia have been described in a variety of conditions. Others will discuss platelet aggregation from the standpoint of prevention and therapy. We have examined one mechanism which may help to explain the basic response of platelet aggregation to these multiple stimuli. It is well known that aggregation of blood platelets occurs upon contact of platelets with exposed collagen. This may be a protective phenomenon, which partially explains the intravascular aggregation in the experiments described above. Taking advantage of this reaction between platelets and collagen, we studied the ability of connective tissue to aggregate blood platelets after hemorrhage and burn shock in rats. In both of these experimental situations, blood SFP rises markedly, indicating intravascular microaggregation. Also, both clinical entities are frequently associated with severe pulmonary insufficiency. The results thus far in this study indicate that the basic ability of connective tissue of these shocked animals to aggregate blood platelets is enhanced. Indeed, incubation of platelets with connective tissue from these animals results in platelet aggregation 35% to 40% earlier, with up to 60% greater slope than that observed in controls. These findings are unrelated to changes in connective tissue water content and suggest a common mechanism in the pathogenesis of intravascular microaggregation in these related conditions.

The pulmonary capillary bed is known to be composed of a vast network of capillaries capable of filtering blood elements larger than normal red cells. In addition, the lung serves normally as an organ for storage and for filtration of blood platelets. Hence, this organ is the natural trap for particulate matter in the venous blood. We have therefore supported the following chain of events as a unified mechanism to explain the pulmonary lesion of these related conditions (Fig. 3). Hemorrhage, trauma, and massive transfusion may all lead to the development of intravascular aggregates and pulmonary microembolism. It is likely that severe acidosis, tissue ischemia, and transfusion of old blood may contribute to intravascular aggregation. In addition, it is attractive to postulate that the occurrence of this phenomenon is further increased by a fundamental enhancement in the natural ability of connective tissue to aggregate blood platelets. Once aggregates have reached the lung, pulmonary function may be altered on the basis of a mechanical obstruction (*i.e.*, microvascular) and/or active vasoconstriction, the latter being due to release of vasoactive amines from aggregated blood platelets. Finally, in some patients, release of lysosomal enzymes or other vascular permeability factors from aggregated platelets may supersede and may contribute to transudation from the pulmonary capillary bed and pulmonary interstitial edema.

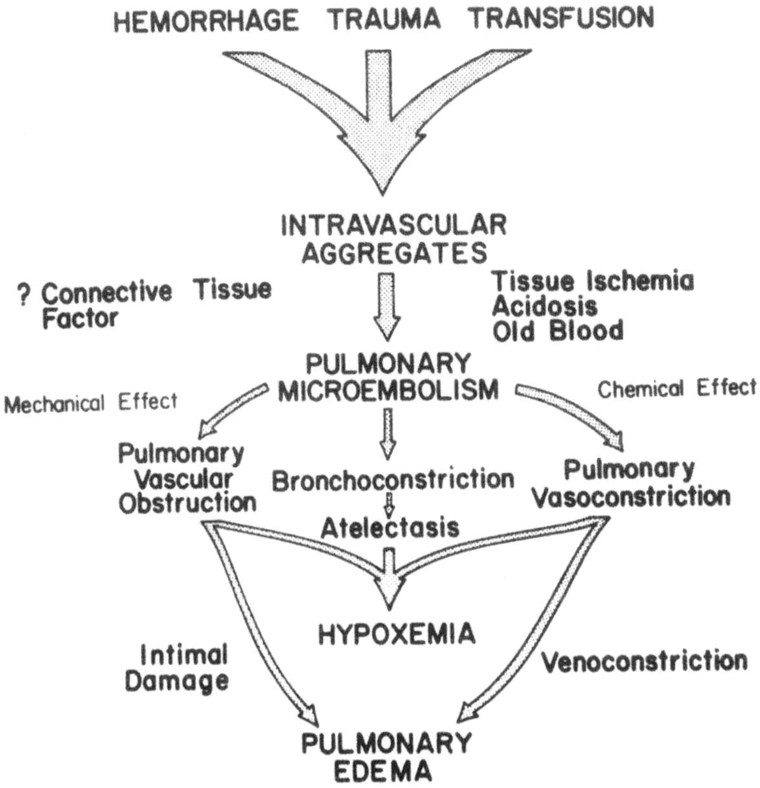

FIG. 3. Hypothetical sequence of events in the development of pulmonary insufficiency after shock and trauma.

REFERENCES

1. Berman, I.R., V.S. Gutierrez, A.L. Burran, and R.D. Boatright. Intravascular microaggregation in young men with combat injuries. Surg. Forum 20:14, 1969.

2. Berman, I.R., M.E. Smulson, P. Pattengale, and S.F. Schoenbach. Pulmonary microembolism after soft tissue injury in primates. Surgery 70:246, 1971.

3. Zucker, M.B. Platelet agglutination and vasoconstriction as factors in spontaneous hemostasis in normal, thrombocytopenic, heparinized and hypoprothrombinemic rats. Am. J. Physiol. 148:275, 1947.

PHYSIOLOGIC MECHANISMS IN CLINICAL SHOCK[1]

William C. Shoemaker, M.D.

Department of Surgery, Mount Sinai School of Medicine,
City University of New York, New York

In clinical terms, shock has been defined as hypotension, tachycardia, cold and clammy extremities, oliguria, stupor, and collapse. In physiological terms, it has been defined as low cardiac output with high resistance. These definitions have been based on data obtained in the dog subjected to the Wiggers' type of experimental hemorrhagic shock and in patients with hemorrhagic and cardiogenic shock (3-5,9,19,20). Moreover, the concept of shock as low output-high resistance appears intuitively attractive since, experimentally, pressure and flow diminish as blood volume decreases and flow ceases when pressure falls to zero.

However attractive this conventional concept of shock may be, it does not adequately explain the majority of clinical shock problems which we have encountered (8,12). We contend that data of hemorrhagic and cardiogenic shock have been erroneously extrapolated to all forms of shock. Obviously, when the low-output concept is diametrically opposed to observed data, therapy based upon the incorrect concept may be inappropriate and ineffectual.

The body's responses to the primary etiologic event produce secondary effects which, together with the underlying physiologic mechanisms, may be complex. Nevertheless, these effects, their underlying mechanisms, and their interactions may be systematically approached by analyzing data obtained in a sequential fashion.

[1]This research was supported by United States Army Contract DADA 17-71-C-9089.

The present study was undertaken to elucidate some of the physiologic mechanisms in clinical shock by description of sequential cardiorespiratory events based on more than 10,000 sets of measurements in 180 patients. Physiologic alterations were divided into the normal control, early, middle, and late periods using arbitrary but rigorously applied criteria. It was assumed that physiologic mechanisms underlying the early events may have pathogenic significance. Physiologic mechanisms underlying hemodynamic changes of the middle period of shock may intensify and prolong the shock state. They may contribute to the ultimate demise of the patient, but they probably should not be considered pathogenic in the strict sense of the word. It is also assumed that some mechanisms represent compensatory responses of the body and may be of advantage, while some are counterproductive and may jeopardize survival. Mechanisms operating in the late stage represent the terminal mechanisms, without pathogenic relevance. The present paper summarizes prior studies in this field (13) and describes work from this institution, with emphasis on the initial reactions to stress rather than the terminal mechanisms.

MATERIALS AND METHODS

Clinical Material

Sequential physiologic measurements were made in a series of 180 shock patients who had sustained: (a) uncomplicated hemorrhage, (b) uncomplicated sepsis, (c) accidental trauma, *i.e.*, without hemorrhage or anesthesia, (d) surgical trauma, (e) sepsis plus hemorrhage and trauma, and (f) cardiac tamponade. The observations reflect the natural history of various types of clinical shock from the physiologic point of view. A search was made for patterns (*e.g.*, specific events as well as time course) which were distinctive for each form of shock. Measurements were made during periods of relative stability when the patient showed no anxiety, restlessness, or agitation. All measurements were taken before therapy, or after the immediate effects of therapy had worn off.

Criteria for Separation of Data into Stages

Since events unfold in time, but not necessarily at the same rate, the data for each group of patients were separated into normal control, early, middle, and late periods to describe the cardiorespiratory patterns. The mean arterial pressure provided an objective, although arbitrary, criterion. The control period prior to onset of the etiologic event or in the post-trauma recovery period was defined as stage A. Usually these data were consistent with control values obtained from 17 healthy volunteer subjects with no evidence of circulatory disorders (18). Stage B was defined as the early period of falling arterial pressure immediately after the etiologic event. The lowest recorded arterial pressure (stage *low*) separated this early period from stage C, the middle period. The latter was divided into stages C_1 and C_2 by the point in time when arterial pressure returned halfway to control values. Stage D was defined as the late (*i.e.*, recovery) period when the patient had normal or nearly normal arterial pressures. Stage E was defined as the preterminal period in patients who subsequently died; it covered the time up to about 1 hour before death, but not the final terminal event, stage F.

Techniques of Hemodynamic, Blood Gas and pH Measurements

The methods used in these studies had been reported previously (8,12,18). For measurement of arterial pressure and cardiac output, polyethylene catheters were inserted into the femoral artery by percutaneous puncture. Central venous pressure was measured through a 36-inch catheter via a brachial vein cutdown or percutaneous puncture of brachial or subclavian veins. Intravascular pressures were measured with Statham pressure transducers and recorded on an Offner multiple-channel recorder.

The standard indicator dilution technique with indocyanine green was used for measuring cardiac output. Blood, withdrawn from the artery, was passed through a Gilford densitometer. Cardiac output was calculated from the dye curve by the Stewart-Hamilton formula (6). Mean transit time, stroke volume, central blood volume, systemic vascular resistance, and left ventricular stroke work were calculated from standard formulas (3-5,8,9,12,13,18-20). All measurements were divided by the patient's body surface area and expressed as indexed values.

Arterial and mixed venous blood samples were obtained anaerobically at the time of cardiac output determinations. Samples were stored in ice water and analyzed as soon as possible. Arterial and mixed venous pO_2, pCO_2, and pH were determined at 37°C by an IL-113 gas analyzer with micro-blood pH assembly. Rectal temperatures were taken at frequent intervals. Hematocrit was measured by the standard microhematocrit technique on aliquots of the samples drawn for blood gas analysis. Arterial and mixed venous oxygen saturation values were measured directly and also calculated using the Severinghaus calculator (10). The oxygen contents were obtained from the oxygen saturation and hemoglobin values.

Oxygen extraction was expressed as the ratio of the arteriovenous oxygen content difference/arterial oxygen content. The

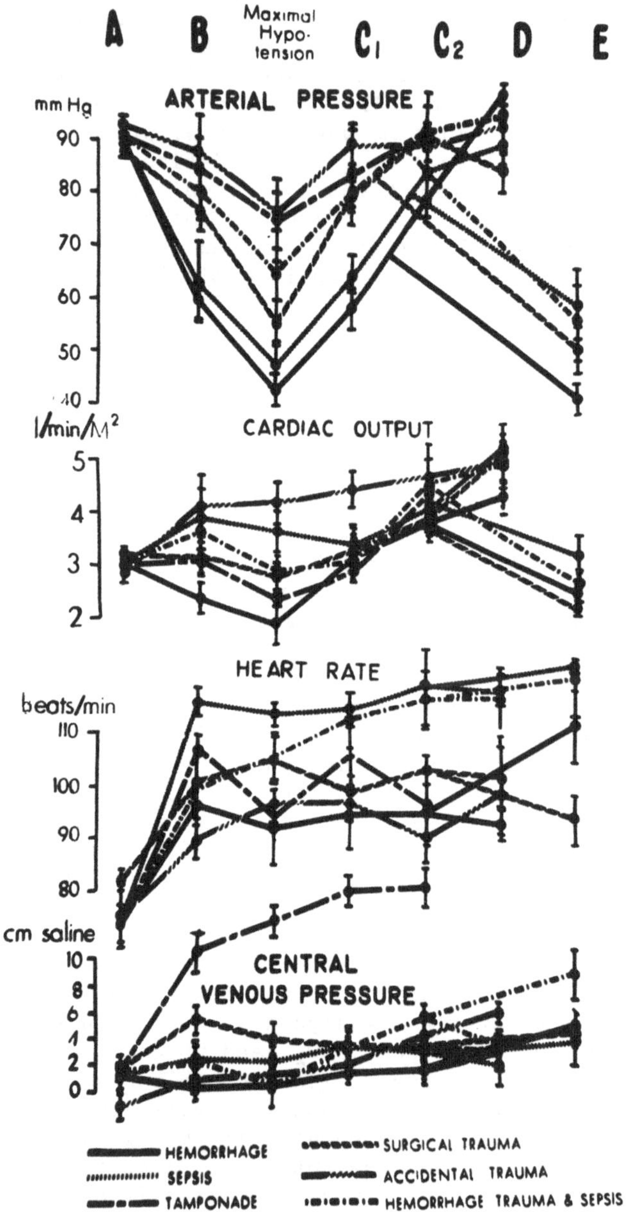

FIG. 1. (For figure legend, see top of next page.)

FIG. 1. Sequential hemodynamic changes in various types of shock. Data include means and SE for arterial pressure, cardiac index, heart rate, and central venous pressure. Note the fall in cardiac index in the B and *low* stage after hemorrhagic shock and to a lesser extent after cardiac tamponade. Other cardiac indices were normal or increased. Heart rates increased in all groups but were greatest in the two groups with sepsis. Venous pressures were within normal range except in the tamponade patients.

oxygen availability was calculated as the product of the cardiac index and the arterial oxygen content. Oxygen consumption was calculated as the product of cardiac index and arteriovenous oxygen content difference. Previously, oxygen consumption was measured concomitantly by this method and the direct Fick method under carefully controlled experimental conditions (8) as well as in clinical circumstances (7). The results of the simultaneous measurements by these two independent methods were in satisfactory agreement.

For purposes of this analysis, the patients were classified into groups with single, uncomplicated etiologic events and those with multiple causes. This was done so that the primary effect of the etiologic event could be defined in terms of the simplest and most obvious immediate action (*e.g.*, hypovolemia after hemorrhage). With this approach, the patients' physiologic responses to the primary effect (*e.g.*, tachycardia from neural mechanisms), as well as the secondary cardiorespiratory effects, could be more easily identified. Decompensations were defined as the physiologic changes which occurred in the preterminal and terminal period. Finally, the mechanisms underlying the observed responses were defined as those physiologic mechanisms most likely to operate under the observed conditions.

RESULTS

The data from 180 patients are summarized in Figures 1-3. There were 22 patients with uncomplicated hemorrhage, 18 with accidental blunt abdominal trauma, 57 with operative trauma, 18 with uncomplicated sepsis, 11 with cardiac tamponade, and 54 with the combination of hemorrhage, trauma, and sepsis. No striking differences emerged between the groups in terms of age, sex, race, or predisposing conditions.

Sequential cardiorespiratory data were analyzed and interpreted according to effects of the etiologic agents and the body's response to them. That is, physiologic alterations were considered

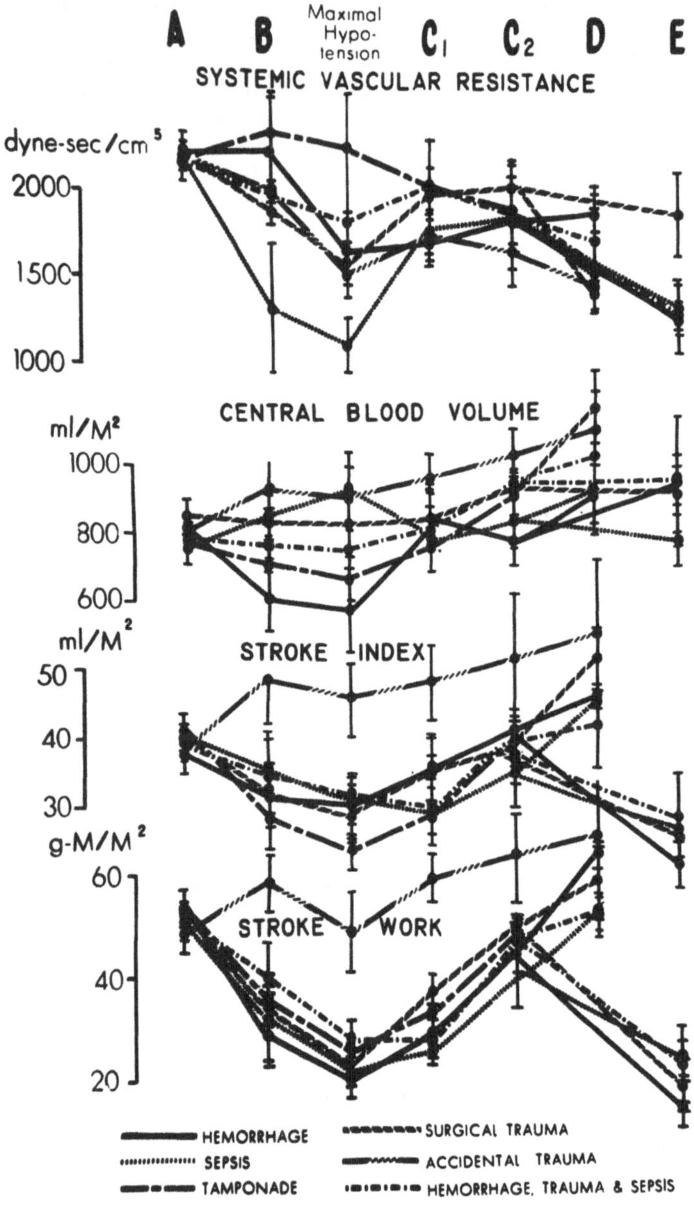

FIG. 2. (For figure legend, see top of next page.)

FIG. 2. Sequential hemodynamic changes including the derived calculations of peripheral resistance, central blood volume, stroke index, and left ventricular stroke work. Note the slight rise in peripheral resistance in the B stage after hemorrhage and tamponade; the resistance values tended to decrease progressively with time. In the B and *low* stages in hemorrhage and tamponade, central blood volume values tended to be low; the other values were normal or high. The stroke volume and stroke work increased progressively in accidental trauma, but these variables decreased in the B, *low* and C_1 stages in the other groups.

---

as: (a) the primary or direct effects of the etiologic agent, (b) compensatory responses by the body to these physiologic effects, (c) the secondary physiologic effects of the agent, and (d) circulatory decompensations. These evaluations are summarized in Tables 1-4.

Some of the physiologic responses and their controlling mechanisms which may operate in early stress are listed in Table 5.

DISCUSSION

This tentative analysis of the early physiologic mechanisms is based on descriptions of physiologic events and depends upon the accuracy of the methods and their reproducibility under conditions of study. Documentation and discussion of the magnitude of the errors of the method have previously been presented (2). The present approach also depends on the use of arterial pressure measurements at definite periods to separate the physiologic data into stages. Those mechanisms which may exert controlling influences on the disturbed circulatory state occurring immediately after the etiologic event are considered potentially pathophysiologic factors. Identification of possible physiologic mechanisms depends upon experimental data as well as certain hypotheses.

Those mechanisms which are compensatory and act in the direction of survival value are inferred from the data of patients who survived. Those changes observed in the preterminal and terminal cases are assumed to reflect decompensatory reactions. Despite the theoretical uncertainties of this approach, principles so derived may be applied to shock patients and tested prospectively.

The body's initial responses to different types of stress are often quite variable, but within each etiologic category, the

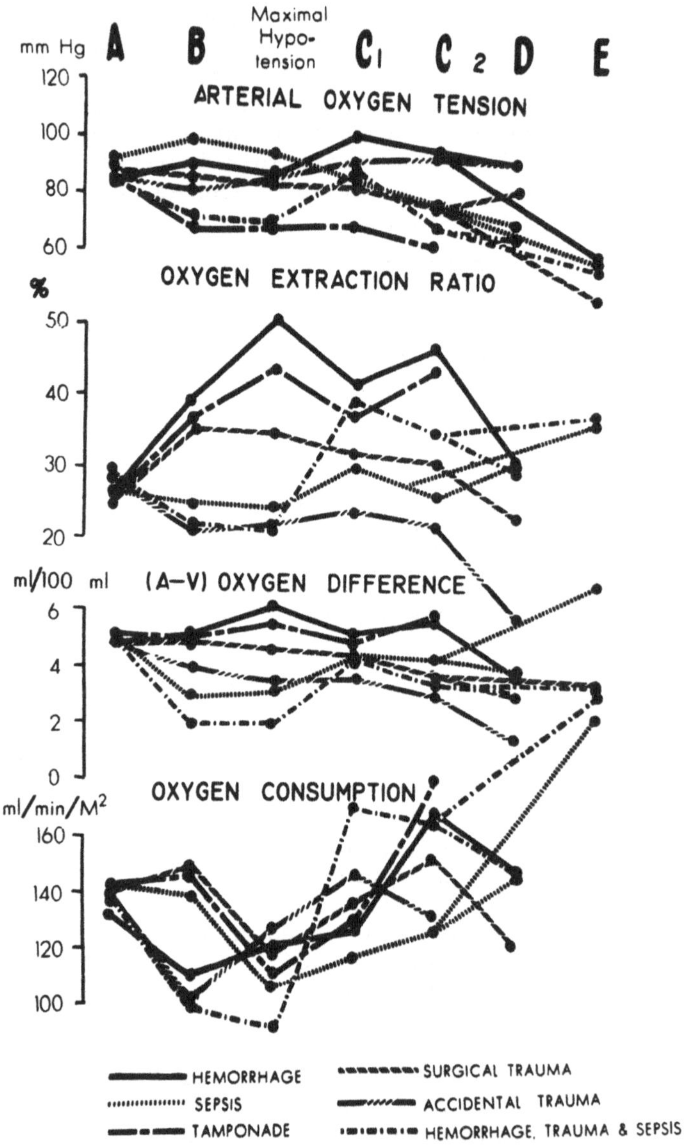

FIG. 3. (For figure legend, see top of next page.)

FIG. 3. Sequential changes in oxygen metabolism including arterial pO_2, oxygen extraction ratio, arteriovenous oxygen content differences, and oxygen consumption in the various types of shock. Note that arterial pO_2 tended to remain normal or somewhat low, but did not fall alarmingly until the late stages. The oxygen ratios and to a lesser extent the arteriovenous oxygen content differences rose in the hemorrhage and tamponade patients. The arteriovenous oxygen content differences fell in accidental trauma, sepsis, and hemorrhage-trauma-sepsis groups. Oxygen consumption fell at some time in the early (B or *low* stage) period and rose in the middle and late periods in all groups.

responses were rather similar. The common compensatory responses to hemorrhage are increased heart rates, vasoconstriction, and increased myocardial contractility (1,3,9,12,19,20). During hypovolemia and low blood flow states, the normal distributions of blood volume and flow are not necessarily maintained (11). Greater fractions of blood volume and cardiac output go to liver, heart, and brain; lesser fractions in differing proportions go to kidney, gut, and skin. The tissues extract oxygen more completely, because less blood is flowing more slowly through them. Metabolic acidosis occurs with hypovolemia and reduced blood flow; under these conditions, respiratory alkalosis is a compensatory mechanism.

Acute injury produces a generalized increase in autonomic neural activity. This stimulates the cardiac and respiratory centers of the brain to increase heart rates, myocardial contractility, and ventilation (14,16). When blood volume deficit is absent, the stroke volume and cardiac output increase—the former because of myocardial stimulation, the latter because of increased stroke volume and heart rate. The increased ventilation leads to respiratory alkalosis. Metabolic influences and the cellular breakdown products of direct tissue injury usually tend to intesify and prolong the circulatory changes provoked by the neural and hormonal mechanisms.

The initial physiologic responses to the various types of trauma and hemorrhage are primarily mediated by neural mechanisms. That is, the generalized autonomic neural tone may stimulate cardiac and respiratory centers of the brain stem to produce most of the observed hemodynamic effects. But the duration and magnitude of these effects depends on other factors. For example, the stimulation of cardiac function increases cardiac output after trauma and sepsis, but this response may be limited by hypovolemia and impaired myocardial function.

TABLE 1

CARDIORESPIRATORY ALTERATIONS AFTER HEMORRHAGE

Physiologic effects	Compensatory responses	Physiologic changes with decompensation
Primary effect	Increased heart rate	Further decreased art. press.
Decreased blood volume	Increased systemic vasc. resist.	Decreased heart rate
Secondary effects		
Decreased mean art. press.	Increased pulmonary vasc. resist.	Further decreased cardiac output
Decreased cardiac output	Redistribution of blood vol.	Increased central venous press.
Decreased central venous press.	Increased myocardial contractility, tendency to increased cardiac output	Increased mean transit time
Increased mean transit time		Decreased systemic vasc. resist.
Decreased central blood vol.	Increased O_2 extraction	Decreased stroke index
Decreased left vent. stroke work	Hyperpnea, tachypnea, respiratory alkalosis	Decreased left stroke
Decreased O_2 availability		Decreased myocardial contractility
		Decreased art. pO_2
Decreased O_2 consumption		Decreased oxygen avail.
Metabolic acidosis		Decreased oxygen consumption
		Metabolic acidosis

TABLE 2

CARDIORESPIRATORY ALTERATIONS AFTER TRAUMA

Physiologic effects	Compensatory responses	Physiologic changes with decompensation
Primary effects	Increased heart rate	Further decreases in art. press.
Tissue injury	Increased cardiac output	Decreased heart rate
Breakdown of damaged tissues, release of breakdown products and intracellular components into the circulation	Increased stroke work	Further decreases in cardiac output
Secondary effects	Increased left vent. stroke work	Increased central venous press.
Decreased mean art. press.	Increased myocardial contractility	Increased mean transit time
Increased O_2 requirements	Increased pulmonary vasc. resist.	Decreased systemic vasc. resist.
Propagation of afferent neural (pain) stimulation	Hyperpnea and tachypnea	Decreased stroke index
	Respiratory alkalosis	Decreased left vent. stroke
	Increased O_2 consumption	Decreased myocardial contractility
		Decreased art. pO_2
		Decreased O_2 avail.
		Decreased O_2 consumption
		Metabolic acidosis

TABLE 3

CARDIORESPIRATORY ALTERATIONS AFTER SEPSIS

Physiologic effects	Compensatory responses	Physiologic changes with decompensation
Primary effect	Alteration in temp. regul. centers	Decreased art. press.
Bacterial infection	Increased heart rate	
Secondary effects		Decreased heart rate
Hyperthermia	Increased cardiac output	Decreased cardiac output
Increased O_2 requirements	Decreased systemic vasc. resist.	Increased mean transit time
	Increased myocardial contractility	Decreased stroke index
	Hyperpnea and tachypnea	Decreased left vent. stroke work
	Respiratory alkalosis	Decreased art. pO_2
	Increased O_2 consumption	Decreased O_2 avail.
		Decreased O_2 consumption
		Metabolic acidosis

TABLE 4

CARDIORESPIRATORY ALTERATIONS AFTER CARDIAC TAMPONADE

Physiologic effects	Compensatory responses	Physiologic changes with decompensation
Primary effects	Increased heart rate	Decreased art. press.
Increased intrapericardial press.	Increased systemic vasc. resist.	Decreased heart rate
Decreased effective filling press.	Increased central venous press.	Relative decrease in central venous press.
Decreased stroke vol.	Increased myocardial contractility	Further decrease of cardiac output
Secondary effects		
Decreased art. press.	Increased O_2 extraction	Increased mean transit time
Decreased cardiac output	Redistribution of blood vol.	Decreased systemic vasc. resist.
Increased central venous press.		Decreased left vent. stroke work
Increased mean transit time		Decreased myocardial contractility
Decreased left vent. stroke work		Decreased art. pO_2
Decreased O_2 avail.		Decreased O_2 avail.
Decreased O_2 consumption		Decreased O_2 consumption
		Metabolic acidosis

TABLE 5

MECHANISMS UNDERLYING CARDIORESPIRATORY RESPONSES OF THE BODY

Mechanisms	Physiologic responses
I. Increased autonomic nervous activity	
A. Increased cardiac drive	A. Increased heart rate Increased myocardial contractility, *i.e.*, increased stroke vol. and stroke work relative to inflow press. Tendency to increase or maintain art. press.
B. Increased respiratory drive	B. Tachypnea, hyperpnea; *i.e.*, increased alveolar ventilation Respiratory alkalosis with decreased pCO_2
C. Stimulation of systemic vasculature	C. Increased metarteriolar tone, *i.e.*, peripheral resist. Increased venous tone Redistribution of blood vol. Redistribution of blood flow
D. Stimulation of pulmonary vasoconstriction	D. Pulmonary art. hypertension Increased pulmonary vasc. resist. Redistribution of pulmonary blood flow Redistribution of pulmonary blood vol. Increased ventilation-perfusion ratio (V_e/Q)
II. Hormonal	
A. Increased release of catecholamines	A. Increased heart rate

Mechanisms	Physiologic responses
II. Hormonal (cont.)	A. (cont.) Increased myocardial contractility Tendency to increase or maintain arterial and venous press. Increased ventilation Increased lipolysis
B. Increased release of glucosteroids	B. Glycogenolysis Release of intracellular K^+ Retention of salt and water Increased protein breakdown
C. Increased release of aldosterone	C. Retention of Na^+ and water
D. Increased release of renin-angiotensin	D. Increased art. press. Increased metarterial tone and peripheral resist.
E. Increased release of vasopressin	E. Increased art. press. Increased metarterial tone and peripheral resist. Oliguria, water retention Increased Na^+ excretion
III. Metabolic	
A. Accumulation of CO_2, lactic acid, pyruvic acid, and other organic acids	A. Metabolic acidosis Reduced peripheral resist. Compensatory respiratory alkalosis
B. Bacterial end-products, endotoxemia	B. Hyperpyrexia Reduced peripheral resist.
C. Release of vasoactive polypeptides, activation of kallikrein system	C. Hyperpyrexia Changes in local pressure-flow relations and redistribution of cardiac output
D. Release of cellular breakdown products from tissue injury and inadequate circulation	D. Hyperpyrexia Reduced peripheral resist.

In sepsis, neural mechanisms stimulate heart rate, myocardial contractility, and ventilation (17). When blood volume is not reduced by dehydration, cardiac index increases as heart rate and myocardial contractility are stimulated. Hyperpnea, tachypnea, and respiratory alkalosis are best explained on the basis of increased respiratory drive. Alternatively, the central nervous system could be acidotic, and this localized acidosis of the cells regulating respiration may alter the physiologic set, such that the extracellular fluid becomes more alkalotic to neutralize the intracellular acidosis of the brain stem.

Metabolic requirements may influence cardiorespiratory functions, but the mechanisms underlying these interactions are unknown. Possibly the cardiorespiratory centers in the brain stem may be triggered directly or indirectly by intracellular hypoxia, hyperthermia, neuroendocrine stimuli, endotoxins, vasoactive polypeptides, metabolic breakdown products, *etc.* In some subtle, unknown manner, increased metabolic needs are translated by the body so as to raise oxygen consumption and increase cardiac output and thus supply the additional required oxygen (17).

In cardiogenic shock, increased neural activity can account for tachycardia and increased vascular resistance. Increased central venous pressures may result from failure of the heart to keep pace with the venous return as well as increased venomotor tone from neural mechanisms. In the early period after cardiac tamponade, the tendency for increased myocardial contractility may be transient and give way to rapid deterioration from progression of the underlying disease and the failure of compensatory responses (15).

Thus, the striking physiologic response to the various etiologic events is the initial tendency toward increased cardiorespiratory function manifest by increased heart rate, myocardial contractility, and ventilation. The first two increase cardiac output, unless limited by reduced blood volume or by reduced myocardial function. Metabolic acidosis occurs when hypovolemia is present; respiratory alkalosis occurs when it is not. The increased cardiorespiratory function arises from: (a) stimulation of cardiac centers of the brain stem by the stress response which produces a generalized increase in autonomic nervous system activity; (b) cellular breakdown products, hyperthermia, vasoactive peptides, metabolic end-products, and endotoxins; and (c) increased metabolic needs of the peripheral tissues. The metabolic requirements are reflected by increased oxygen consumption, as well as other factors.

In summary, shock syndromes result from either the overwhelming stress of the etiologic event or the failure of compensatory mechanisms to provide adequate circulatory drive to meet physiologic needs, be they normal or increased. Death occurs with the advent of terminal mechanisms, some of which may represent decompensations. The latter, to be lethal, need not be enormous influences; they may resemble the proverbial straw that broke the camel's back, coming as they often do behind a long sequence of complications.

SUMMARY

Cardiorespiratory measurements were made throughout the course of six types of shock in 180 patients. The data were separated into early, middle, and late periods by objective criteria based on time and arterial pressure. The early cardiorespiratory changes were evaluated in terms of primary and secondary physiologic effects, compensatory responses, and their possible physiologic mechanisms. The late decompensatory reactions were thought to reflect terminal mechanisms. The shock states, therefore, are the clinical manifestations of the etiologic events and the bodily responses to them. The present studies suggest that the cardiorespiratory patterns are quite varied because they represent many different combinations of stresses and responses, but they have, as an underlying common denominator, activation of autonomic neural and hormonal mechanisms which tend to increase cardiac and respiratory functions. When these compensatory responses are inadequate or overwhelmed by the magnitude of the etiologic events or subsequent complications, decompensations occur. Physiologic mechanisms underlying terminal events are the influences immediately responsible for death. They are not to be confused with the pathogenic mechanisms which contribute to the development of the shock states. Therapy, to be maximally effective, should take cognizance of these factors.

REFERENCES

1. Bassin, R., B.C. Vladick, A.E. Kark, and W.C. Shoemaker. Rapid and slow hemorrhage in man. Ann. Surg. 173:325, 1971.

2. Carey, J.S., R.S. Brown, P.A. Mohr, D.O. Monson, S.T. Yao, and W.C. Shoemaker. Cardiovascular function in shock. Circulation 35:327, 1967.

3. Cournand, A., R.L. Riley, S.E. Bradley, E.S. Breed, R.P. Noble, H.D. Lauson, M.I. Gregersen, and D.W. Richards. Studies of the circulation in clinical shock. Surgery 13:964, 1943.

4. Fries, E.D., H.W. Schnaper, R.L. Johnson, and G.E. Schreiner. Hemodynamic alterations in acute myocardial infarction. J.

Clin. Invest. 31:131, 1952.

5. Hopkins, R.W., G. Sabga, I. Penn, and F.A. Simeone. Hemodynamic aspects of hemorrhagic and septic shock. JAMA 191: 127, 1965.

6. Hamilton, W.F., J.W. Moore, J.M. Kinsman, and R.G. Spurling. Studies on the circulation. Am. J. Physiol. 99:534, 1932.

7. Kho, L.K., and W.C. Shoemaker. Evaluation of therapy in clinical shock by cardiorespiratory measurements. Surg. Gynecol. Obstet. 127:81, 1968.

8. Kim, S.I., J.M. Desai, and W.C. Shoemaker. Sequence of cardiorespiratory alterations after gradual prolonged hemorrhage in conscious dogs. Am. J. Physiol. 216:1044, 1969.

9. Richards, D.W., Jr. Circulation in traumatic shock in man. Harvey Lectures 39:217, 1943-44.

10. Severinghaus, J.W. Oxyhemoglobin dissociation curve correction for temperature and pH variation in human blood. J. Appl. Physiol. 12:485, 1958.

11. Shoemaker, W.C. *Shock: Chemistry and Therapy*. Springfield, Ill.: Charles C Thomas, 1967.

12. Shoemaker, W.C. Sequential hemodynamic patterns in various causes of shock. Surg. Gynecol. Obstet. 132:411, 1970.

13. Shoemaker, W.C. Analysis of physiologic mechanisms in various etiologic types of clinical shock from sequential cardiorespiratory measurements. Excerpta Med., in press.

14. Shoemaker, W.C., D.M. Boyd, S.I. Kim, R.S. Brown, D.A. Dreiling, and A.E. Kark. Sequential oxygen transport and acid-base changes after trauma to the unanesthetized patient. Surg. Gynecol. Obstet., in press.

15. Shoemaker, W.C., J.S. Carey, S.T. Yao, P.A. Mohr, J.J. Amato, K.J. Printen, R.D. Corley, and D.O. Monson. Hemodynamic alterations in acute cardiac tamponade after penetrating injuries of the heart. Surgery 67:754, 1970.

16. Shoemaker, W.C., L. Lim, D.M. Boyd, R.S. Corley, J.M. Reinhard, D.A. Dreiling, and A.E. Kark. Sequential hemodynamic events after trauma to the unanesthetized patient. Surg. Gynecol. Obstet. 132:651, 1971.

17. Shoemaker, W.C., P.A. Mohr, K.J. Printen, R.S. Brown, J.J. Amato, J.S. Carey, S. Youssef, J. Reinhard, S.I. Kim, and A.E. Kark. Treatment of uncomplicated septic shock: Use of sequential physiologic measurements as guides to therapy. Surg. Gynecol. Obstet. 131:245, 1970.

18. Shoemaker, W.C., K.J. Printen, J.J. Amato, D.O. Monson, J.S. Carey, and K. O'Connor. Hemodynamic patterns after acute anesthetized and unanesthetized trauma. Arch. Surg. 95: 492, 1967.

19. Weil, M.H., and H. Shubin. *Diagnosis and Treatment of Shock.* Baltimore: Williams & Wilkins, 1966.

20. Wiggers, C.J. *Physiology of Shock.* New York: Commonwealth Fund, 1950.

ROLE OF LEUKOCYTES IN THE LUNG AFTER ENDOTOXIN ADMINISTRATION

Clarence A. Guenter, M.D.

Department of Medicine, University of Oklahoma Medical Center, Oklahoma City, Oklahoma

Informal Presentation[1]

One of the conspicuous things about shock research is the large number of department heads and deans who have previously dabbled in this area. As a young investigator looking for areas in which to design studies, I quickly recognized this. With the assurance that such research would certainly be fruitful in terms of career development, if not in solving problems, I forged ahead, and I am proud to be a member of this group today. The field of shock research is conspicuous not only because of the large number of carefully controlled, double-blind, or well-designed randomized studies in experimental models of several species (most of which produce different results in the next investigator's laboratories). The field is also notable for the large volume of incredibly unscientific clinical reports, based on studies of patients with incomprehensibly complex illnesses, which have been published and accepted by the medical community.

I would be particularly pleased if, as a result of this symposium, we were able not only to identify what mechanisms are important in the genesis and sequelae of shock but, perhaps, even agree about a few mechanisms that are not important. It is quite clear and generally accepted, for example, that the patient in septic shock usually does not die as a result of his fever—this being in all likelihood an incidental manifestation of his illness.

[1]This manuscript appears here as presented at the symposium, with minor editorial revisions.

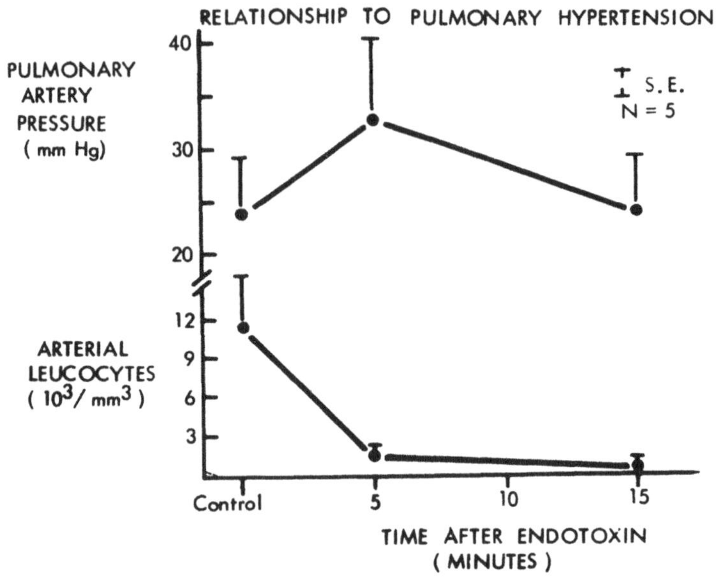

FIG. 1. Mean peripheral blood leukocyte count in animals before and after rapid infusion of 4 mg of *E. coli* endotoxin (Difco) per kilogram of body weight. Note the rapid decrease in leukocyte count, approximately a mirror image of the change in pulmonary artery pressure (and pulmonary vascular resistance). The decrease in leukocyte count and increase in pulmonary artery pressure are both significant ($P < 0.01$).

There must be a host of other manifestations of the shock state which also are incidental rather than fundamental, and these need to be clarified.

We have been interested in the pulmonary lesion in shock, and I would like to briefly consider one postulated mechanism which I think is relatively unimportant in its genesis. As Dr. Berman pointed out, the platelets aggregate in the pulmonary circulation after endotoxin administration, and they may be important. It intrigued us to note, however, that leukocytes also aggregate in the pulmonary circulation. Several years ago, we became interested in the fate of leukocytes during the leukopenia which follows endotoxin administration. Figure 1 summarizes the effects of endotoxin on the peripheral leukocyte count and on the pulmonary artery pressure in a group of five baboons. Within a short time after an appropriate dose of endotoxin, the peripheral leukocyte count drops dramatically; this takes place almost as a mirror image of the rise in pulmonary pressure. I hasten to point out

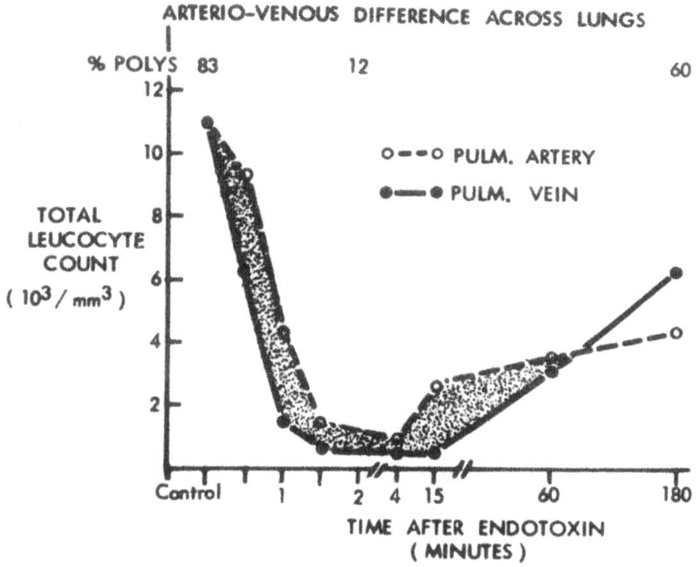

FIG. 2. Leukocyte counts performed on samples collected simultaneously from catheters in the pulmonary artery and pulmonary vein in an open-chest dog, before and after the injection of endotoxin. Note the large arteriovenous difference across the lung during the development of leukopenia.

that this precedes by minutes the decrease in systemic pressure and drop in cardiac output, and therefore is not a result of a low-flow state, at least in the baboon and the rhesus monkey. We were interested in learning whether this rise in pulmonary pressure was related to mechanical occlusion of pulmonary vessels by leukocytes. Figure 2 demonstrates that the leukocytes are, in fact, sequestered in the pulmonary circulation, as indicated by the arteriovenous difference across the lungs. (If one calculates from the cardiac output and the flow through the lungs and the leukocyte count at these various times, one could calculate as many as 10-18 leukocytes per alveolus in the lung, if one figures that there are 300,000,000 alveoli; this is an enormous volume of formed elements in the vascular bed). Furthermore, the possibility has been raised that these leukocytes subsequently degranulate, and that their lysosomes released within the circulation might cause capillary damage in the pulmonary vascular bed.

Dr. Jacque Coalson has played a major investigative role in our studies. She demonstrated (Exptl. Molec. Pathol. 12:84-103,

1970) that a large number of leukocytes can be seen in the pulmonary capillaries by light or electron microscopy, and that they appear to degranulate and disintegrate in the pulmonary capillaries with release of lysosomal granules into the capillary lumen.

Since these initial observations, we have explored the significance of the leukocytes in several ways: (a) in experiments involving animals previously rendered leukopenic by irradiation; (b) in studies on isolated lobes perfused with normal blood or blood which had been depleted of leukocytes; and (c) by attempts to stabilize leukocyte lysosomes by pretreatment with steroids or salicylates. It is particularly noteworthy that leukopenia did not prevent the early pulmonary hypertension or the late histological changes in the "shock lung", and that attempts at stabilizing leukocyte lysosomes were ineffective in preventing the histological lesion of the shock lung.

I would like to suggest, then, that leukocytes in the pulmonary vascular bed are another not very important, but intriguing, phenomenon which occurs in shock.

FATE OF ENDOTOXIN IN THE CIRCULATION

Geoffrey Evans, M.D.

Department of Surgery, McMaster University, Hamilton, Ontario, Canada

Informal Presentation[1]

We have been conducting studies to examine the fate of endotoxin in the circulation. For this, we labeled endotoxin with chromium and showed that the endotoxin was present essentially in the whole blood after injection, with very little in the plasma. When we then looked at the formed elements of the blood, we found that the chromium-labeled endotoxin was related to the platelet component of the formed elements, in contradistinction to free chromium which is related to the red cell.

We know that endotoxin can cause platelet aggregation, and we have demonstrated that endotoxin requires a serum factor (probably antibody) to cause platelet aggregation. Therefore, it is probably an antigen-antibody complex; when one infuses endotoxin into rabbits, one observes platelet aggregates. On 1-2 micra sections for electronmicroscopy, a pulmonary vessel can be seen plugged full of platelet aggregates, with an occasional white cell. Under high power, platelets are seen in the small pulmonary vessels, with very few white cells. The lung is not the only organ involved. In the kidney, the renal glomerulus shows platelet aggregates which are abnormal. They have pseudopod formation and they are, indeed, aggregates of platelets.

[1]This manuscript appears here as presented at the symposium, with minor editorial revisions.

Endotoxin-induced platelet aggregation can be inhibited by substances such as acetylsalicylic acid, other anti-inflammatory drugs such as indomethacin, phenylbutazone, steroids, and sulfinpyrazone. In animals pretreated with sulfinyprazone, there is very little change in platelet count or white blood cell count, and there are no changes in arterial or venous pressures.

We attempted to make animals thrombocytopenic, and to do this, we treated them with ^{32}P. The animals so treated showed far less fall in arterial pressure or rise in venous pressure after the administration of endotoxin.

If this, then, is an endotoxin interaction with antibody (*i.e.*, an antigen-antibody complex interaction), one should be able to produce the same degree of shock with preformed antigen-antibody complexes. Our experiments show that, with preformed antigen-antibody complexes in animals, a fall occurs in the platelet count, there is a decrease in arterial pressure, and a rise in venous pressure occurs. After treatment with sulfinpyrazone, the platelet fall is prevented, and correspondingly there is no change in arterial or venous pressures. In all these experiments, the animals died within 2 hours of administration of either endotoxin or antigen-antibody complexes unless they were pretreated with these drugs which prevent platelet aggregation induced by the endotoxin.

DISCUSSION[1]

DR. W. C. SHOEMAKER, *Panel Moderator (New York, N.Y.)*: I'm sure there will be questions on this and the preceding paper. I don't see how the small platelets do so much damage when there are fewer of them than the large white cells, which are more capable of plugging up the circulation. Does anyone choose to answer?

DR. EVANS: In the experiments with platelets in the peritoneal cavity, one finds that if one does aggregate platelets large quantities of white cells are associated with this. If you embolize platelet aggregates in the pulmonary circulation, you get masses and masses of white cells associated with these platelet aggregates. If you embolize something like pre-formed fibrin, you get relatively few white cells related to the fibrin.

DR. SHOEMAKER: The question that Dr. Schilling posed was whether the platelet aggregate has to do with some changes on the pulmonary capillary wall, as opposed to mechanical features or

[1]This discussion also covers the presentation of Dr. Guenter (see preceding paper).

other neurological features.

DR. EVANS: I think that's a difficult question to answer. Does endotoxin have a direct effect on the vessel wall, or does it work indirectly through the release of platelet constituents? These, as you know, include a platelet permeability factor which is probably the same as the leukocyte permeability factor. I think that is an open question that really hasn't been answered yet.

DR. B. D. LOWERY *(Baltimore, Md.)*: The basic platelet physiologist has demonstrated several specific receptor sites on the platelet surface for different things, such as ADP, catecholamines, and serotonins, so that aggregating platelets by ADP does not prevent further aggregation of platelets by other vasoactive agents. Which of these agents, do you think, may be most important in causing platelet aggregation, either released from a site of injured tissue or released from cells which are damaged by low perfusion? Or do you think that all of them may be important, or none of them?

DR. EVANS: I think that all of them are important. After endotoxin, I think it's the antigen-antibody complex which is causing platelet aggregation. As you know, in these lesions, especially in the kidney, although the initiating mechanism appears to be a platelet antigen-antibody complex interaction, later one gets different sorts of platelets. These are platelets with intact granules; the initial platelets appear to have lost their granules. They may release ADP or ADP may be released from the membrane, which also contributes to the generation of the platelet mass.

DR. LOWERY: Do you believe that an endothelial lesion in the lung may procede the platelet problem?

DR. EVANS: I said that was an open question, because we haven't proved it yet. The other interesting thing is that, if you give ADP to animals and produce the same shock, exactly the same white count fall is observed as in these experiments.

DR. SHOEMAKER: It seems that there are at least four different cellular factors: red cells, platelets, white cells, and capillary membranes. Now, the question that I would like to propose not only to you, Dr. Evans, but to Dr. Guenter is, where does this block occur? Does it occur at the capillary or does it occur on the venous side? And if it is on the venous side, is this how we can explain the appearance of pulmonary edema and increase in extracellular water which is so characteristic of the lesion? In other words, is there something here that can tie the whole thing up into one ball of wax?

DR. GUENTER: I don't know where the lesion occurs. The experiments we designed to resolve this were conducted in two ways. One was an isolated perfused lung lobe (about which Dr. Massion and Dr. Kux have a paper in press), in which we rendered the blood perfusing the lobe leukopenic by passing it through filters and filtering out the white cells and platelets. We were able to reproduce at least as severe pulmonary lesions after endotoxin in this leukopenic and thrombocytopenic lobe as we were in the animals perfused with blood with normal leukocytes and thrombocytes. About that time, we realized that this might be an antigen-antibody reaction, and that perhaps depleting a perfusate of calcium would make a difference. If we took blood with normal counts of leukocytes and platelets and used acid-citrate-dextrose as our anticoagulant solution in this isolated perfused lobe, we got the best protection of the lung in terms of histological changes and vasomotor responses of any preparation we've had. I think that offers evidence that the actual aggregates of either of those cell types may not be as critical as whatever causes them to aggregate. Even in the leukopenic animals, both in intact animals radiated to the extent where their white cells are below 1,000 and in the animals perfused with leukopenic blood, we observed similar kinds of endothelial changes and perivascular edema.

DR. SHOEMAKER: Do you have any additional comment, Dr. Evans, on this particular problem?

DR. EVANS: I think the problem in all these experiments is to render these animals thrombocytopenic. We have extreme difficulties in rendering animals thrombocytopenic. In the ^{32}P experiments we did, the white count was high. Now, whether these white cells were working well, I don't know. Certainly, though, the white cell count was high because of the different half-lives of platelets and white cells. The other problem about your perfusing with acid-citrate-dextrose—did you actually prove that the platelets were functional?

DR. GUENTER: I have no idea about function. I just know we hadn't depleted the blood of them, and the counts of leukocytes and platelets decreased after endotoxin, just as they had in heparin-anticoagulated blood. I don't know anything about the function of either of the cell types.

DR. J. H. DUFF *(Montreal, Canada):* I'd like to ask Dr. Evans to clarify the species differences between the lung lesions. He has worked with rabbits, in which the target organ in endotoxin shock is the lung. I think Dr. Guenter has probably used dogs. Dr. Lowery has studied the lung lesion in pigs. Now, is there a species difference with respect to platelets causing lung pathology?

DR. EVANS: I can't answer that question. We've done preliminary work in the dog, and it does appear that, even in the dog, one gets these platelet aggregates in the lungs, but this is merely preliminary work.

DR. G. L. HABERLAND *(Wuppertal-Elberfeld, Germany):* The question of whether it's the thrombocytes, leukocytes, or erythrocytes, I think, leads to a more mechanistic thinking of the whole matter. But what I would like to mention are some findings which I recall, in which one group went as far as to separate the various plasma fractions. They found out that, with a plasma fraction with a molecular weight between 1,000 and 10,000, they were able to produce these lesions. In other words, these lesions are produced by constituents of these cells but not by the cells themselves, directly.

SPLANCHNIC BLOOD FLOW IN EXPERIMENTAL SHOCK

Kenneth G. Swan, LTC, MC, Randall W. Barton, SP4, and
David G. Reynolds, LTC, MSC

Department of Gastroenterology, Division of Medicine,
Walter Reed Army Institute of Research, Walter Reed
Army Medical Center, Washington, D.C.

This paper will examine the role of the splanchnic circulation in experimental shock and reassess the so-called "target organ" or "adrenergic" theories in the pathogenesis of irreversible shock. In the dog, the endogenous catecholamines are mesenteric vasoconstrictors whether injected or infused into the superior mesenteric artery or inferior vena cava. This response appears to be independent of the dose given. Infusion of catecholamines causes vasoconstriction characterized by autoregulatory escape from the adrenergic agonist within minutes of drug administration. In the baboon, the responses to norepinephrine and epinephrine are similar, with one exception: low-dose epinephrine injected or infused into the superior mesenteric artery causes vasodilation. In contrast to the canine models of experimental shock (10), the baboon responds to neither endotoxic or hemorrhagic shock with mesenteric or hepatic ischemia over many hours of observation. Likewise, the subhuman primate exhibits no evidence of pathological change in the intra-abdominal viscera, in contrast to the dramatic changes observed in canine shock. Catecholamine concentrations are equally elevated in both species during either form of experimental shock. The amount of epinephrine elaborated by either species during experimental shock would be unlikely to evoke significant mesenteric ischemia. In fact, in the subhuman primate it might well act as a vasodilator and increase organ perfusion. The findings suggest that the adrenergic or target organ theory of shock is invalid in primate shock models and is thus unlikely to find application to human shock therapy.

In the search for fundamental mechanisms in shock, considerable efforts have been expended to identify a specific defect or abnor-

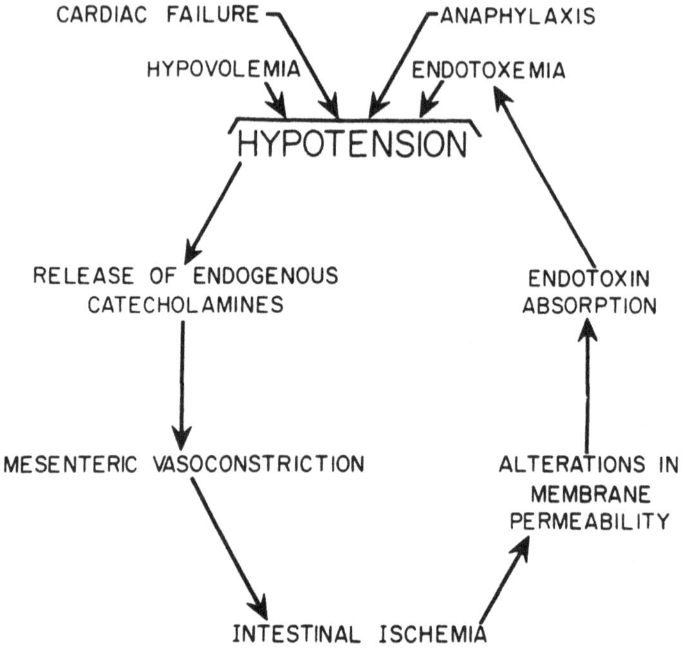

FIG. 1. Schematic diagram of the "target organ" theory as applied to the gut.

mality in a tissue or system, which, when once elicited, causes irreversibility. "Target organs" have been impugned, and experimental evidence has been accumulated both for and against the concept. A target organ discussed extensively in the literature is the gut. In this discussion, we shall review the evidence on both sides of the question, as it relates to the pathogenesis of shock. Species differences in response to shock will be considered, with particular emphasis on the limitations of the canine model. We will consider the major splanchnic hemodynamic events accompanying different forms of shock in the experimental animal. The "target organ" or "adrenergic theory" of shock (Fig. 1) will be evaluated in terms of the effects of alpha- and beta-adrenergic stimulation upon splanchnic blood flow, as well as the predictable effects of endogenous vasoactive agents (*e.g.*, catecholamines) upon this circulation.

The endogenous catecholamines, norepinephrine and epinephrine, have generally been considered vasoconstrictors in the gut, although this point has been debated (22). Their effects, after intravenous or intra-arterial injection or infusion, are primarily vasoconstric-

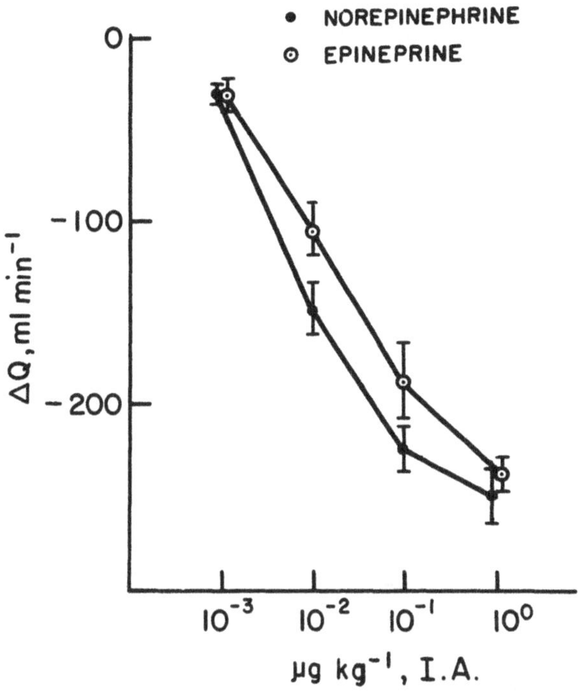

FIG. 2. Effects of norepinephrine and epinephrine injections upon canine mesenteric arterial blood flow. Log dose is represented on the abscissa and absolute change in blood flow (ΔQ) on the ordinate. Control blood flow is indicated by the zero. Each point indicates the mean ±SE of five experiments in five dogs.

---

tive on the superior mesenteric artery of most species studied. In the dog (Fig. 2), progressively increasing doses of either norepinephrine or epinephrine, injected into the superior mesenteric artery, progressively intensify vasoconstriction over a wide dosage range. At intermediate doses, norepinephrine is a more potent vasoconstrictor than epinephrine. When the same drugs are infused (Fig. 3), there is vasoconstriction characterized by autoregulatory escape; in the case of epinephrine, the effects are more complete as well as more rapid. Alpha-adrenergic blockade with phenoxybenzamine reverses the vasoconstrictor effects of intra-arterially injected and infused epinephrine at all doses studied (22,23). The same antagonist attenuates but does not reverse the vasoconstrictor effects of norepinephrine (22,23). Beta-adrenergic blockade with propranolol potentiates the vasoconstrictor effects

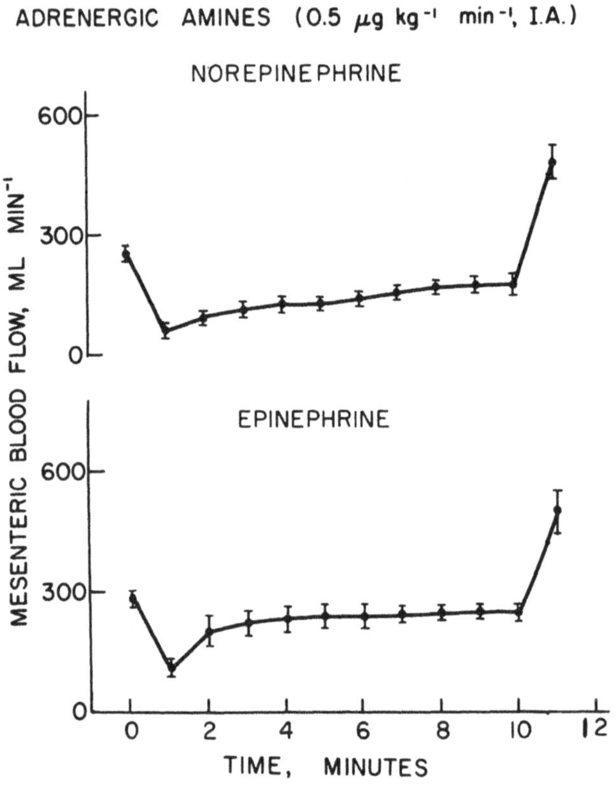

FIG. 3. Effects of norepinephrine and epinephrine infusions upon canine mesenteric arterial blood flow. The 10-minute infusions begin at zero minutes (mean ±SE of five experiments in five animals).

---

of both drugs, whether injected (23) or infused (22), and appears to attenuate the escape from infused drugs (22).

Similar experiments in the subhuman primate yield comparable results with norepinephrine; with epinephrine, more of a disparity exists. Injection of norepinephrine into the superior mesenteric artery causes vasoconstriction at all doses studied (Fig. 4), the degree being directly proportional to the dose. Epinephrine causes no significant vasoconstriction at a comparably low dose. In fact, there is the hint of a vasodilator effect. At higher doses, the effects of the two catecholamines become indistinguishable. Infused norepinephrine causes vasoconstriction followed by autoregulatory escape in the subhuman primate (Fig. 5), which is slightly delayed in time and is also somewhat less marked in terms

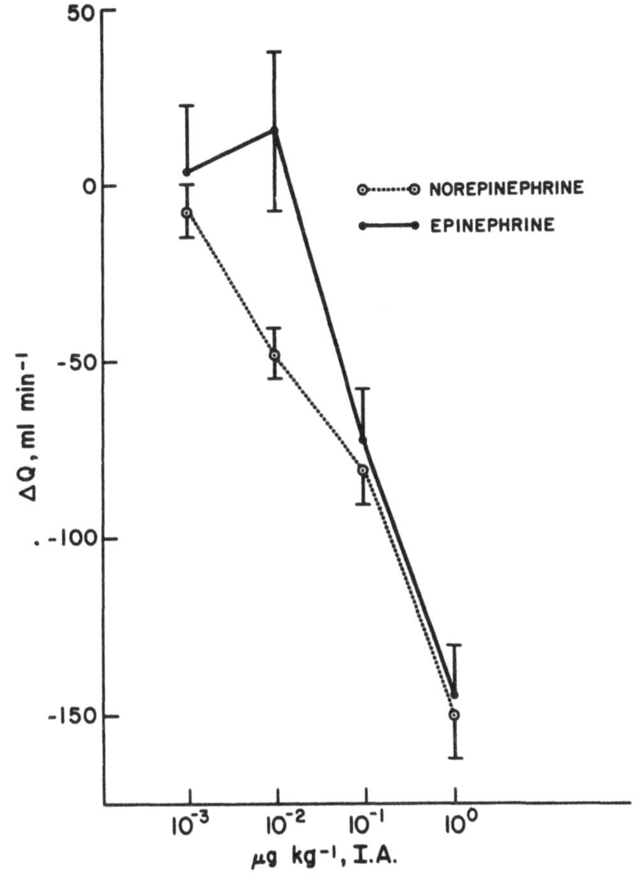

FIG. 4. Effects of norepinephrine and epinephrine injections upon mesenteric arterial blood flow in the baboon. Abscissa denotes log dose; ordinate shows change in blood flow (ΔQ) in milliliters per minute (mean ±SE of five experiments in five animals).

of absolute flow values, when compared to autoregulatory escape in the dog. Infusion of epinephrine sustains the vasoconstrictor response. In our experience, autoregulatory escape does not occur at this dose, for reasons unknown at present. Interestingly enough no "overshoot" follows cessation of the infusion. While the significance of this observation also awaits explanation, we should mention that we have not observed autoregulatory escape in the absence of the "overshoot" phenomenon and *vice versa*. The only exception is the observation that transient mechanical occlusion of an artery is followed by an overshoot. The underlying mechanism remains unknown, despite many proposed theories (23).

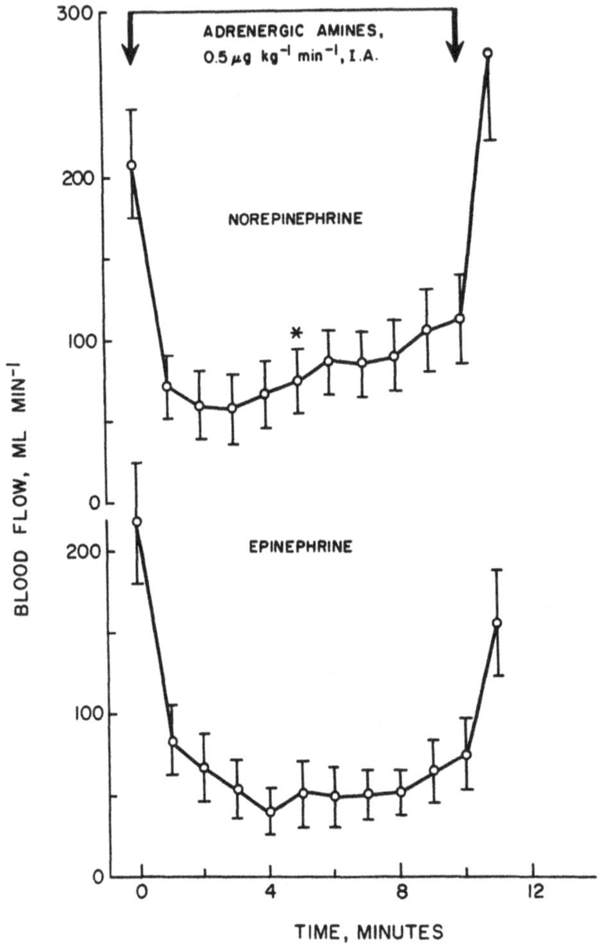

FIG. 5. Effects of norepinephrine and epinephrine infusions upon mesenteric arterial blood flow in the baboon. The start of the 10-minute infusion is at zero minutes (mean ±SE of five experiments in five animals).

In both the dog and the monkey, higher doses of infused catecholamines cause greater vasoconstriction and lower doses cause less, with one exception. At a dose of 0.05 $\mu g\ kg^{-1}\ min^{-1}$, intra-arterially administered epinephrine produces a vasodilation in the baboon gut. We have observed no vasodilator response to infused norepinephrine at any dose in the gut of either species. Thus, we conclude that the endogenous catecholamines, under most circumstances tested, are vasoconstrictors in the gut of dog and monkey and, by inference, in the gut of man as well. The ability of epinephrine to exert opposite and dose-dependent effects upon the mesenteric circulation has not been described before, although this characteristic of epinephrine, with respect to other circulations, has been known for many years (1). Quite possibly, the low dose of epinephrine which dilates vessels in the primate gut most closely approximates the level which might be achieved through endogenous elaboration. Thus, we would have to modify our earlier conclusion and suggest that endogenous epinephrine may well prove to be a mesenteric vasodilator in man.

The catecholamines have been implicated in the pathogenesis of shock in both man and the experimental animal. Surprisingly enough, within the past 3 years reports have appeared in the literature championing the use, based upon "experimental evidence", of alpha-adrenergic agonists (5), alpha-adrenergic antagonists (7), beta-adrenergic agonists (18), and beta-adrenergic antagonists (3)—either alone or in various combinations, for the specific amelioration of hypotensive syndromes in man.

The readily demonstrable vasoconstrictor effects of the endogenous catecholamines upon most vascular beds have led to the general discredit of norepinephrine and epinephrine in shock therapy. It is our premise, however, that the catecholamines probably play an insignificant role in the pathogenesis of experimental shock. We base this upon the contrast between the responses of the dog *vs.* those of the monkey to various forms of shock. For example, a near-lethal dose of endotoxin in the dog (Fig. 6) profoundly disturbs mesenteric hemodynamic events. Portal venous pressure rises dramatically within minutes and gradually returns to control levels. At the same time, both arterial pressure and mesenteric blood flow fall abruptly. Their initial recovery at about 30 minutes is followed by a second decline, which is sustained for many hours and is associated with a progressive rise in mesenteric vascular resistance. These observations coincide with the cyanotic appearance of the bowel as well as the development of bloody diarrhea. Hemorrhagic shock produces a similar sequence of events in the dog (28). Plasma catecholamine concentrations are reportedly elevated in all forms of experimental canine shock (20); however a wide range in values is cited from different laboratories (6,14,20,24,29), as well as within the same laboratory (6,16).

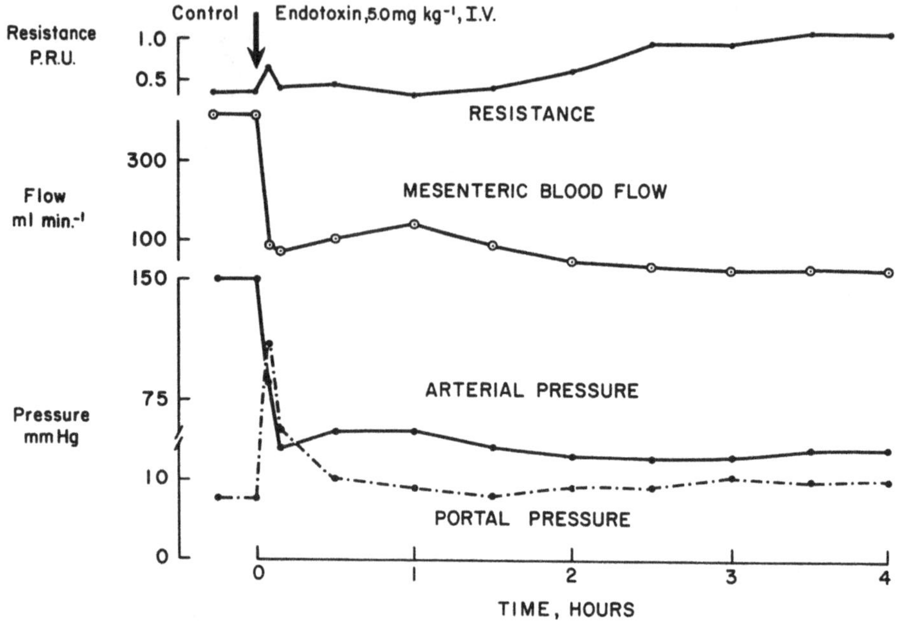

FIG. 6. Effects of *E. coli* endotoxin upon canine mesenteric hemodynamics.

While some investigators have reported beneficial effects from the use of adrenergic antagonists in experimental shock (25,26), their data have been challenged with contrary evidence (21,30).

In contrast to the dog, the subhuman primate responds to a near-lethal dose of endotoxin (Fig. 7) with fall in arterial pressure that is unaccompanied by any change in either mesenteric blood flow or portal venous pressure. Thus calculated mesenteric vascular resistance falls over the course of a 4-hour experiment. If the source of hypotension in the monkey is hypovolemia (Fig. 8), mesenteric blood flow declines profoundly. This hemodynamic pattern resembles that observed in the dog, although the monkey can tolerate this degree of hypotension, as well as mesenteric ischemia, for many hours without evidence of intestinal damage or death if the shed blood is reinfused (2). Inspection of the intra-abdominal viscera of the monkey, in contrast to the dog (16), reveals no gross changes in any organ (3,24) upon termination of the experiment. Bloody diarrhea is not associated with endotoxic or hypovolemic shock in the subhuman primate (8,19,24). The only similarity between the two species, then, is hypotension and death. Added to this comparison, however, is a progressive rise in plasma catecholamine levels in the monkey (19,24). The values we have

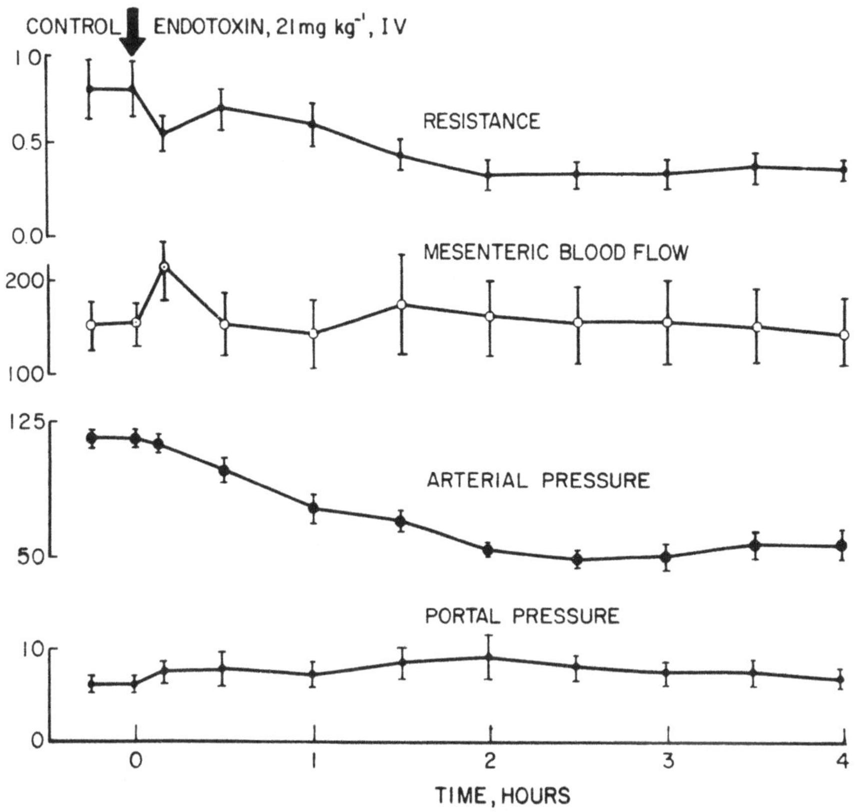

FIG. 7. Effects of *E. coli* endotoxin on mesenteric hemodynamics in the baboon. Each point is the mean ±SE of five experiments in five animals.

recorded in the anesthetized baboon subjected to either hemorrhagic (2) or endotoxic (24) shock are quite similar and increase progressively as the experiment continues. In each series, the maximum value is less than 10.0 µg of epinephrine per liter of plasma. We have not recorded higher values for epinephrine during lethal endotoxin shock in the dog. In both baboon and dog, norepinephrine is present in considerably lower concentrations.

Calculating for hematocrit (40%) and blood flow (10-20 ml min^{-1} kg^{-1}) through the superior mesenteric artery of either monkey (24) or dog (23), this concentration of epinephrine (approximately four times the concentration of norepinephrine) would deliver to the gut 0.06-0.12 µg min^{-1} kg^{-1}. As we have observed in canine experiments, infusion of five to ten times this quantity of either

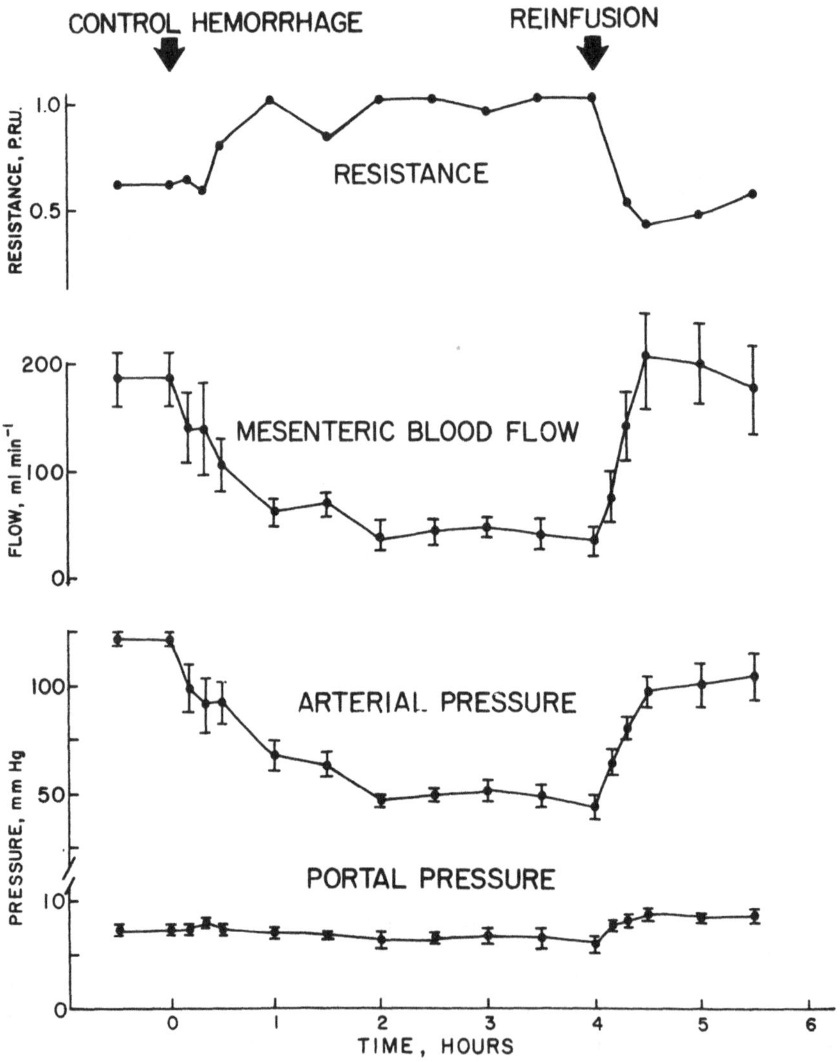

FIG. 8. Effects of hemorrhagic shock upon mesenteric hemodynamics in the baboon (mean ±SE of five experiments in five animals).

norepinephrine or epinephrine causes a vasoconstrictor response characterized by autoregulatory escape within minutes. The amount of endogenously released catecholamine discovered in the circulating plasma of experimental shock models does not begin to approach known concentrations of exogenously delivered catecholamines which are required to evoke significant and sustained vasoconstriction in the gut of either dog or subhuman primate. In fact, this amount of epinephrine probably acts to dilate the primate gut.

These findings cast considerable doubt upon the validity of the so-called "adrenergic theory" of shock. They also help shed some light upon the finding that adrenergic antagonists fail to alter the irreversible progression of the hemodynamic events accompanying experimental shock (21,30). The obvious similarities between the degree of hypotension, concentration of plasma catecholamines, and survival rate in dogs and monkeys receiving endotoxin is contrasted by the obvious discrepancy between the hemodynamic and pathologic changes in the gut of these two species. Thus, the hemodynamic as well as the pathologic differences between dogs and subhuman primates are of sufficient magnitude to warrant the conclusion that experimental shock studies must consider obvious species differences. For example, the cat and rabbit (15) behave more like the monkey than the dog in both hemodynamic as well as pathologic responses to endotoxic shock. On the other hand, responses of the rat (30) simulate those of the dog. It seems justified, then, that the burden of proof that the dog responds to shock more like the human than does the monkey should rest upon those who advocate the use of the canine shock model and accept the conclusion drawn therefrom. One might even venture to suggest that the dog is an unusually poor model for studies of experimental shock.

Since our concern lies not with the mesenteric circulation to the exclusion of other splanchnic viscera, it is appropriate here to consider the hepatic circulation. At least one investigator has maintained over the years that mesenteric ischemia is not the most important event in the pathogenesis of irreversible shock. Rather, the ischemic and hence inadequate reticuloendothelial system of liver and spleen (17) produces the greatest damage because endotoxin (normally found in the portal venous blood of the dog) escapes into the systemic circulation due to the fact that it is not detoxified by the reticuloendothelial system. Thus, hypotension, regardless of its etiology, ultimately leads to endotoxemia and irreversible shock. Supporting this reasoning are studies which have quantitated the levels of circulating plasma endotoxin in experimental shock (12,19); however, their validity has been questioned (9). Invoked in support of the same theory are studies of canine hepatic blood flow (Fig. 9), which simulates superior mesenteric arterial blood flow in endotoxic shock.

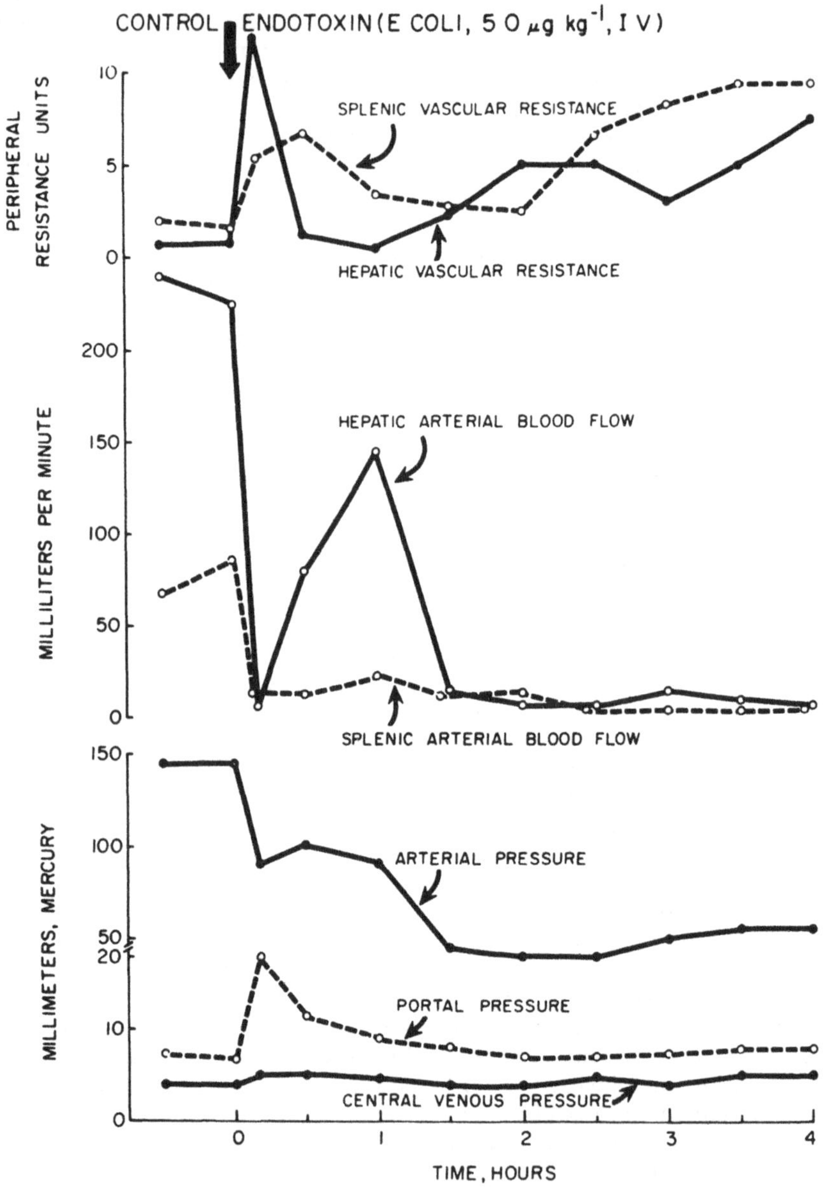

FIG. 9. Effects of endotoxin on blood flow to the liver and spleen of the dog.

Splenic arterial blood flow is also severely depressed in endotoxic shock (Fig. 9). Four hours later, liver, spleen, stomach, and intestines appear grossly infarcted.

In contrast, hepatic blood flow of the baboon in endotoxic shock (Fig. 10) remains unchanged despite severe hypotension over many hours and ultimate death. In the baboon, then, hepatic blood flow during endotoxemia is as unchanged as gut blood flow. Since most blood flow in the portal vein is derived from the superior mesenteric artery (13), little evidence exists to suggest any significant hepatic ischemia of the baboon during endotoxic shock. Not surprisingly, then, after many hours of septic (24) or hemorrhagic shock (19), the baboon's liver, like his other intra-abdominal viscera, appears grossly unremarkable (and histologically, as well).

Blood flow to the spleen of the baboon falls significantly during endotoxic shock (Fig. 10), resembling the canine response (Fig. 9). Thus, both the spleen and kidney (4) of the subhuman primate can be causally associated with hypotension as possible "target organs". The explanation of these organ-specific responses remains obscure. This small percentage of reticuloendothelial potential seems very unlikely to explain the postulated irreversibility in shock. It is not surprising, then, that splenectomy *per se* does not increase the mortality of guinea pigs in endotoxin shock (9).

We are left to conclude that very little valid evidence supports a "target organ" or "adrenergic" theory for the pathogenesis of irreversible shock in the subhuman primate, and therefore in man. Although the extensively studied and still-popular canine shock model has value in terms of comparative biology, it serves only to confuse an already-difficult area of investigation in terms of clinical application. Recent studies in our laboratory indicate that the canine gut is sensitive to sublethal effects of endotoxin injected directly into the superior mesenteric artery at a dose which does not change arterial blood pressure. Whether this finding adequately explains the obvious pathology in the canine gut during endotoxin shock is unclear, but it does support the possibility that the canine gut is a target organ. We have also recently completed a study of catecholamine responses in the mesenteric circulation of dogs pretreated with a sublethal dose of endotoxin. The absolute values for mesenteric blood flow and resistance changes in response to either norepinephrine or epinephrine administration decreased when compared to control values. However, when percent change was calculated, the effects of the endogenous catecholamines upon mesenteric hemodynamics before and after sublethal endotoxin administration were indistinguishable. Thus, at least in the canine shock model, endotoxin does not appear to sensitize the gut to the vasoconstrictor effects of endogenous catecholamines, as has been suggested (11).

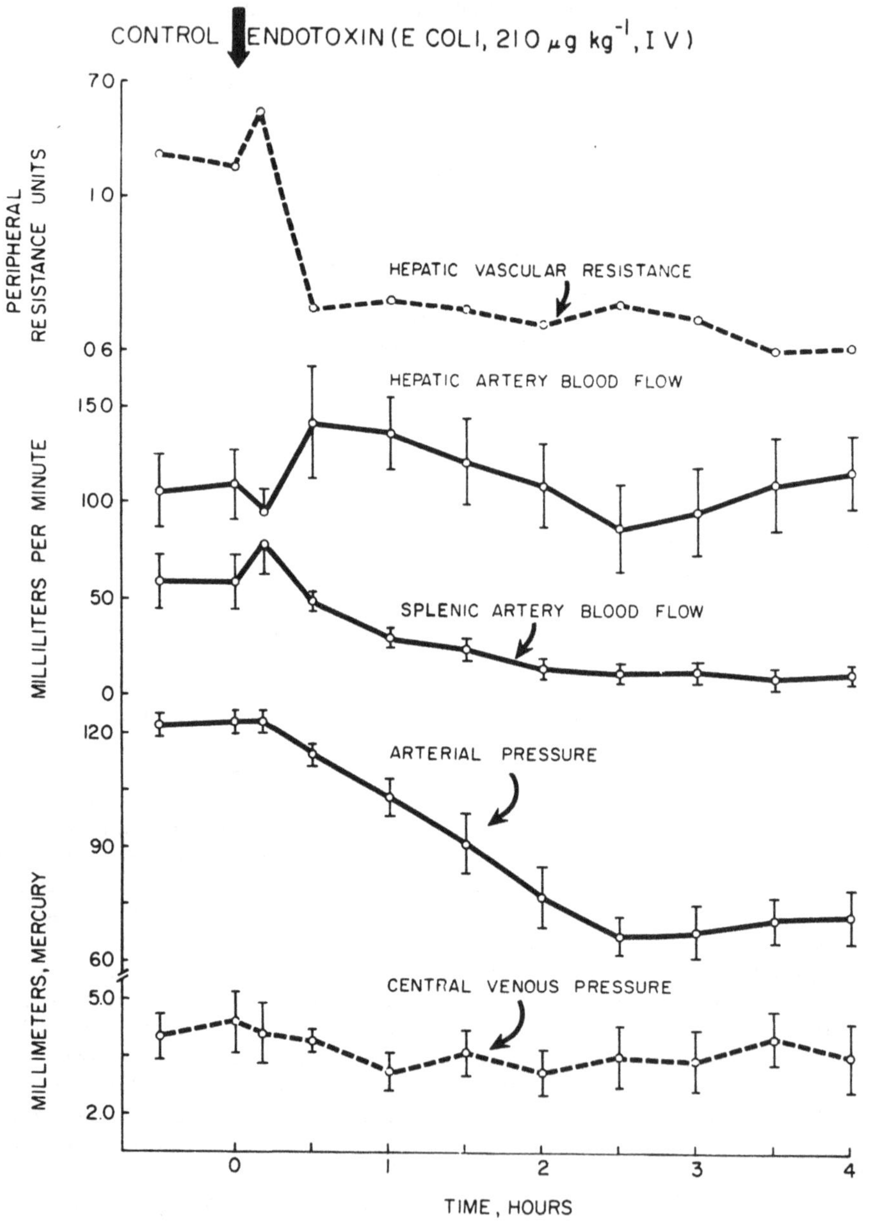

FIG. 10. Effects of endotoxin upon blood flow to liver and spleen of the baboon. Each point is the mean ±SE of seven experiments in seven animals.

Of final interest to those concerned with the possible existence of a target organ in the splanchnic viscera are studies designed to test this hypothesis directly. If the gut or any other splanchnic organ is a target organ which adversely affects the course of hypotensive syndromes, ablation of the organ should confer a protective effect upon the shock model. Some workers have reported this in dogs (16), but other investigators have failed to confirm the finding in enterectomized rats (30) or in dogs undergoing enterectomy or stepwise total evisceration (27).

REFERENCES

1. Barcroft, H. Circulation in skeletal muscle. In: *Handbook of Physiology: Circulation.* Washington, D.C.: American Physiological Society, 1963, sect. 2, vol. II, pp. 1353-1385.

2. Barton, R.W., D.G. Reynolds, and K.G. Swan. Mesenteric circulatory responses to hemorrhagic shock in the baboon. Ann. Surg., in press.

3. Berk, J.L., J.F. Hogen, W.H. Beyer, M.J. Gerber, and G.R. Dochat. The treatment of endotoxic shock by beta-adrenergic blockade. Ann. Surg. 169:74-81, 1969.

4. Cavanagh, D., and P.S. Rao. Endotoxin shock in the subhuman primate. Arch. Surg. 99:107-112, 1969.

5. Corday, E. Pressor agents in cardiogenic shock. Am. J. Cardiol. 23:900-902, 1969.

6. Dietzman, R.H., J.H. Block, J.A. Feemster, Y. Idezuka, and R.C. Lillehie. Mechanisms in the production of shock. Surgery 62:645-654, 1967.

7. Dietzman, R.H., and R.C. Lillehei. The treatment of cardiogenic shock. IV. The use of phenoxybenzamine and chlorpromazine. Am. Heart J. 75:136-138, 1968.

8. Einheber, A., and G.J. Cerilli. Hemorrhagic shock in the monkey. Am. J. Physiol. 202:1183-1187, 1962.

9. Farrar, W.E., and L.M. Corwin. The essential role of the liver in detoxification of endotoxin. Ann. N.Y. Acad. Sci. 133:668-684, 1966.

10. Fine, J. Shock and peripheral circulatory insufficiency. In: *Handbook of Physiology: Circulation.* Washington, D.C.: American Physiological Society, 1965, sect. 2, vol. III, pp. 2037-2067.

11. Gilbert, R.P. Mechanisms of the hemodynamic effects of endotoxin. Physiol. Rev. 40:245-279, 1960.

12. Green, R., T. Wiznitzer, S. Ruberberg, E. Frank, and J. Fine. Hepatic clearance of endotoxin absorbed from the intestine. Proc. Soc. Exptl. Biol. Med. 108:261, 1961.

13. Grim, E. The flow of blood in the mesenteric vessels. In: *Handbook of Physiology: Circulation.* Washington, D.C.: American Physiological Society, 1963, sect. 2, vol. II, pp. 1439-1456.

14. Jacobson, E.D., B. Mehlman, and J.P. Kalas. Vasoactive mediators as the "trigger mechanism" of endotoxin shock. J. Clin. Invest. 43:1000-1013, 1964.

15. Kuida, H., R.P. Gilbert, L.B. Hinshaw, J.G. Brunson, and M.B. Visscher. Species differences in effect of gram-negative endotoxin on circulation. Am. J. Physiol. 200:1197-1202, 1961.

16. Lillehei, R.C., J.K. Longerbeam, and J.C. Rosenberg. The nature of irreversible shock: Its relation to intestinal changes. In: *Shock: Pathogenesis and Therapy,* edited by K.D. Bock. Berlin: Springer-Verlag, 1962, pp. 106-129.

17. Nickerson, M. Drug therapy of shock. In: *Shock: Pathogenesis and Therapy,* edited by K.D. Bock. Berlin: Springer-Verlag, 1962, pp. 356-370.

18. O'Connell, T., and D.W. Fonkalsrud. Hepatocellular response to hypovolemic shock and vasoexcitor drugs. Surgery 69: 373-379, 1971.

19. Ravin, H.A., D. Rowley, C. Jenkins, and J. Fine. On the absorption of bacterial endotoxin from the gastrointestinal tract of the normal and shocked animal. J. Exptl. Med. 112:783-792, 1960.

20. Richardson, J.A. Catecholamines in shock. In: *Twelfth Hahnemann Symposium on Shock.* New York: Grune & Stratton, 1965, pp. 340-346.

21. Swan, K.G., and E.D. Jacobson. Hemodynamics of endotoxin shock in the conscious animal. Surg. Gynecol. Obstet. 125: 1041-1046, 1967.

22. Swan, K.G., and D.G. Reynolds. Effects of catecholamine infusions on the canine mesenteric circulation. Gastro-

enterology, in press.

23. Swan, K.G., and D.G. Reynolds. Adrenergic mechanisms in the canine mesenteric circulation. Am. J. Physiol. 220: 1779-1785, 1971.

24. Swan, K.G., and D.G. Reynolds. Mesenteric hemodynamics of endotoxin shock in the baboon. Gastroenterology, in press.

25. Vick, J.A. Endotoxin shock in the primate: Treatment with phenoxybenzamine. J. Clin. Invest. 43:279, 1964.

26. Vick, J.A., H.P. Ciuchta, J.H. Merikel, and E.O. Lindseth. Vasodilator therapy in acute hemorrhagic shock. Circ. Res. 16:58-64, 1965.

27. Vick, J.A., L.E. Wittmers, M.M. Jordan, and L.B. Hinshaw. Role of the intestine in endotoxin shock. Proc. Soc. Exptl. Biol. Med. 109:200-202, 1962.

28. Waldhausen, J.A., F.L. Abel, and W.L. Pearce. Portal systemic venous shunts in hemorrhagic shock in the dog and monkey. Ann. Surg. 166:183-189, 1967.

29. Watts, D.T., and V. Westfall. Studies on peripheral blood catecholamine levels during hemorrhagic shock in dogs. Proc. Soc. Exptl. Biol. Med. 115:601-604, 1964.

30. White, F.N., G. Ross, L. Barajas, and E.D. Jacobson. Hemodynamics of endotoxin shock in the rat and the effects of phenoxybenzamine. Proc. Soc. Exptl. Biol. Med. 122: 1025-1029, 1966.

DISCUSSION

DR. A. M. LEFER *(Jerusalem, Israel):* There are a couple of things I would like to raise about this; one is that you're not measuring distribution of blood flow within the splanchnic circulation, and you're certainly not measuring nutritive blood flow. As several people have shown, both in humans and in subhuman primates, there is a dramatic decrease in pancreatic blood flow during a variety of forms of shock. This is emerging now as quite a crucial finding in the early stages of the pathogenesis of shock. So I submit, don't write off the splanchnic circulation on the basis of gross hemodynamic studies.

DR. SWAN: The blood supply to the pancreas is derived from branches of the splenic artery and from the pancreaticoduodenal branches of the gastroduodenal and superior mesenteric arteries. During endotoxic shock, in the baboon, splenic artery blood flow does fall, but the other circulations are unchanged. We have not measured renal blood flow under these circumstances. Aside from this parameter, certainly the major portion of the splanchnic visceral circulation is unchanged during the early phase of endotoxic shock, in terms of arterial inflow to organs. As you have mentioned, this does not prove that the microcirculation is not impaired. We have recently accumulated evidence, that Dr. Reynolds will present tomorrow, suggesting that there is no abnormality in the intestinal microvasculature of the monkey during endotoxic shock, as opposed to findings of marked changes in the canine model. We have not studied the microcirculation of the pancreas. As we have discussed privately in the past, I think the techniques for measuring pancreatic blood flow are difficult to validate, let alone calibrate, and the results must be interpreted with caution.

DR. C. M. HERMAN *(Bethesda, Md.):* We haven't been able to measure microcirculatory changes in the splanchnic circulation during shock. We are examining the consequences of changes in splanchnic blood flow during hemorrhagic shock in these same baboons. What we're looking for is the appearance of endotoxin in the portal circulations as well as in the systemic circulation during a 20-30% lethal hemorrhagic shock model, as well as in a fully lethal hemorrhagic shock model. Based on endotoxin concentration and the gross and microscopic appearance of the bowel at the time of sacrifice after the end of the study, I think that the appearance of endotoxin in portal blood coming as a result of ischemic changes in the bowel circulation during hemorrhagic shock, in this particular subhuman primate, is probably not a real issue. We have not been able to find endotoxin with an assay method which, while it has some problems, certainly seems to be the best we have and is a fairly reliable method. So, this is one functional measurement which appears to corroborate what Dr. Swan is talking about.

DR. A. P. THAL *(Kansas City, Kansas):* What is the assay method you used?

DR. HERMAN: This is the limulus method. We're using both techniques: the modification that Dr. Fine made in which he uses a pH adjustment rather than a chloroform extraction in order to get the material out.

DR. W. C. SHOEMAKER, *Panel Moderator (New York, N.Y.):* Dr. Swan, could you elaborate on the effects of the endotoxin, specifically on the catechol responses in the mesenteric circulation under both normal and shocked conditions?

DR. SWAN: Yes. Logarithmically increasing doses of either norepinephrine or epinephrine (10^{-3} to 10^{0} or 1 μg/kg) as an intra-arterial injection cause only a vasoconstrictor response in the dog. We pretreated dogs with a sublethal dose of endotoxin (and the endotoxin we used requires about 5.0 mg/kg for 80% lethality). If we take a twentieth of that amount and pretreat the animal with 0.125 mg/kg and then study the catecholamine effects, we find no change in the response to either injected or infused norepinephrine or epinephrine. The absolute flow values are reduced because endotoxin, even in a tiny dose, decreases mesenteric blood flow; but in terms of percent change, there is no difference.

DR. T. E. EMERSON, JR. *(East Lansing, Mich.)*: We showed some years ago in the monkey that no intra- or extravascular pooling of blood occurred in the foreleg. So, neither the skeletal muscle nor skin seem to serve as a reservoir to explain the intravascular pooling or loss of fluid into the interstitium. If you have any data indicating pooling of blood in the splanchnic region in the monkey, and if this does not occur, can you speculate where the blood might be going in order that venous return is reduced and cardiac output is reduced?

DR. SWAN: In answer to the first part of your question, there is no evidence, either hemodynamically or morphologically, that any degree of pooling of blood occurs in the splanchnic viscera of the monkey. Again, there is a marked species difference between the dog and subhuman primate. The dog, regardless of where endotoxin is injected, responds with an increase in portal venous pressure from a mean of about 5 mm Hg up to about 25 mm Hg within minutes. Then, portal pressure recovers. This is an enormous change in portal pressure and requires a massive dose of epinephrine to duplicate the phenomenon. In the primate (and Jacobson showed this in the rhesus monkey, also), there is no change in portal pressure, either in hemorrhagic shock or in endotoxin shock, despite equivalent lethality. Where the pooling that you referred to is going on, I don't know. We have not measured cardiac output and venous return. We have no evidence of anything below the diaphragm explaining the decreased cardiac output.

DR. A. G. B. KOVÁCH *(Budapest, Hungary)*: Can I ask Dr. Swan about the anesthesia he used in the dog and the baboon experiments?

DR. SWAN: The baboons were immobilized with Sernylan (phencyclidine hydrochloride). Anesthesia was maintained with pentobarbital (Nembutal). The dogs were anesthetized with intravenous pentobarbital.

DR. KOVÁCH: According to our findings it has some sympathicolytic effect, and I would be very anxious to know whether the difference is not related to the anesthesia.

DR. SWAN: Yes, this seems to be something one has to live with. I think there have been some good studies—Greenway and Lawson, for instance, showing that the mesenteric circulatory responses to catecholamines are not affected by pentobarbital as opposed to chloralose, which is supposedly one of our better anesthetic agents, if we want to eliminate effects on the central nervous system. We do get a slight pressor response and a slight tachycardia using pentobarbital in the dog; that's unavoidable. We should, of course, be working toward the chronic model and eliminate the problem.

DR. SHOEMAKER: I would like to take the liberty of taking issue with you. Anesthesia is not a problem that you have to live with. We have, for 15 years, been studying unanesthetized shock models and have observed blood flow methods more recently with labeled microspheres. We have demonstrated an increase in tissue concentrations of chromium-labeled red cells in liver which are about two and three times normal in shock. This type of protocol in an unanesthetized dog simulates what is happening in clinical shock, in contrast to experiments in which the animal is put into late shock, maintained there for a few hours, and then retransfused at the end of 2 hours.

DR. L. D. MACLEAN *(Montreal, Canada):* I hesitate to bring up something that is clinical but I'd like your help on it. It's on a single patient. It's a little like throwing a lead ball out of the balloon: if it goes up, it's significant, and that's the way I've always looked at this. The patient is a man with a cord section very high, who is quadriplegic. We studied his cardiac output, peripheral resistance, and blood pressure. He had a cardiac index of about 5, peripheral resistance of about 500, and normal blood pressure. About 10 days later, the urologist operated on him and diverted his urinary stream. He developed *E. coli* septicemia and went into septic shock. At the time we studied him 10 days previously, his heart rate was around 75; this did not change after he was in septic shock, indicating that a massive outflow of epinephrine or catecholamines, in my interpretation, was not present. His peripheral resistance went up a little, and his cardiac output dropped from 5 down to about the normal level, a little over 3. Our further interpretation was that neurogenic factors were not playing the major role either. We reasoned that, since his lactate was high, his cardiac output wasn't sufficient to meet the needs of his body. With increasing his cardiac output, pharmacologically, he did recover. I'd be interested in your interpretation of this.

DR. SHOEMAKER: I recall the admonition of one of my old professors of medicine: God save us from the man with one of a series.

DR. SWAN: I don't think that sympathectomy *per se* increases flow through the splanchnic viscera. I presume this is a sympathectomized patient. There have been several relevant laboratory studies: Folkow, in particular, in Sweden, studying the effects of sympathetic stimulation, and Greenway and Lawson studying sympathetic denervation through splanchnicectomy. Sympathetic stimulation certainly decreases flow, but sympathetic denervation does not seem to increase flow.

ARE ADRENERGIC OVERACTIVITY AND SPLANCHNIC VASOCONSTRICTION THE PRIME PATHOPHYSIOLOGICAL EVENTS IN SHOCK?

Eugene D. Jacobson, M.D.

Program in Physiology, The University of Texas Medical School at Houston, Texas Medical Center, Houston, Texas

During the past three decades, an hypothesis has evolved to explain the pathophysiology of lethal human shock states. I shall refer to this hypothesis as the "adrenergic theory of shock". The adrenergic theory is widely accepted (2,6,7). In essence, the theory holds that the stress that produces shock—whether by blood loss, sepsis, myocardial infarction, or trauma—activates mechanisms in the body which initially restore arterial pressure and cardiac output back to normal. Among these compensatory mechanisms is stimulation of the sympathetic nervous sytem and release of circulating catecholamines. The adrenergic system is overstressed by the severe and prolonged cause of shock. The result is widespread arteriolar constriction, particularly in the splanchnic region. Poor perfusion of critical abdominal viscera ensues, leading to ischemic damage of tissues in the liver, the reticuloendothelial system, and the gut. Impaired defense processes, deranged metabolic activity, and loss of function of the intestinal barrier are major consequences of splanchnic vasoconstriction. Toxic molecules, such as endotoxins, enter the circulation and cannot be cleared by normal defenses. The toxemia is added to the initial shock state, resulting in a vicious circle which propels the patient into irreversible shock and death.

When one analyzes this theory at face value, two points must be noted: first, the application of this theory to man is theoretical, since our experimental information comes from animal studies; second, much of the hypothesis cannot readily be tested by direct measurements.

A body of evidence fails to support this theory. It is my

intent to summarize the main parts of that evidence.

Is sympathetic overactivity essential to the early development of circulatory shock? If tissue catecholamine stores are depleted with daily administration of reserpine to dogs and the animals are subjected to a shocking dose of endotoxin, one observes typical shock responses such as arterial hypotension, portal hypertension, and splanchnic vasoconstriction (5). Similarly, blockade of alpha- or beta-adrenergic circulatory responses to norepinephrine or isoproterenol fail to prevent typical canine or rat hemodynamic responses to endotoxin (4,5,11). Vascular reactivity to catecholamine declines after onset of shock (5). In dogs and cats, endotoxin produces a profound and persistent reduction in mesenteric blood flow, whereas prolonged stimulation of the splanchnic sympathetic nerves or infusion of norepinephrine causes only a transient decrease in intestinal blood flow. This ability of the circulation of the gut to avoid persistent underperfusion during persistent adrenergic input has been termed "autoregulatory escape" (8).

It appears that interference with adrenergic mechanisms in the shocked animal does not include interference with major splanchnic hemodynamic responses to endotoxin, and the splanchnic responses to catecholamines do not mimic the vascular reactions to endotoxin.

The second major question to ask about the adrenergic theory of shock is this: do the splanchnic circulatory responses in anesthetized dogs apply to primates, including man? Extrapolation from dog to man is dubious if the canine responses fail to occur in monkeys. It should be noted, parenthetically, that the splanchnic circulatory responses of immature anesthetized and mature conscious dogs to endotoxin administration are not identical to those of anesthetized adult dogs (10). The anesthetized monkey shows the following responses to a lethal dose of endotoxin: mild persistent portal hypertension, gradual onset of deepening arterial hypotension, no change in mesenteric artery blood flow, and a decline in mesenteric vascular resistance (1). These responses are apparent for as long as 4 hours after injection of endotoxin. Furthermore, these responses have also been observed in the baboon (9). Thus, as lethal shock develops in the subhuman primate, the mesenteric arterioles dilate to escape ischemic damage. Histopathologic findings of little vascular alteration in the gut of the shocked monkey support the hemodynamic observations. The splanchnic circulatory responses of primates clearly differ from those of the dog. At this point we can ask: which is more representative of the human circulatory response in lethal shock—that of the dog, or that of subhuman primates?

It appears that wide use of a different shock model, namely

the primate, would probably have resulted in an hypothesis quite different from the adrenergic theory of shock. The preceding evidence seems to support a few conclusions. First, we are ignorant of the critical early events in shock and are unlikely to define them while our view remains restricted to simple circulatory events. Second, the primacy of one circulatory region as the special target in shock seems dubious. Third, shock becomes lethal when widespread subcellular processes are impaired. Recently, we have found that a key enzyme, hepatic adenyl cyclase, is activated by endotoxin under both *in vitro* and *in vivo* conditions (3). The finding that endotoxin shock involves cyclic AMP suggests a more profitable avenue of investigation than many previous studies.

SUMMARY

The major evidence against a prime role of the adrenergic system in endotoxin shock is that depletion of tissue catecholamines and adrenergic blockade fail to alter circulatory responses to endotoxin in dogs and rats.

The major evidence against the splanchnic circulation as the prime target of the adrenergic system in endotoxin shock is two-fold: (a) in dogs and cats, the mesenteric circulation responds to prolonged adrenergic overactivity by restoring blood flow to control levels or higher despite continued adrenergic stimulation ("autoregulatory escape"); and (b) in monkeys and baboons, lethal doses of endotoxin fail to decrease intestinal blood flow for hours after induction of profound hypotension.

These findings suggest that the adrenergic system is not the prime mediator of endotoxin shock and that the splanchnic circulation is not the prime target of this disorder.

REFERENCES

1. Brobmann, G.F., H.B. Ulano, L.B. Hinshaw, and E.D. Jacobson. Mesenteric vascular responses to endotoxin in monkey and dog. Am. J. Physiol. 219:1464-1467, 1970.

2. Fine, J. Shock and peripheral circulatory insufficiency. In: *Handbook of Physiology*, edited by W. Hamilton. Washington, D.C.: American Physiological Society, 1965.

3. Gimpel, L.P., D.S. Hodgins, and E.D. Jacobson. Effect of endotoxin on liver adenyl cyclase. Clin. Res. 19:475, 1971.

4. Jacobson, E.D., B. Mehlman, and J.P. Kalas. Vasoactive

mediators as the "trigger mechanism" of endotoxin shock. J. Clin. Invest. 43:1000-1013, 1964.

5. Kalas, J.P., and E.D. Jacobson. The effect of vasoactive antagonists in endotoxin shock. Am. Heart J. 67:764-778, 1964.

6. Lillehei, R.C., J.K. Longerbeam, J.H. Block, and W.G. Manax. Hemodynamic changes in endotoxin shock. In: *Twelfth Hahnemann Symposium on Shock*. New York: Grune & Stratton, 1965.

7. Nickerson, M. Drug therapy in shock. In: *Shock: Pathogenesis and Therapy,* edited by W. Bock. Berlin: Springer-Verlag, 1962.

8. Shanbour, L.L., and E.D. Jacobson. Autoregulatory escape in the gut. Gastroenterology 60:145-148, 1971.

9. Swan, K.G. Circulatory responses of the baboon in endotoxin shock. In: *A Symposium on the Splanchnic Circulation in Shock,* edited by J.P. Kalas, D.G. Reynolds, and K.G. Swan. New York: Prentice Hall, in press.

10. Swan, K.G., and E.D. Jacobson. Hemodynamics of endotoxin shock in the conscious animal. Surg. Gynecol. Obstet. 125: 1041-1047, 1967.

11. White, F.N., G. Ross, L. Barajas, and E.D. Jacobson. Hemodynamics of endotoxin shock in the rat and the effects of phenoxybenzamine. Proc. Soc. Exptl. Biol. Med. 122:1025-1029, 1966.

EFFECTS OF ENDOTOXIN ON THE VASCULAR ARCHITECTURE OF INTESTINAL MUCOSA

David G. Reynolds, LTC, MSC, James M. Brungardt, and Kenneth G. Swan, LTC, MC

Department of Gastroenterology, Division of Medicine, Walter Reed Army Institute of Research, Washington, D.C.

The mesenteric vascular bed has been functionally implicated in the development of irreversible shock (8). Most studies of mesenteric hemodynamics during experimental shock have been performed on dogs and have been designed to characterize changes in superior mesenteric arterial blood flow during the course of shock. The site of the vascular response in these studies presumably would be the microvasculature of the intestinal mucosa. Failure of microcirculatory control has been repeatedly demonstrated to be a factor in the pathophysiology of shock (1,6,14).

Johnson (7) has considered the role of local vascular mechanisms in shock. He describes the intestinal arteriovenous reflex as a possible detrimental mechanism, in that it maintains capillary pressure at the expense of capillary flow. This would be compatible with the observations of Meyer and Visscher (10) that endotoxin causes initial arteriolar constriction and venular dilation in the intestinal serosa, which is followed by relaxation of the arterioles and constriction of the venules. During this secondary response capillary pressure increases, producing hemostasis, edema, and tissue hypoxia. Palmerio *et al.* (11) demonstrated that the ischemic lesion associated with endotoxemia is due to the action of catecholamines released from adrenergic nerve endings in visceral tissue. They further described the lesion as hemorrhage within the arteriolar walls without destruction of the elastic lamina. A direct action of endotoxin on vascular smooth muscle has been described by Delaunay and co-authors (4), who reported strong contractions of mesenteric arteries, arterioles, and metarterioles during the early stages of shock.

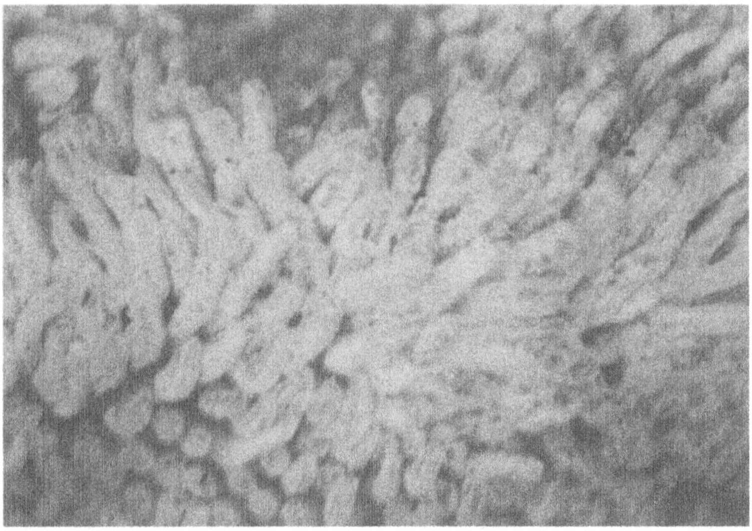

FIG. 1. Surface view of canine jejunal mucosa. Villi are closely packed and are slender cylindrical structures of approximately 1 x 0.2 mm. Magnification X22.5.

Branemark (2) has stated that "in order to delineate qualitatively the problem of microcirculatory disturbances in shock, detailed information about microvascular architecture and flow, as well as interrelation between blood cells, plasma, and endothelium, is required." The purpose of this manuscript is to describe the normal microvascular architecture of the intestinal mucosa and to compare it with that seen in animals during endotoxemia. Marked species variation exists in responses to endotoxin (5). Current concepts of the pathophysiology of shock have been derived largely from mesenteric hemodynamic studies in canine models. The results of these studies differ distinctly from those reported in recent studies of subhuman primates (3,17); *i.e.*, the latter do not respond to endotoxin with mesenteric vasoconstriction. For these reasons, the mucosal vascular architecture of both dog and baboon will be compared before and after endotoxin administration.

The silicone-rubber injection technique, introduced by Sobin (15), was used to study the intestinal vasculature. The nature of the injection compound, the methodology, and validation of the technique have been described in detail elsewhere (12,16). Microfil, MV-118 (Canton Biochemical Products), a low-viscosity silicone-rubber compound with a particle size of 1-3 microns, was

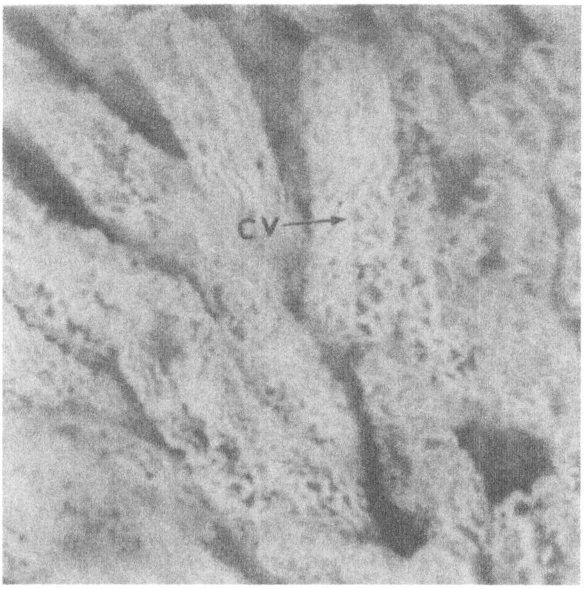

FIG. 2. High magnification (X72) of an area from Figure 1. The subepithelial vascular plexus is shown to extend from the villus base to tip as sinusoidal vascular channels 10-15 microns in diameter. CV = core vessels inside of villus.

used in this study. In the canine experiments, the injection mass was delivered through a polyethylene cannula inserted into an artery in the secondary arcase. In the monkey experiments, the cannula was placed directly in the superior mesenteric artery. Upon polymerization of the injection mass, distal jejunal segments were excised and processed through a glycerin "clearing" procedure. In the clearing process, tissue water is replaced by glycerin, which reduces tissue optical density toward zero. On microscopic examination, one then looks through the intact parenchyma and sees only the solidified rubber filling all the vascular channels.

NORMAL VASCULAR ARCHITECTURE

Canine Intestinal Mucosa

Canine jejunal mucosa viewed through the dissecting microscope appears as closely packed villi that are typically long, slender, and cylindrical (Fig. 1). The mean height of a villus is slightly under 1.0 mm and its width is about 0.2 mm. These estimated

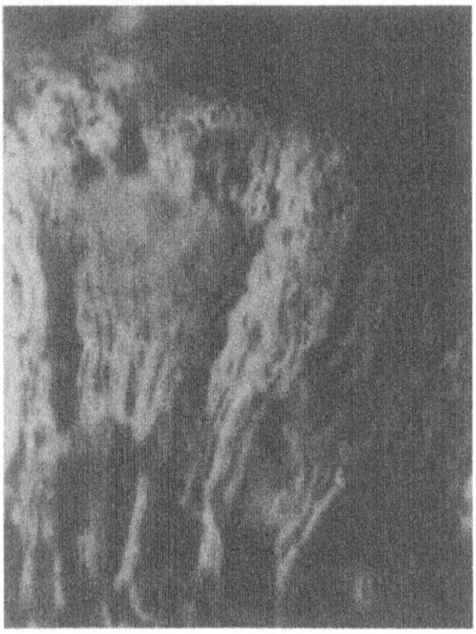

FIG. 3. Cross-section of canine mucosa illustrating the typical morphology of the subepithelial plexus. Core vessels, 25-35 microns, are shown entering at the base of villi. Magnification X50.

dimensions reflect the size of the vascular bed and exclude the epithelial layer covering the villus, making the actual dimensions somewhat greater.

The highly anastomotic and complex nature of the villus subepithelial plexus is readily apparent in Figure 2 (a high magnification of part of Fig. 1). The vessels, measuring approximately 10-15 microns in diameter, form a vascular net that extends to the tip of the villus. These vessels follow a sinusoidal course from villus base to tip. This pattern is also apparent in Figure 3, which shows the extensive, large central or core vessels serving the villi. Microscopic dissection and examination of these tissues suggest that the core vessels consist of a central vein and a pair of marginally located arterioles. The mucosal vascular supply of the dog is depicted in Figure 4. Submucosal arterial branches extend through the cryptic layer of the mucosa and rise laterally in the villi. These arterial branches also provide arteriolar twigs serving the cryptic layer. The villus arterioles extend through the lower half of the structure, at which point they are distributed to the subepithelial plexus. However, it is obvious that an appreciable amount of vasculature, especially in the lower half of the villus, is derived directly from the cryptic layer of the mucosa. Venous drainage of the subepithelial plexus is accom-

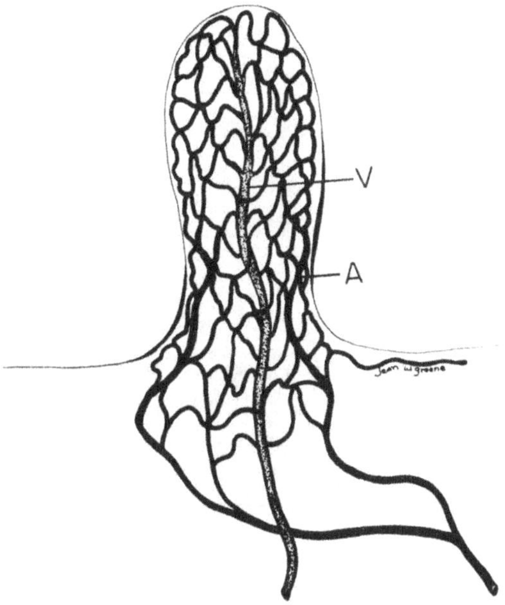

FIG. 4. Schematic representation of the canine mucosal vasculature. Arterioles (A) rise into the lower half of the villus and supply the subepithelial vascular plexus, which is drained via the central venule (V). Arteriolar branches also supply the cryptic layer and, in turn, the lower part of the villus.

plished through the centrally located villus vein.

The above-described vascular pattern might be considered a mirror image or the reciprocal of Mall's original "fountain concept" of villus vascular architecture (9). Mall's description includes arterial supply via a central arteriole and venous drainage by marginal veins.

The vascular architecture described here is not unique to the dog. The same basic pattern is found in the intestinal mucosa of rats, rabbits, and guinea pigs (unpublished observations). However, as we shall see next, the pattern differs markedly from that in two species of subhuman primates.

Rhesus Monkey Intestinal Mucosa

A detailed description of the vascular architecture of the rhesus monkey intestinal mucosa has been published elsewhere (13).

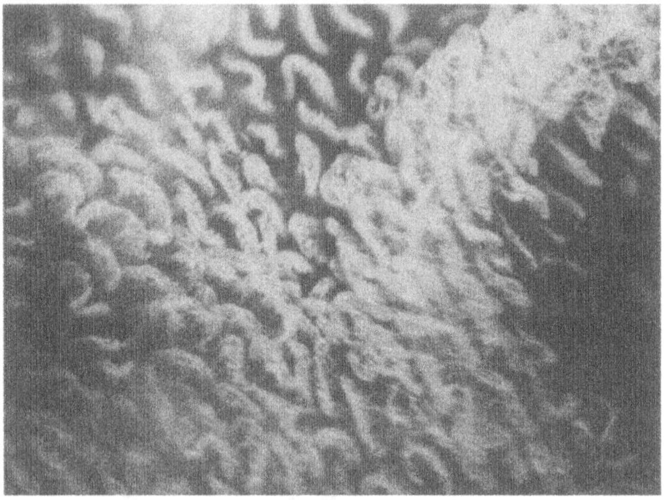

FIG. 5. Jejunal mucosa of the baboon photographed from the same aspect and at the same magnification as Figure 1. The villi are less densely packed than those of the dog and are shorter (0.6 mm), broader (0.5 mm), and flat.

There are several major differences between the canine and primate mucosa. Grossly, the villi are less closely packed and are shorter, wider, and thinner. The subepithelial plexus is composed of smaller-caliber vessels and would be considered sparse compared to that in the dog. The capillary channels rise from the base of the villus to its midlevel as parallel fine vessels and, from these, branch to form the anastomotic plexus. Submucosal arterial branches extend to the base of the mucosa where they branch into fine arteriolar twigs that are distributed directly into the cryptic capillary plexus. No arterial branches penetrate the mucosa, and the vascular supply of the villus is derived directly from the cryptic plexus. Venous return occurs via a single central vein.

Baboon Intestinal Mucosa

The vascular architecture of the intestinal mucosa of the baboon is much like that of the rhesus monkey. Figure 5 shows villi of baboon jejunum from the same aspect and at the same magnification as the villi of canine jejunum shown in Figure 1. Grossly, this tissue resembles that of the rhesus monkey, in that the villi are not closely packed and are flat, broad structures. Under high-power magnification, the resemblances still apply

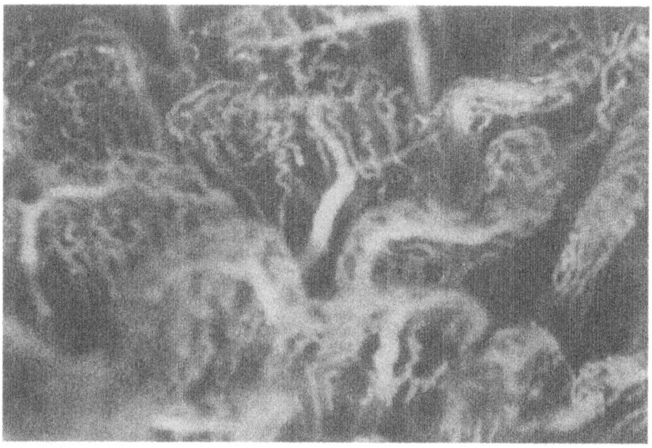

FIG. 6. High magnification (X72) of baboon villi. The subepithelial plexus is sparse and delicate. The single, central vein is readily apparent.

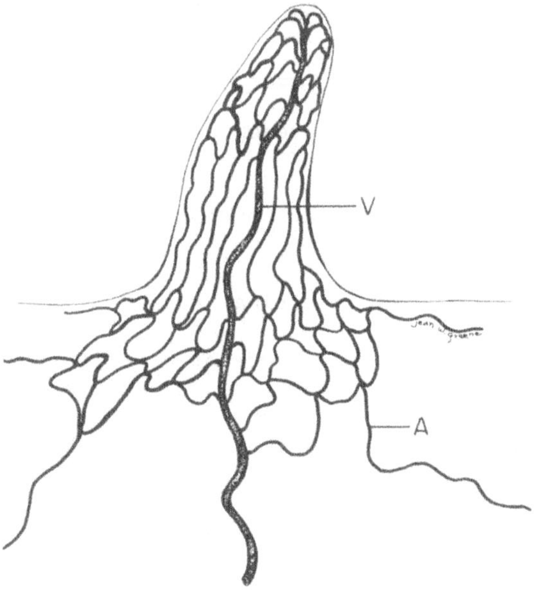

FIG. 7. Schematic diagram of the baboon mucosal vascular architecture. Arteriolar branches (A) are distributed to the base of the mucosa and supply the cryptic plexus. The villus vasculature is derived from the cryptic plexus as parallel vessels that rise and form an anastomotic plexus in the upper half of the villus. These then converge on the centrally located vein.

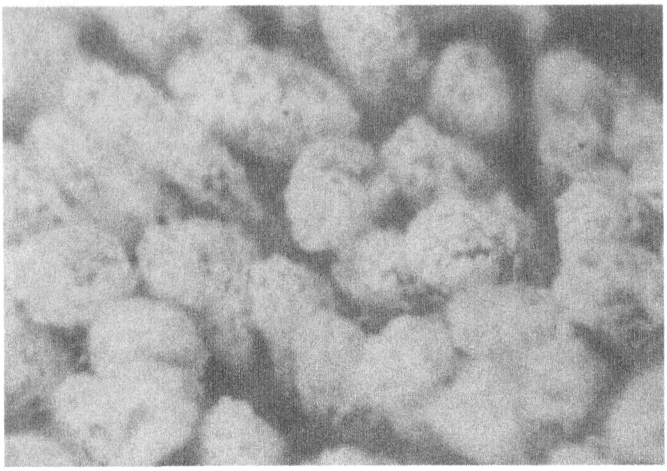

FIG. 8. Mucosal surface, canine jejunum, 4 hours after administration of lethal dose of endotoxin. Photograph was taken from the same aspect and at the same magnification (X72) as Figure 2. Villi are shortened to less than 0.5 mm and the subepithelial plexus is coiled, dilated, and congested.

(Fig. 7). These features are presented schematically in Figure 7.

VASCULAR ARCHITECTURE DURING ENDOTOXEMIA

Canine Intestinal Mucosa

When the intestinal vasculature of dogs is injected with silicone rubber 4 hours after the intravenous delivery of a lethal dose of endotoxin, four noteworthy morphological changes take place (Figs. 8 and 9). First, the villi decrease in height from almost 1.0 mm to less than 0.5 mm. Second, the subepithelial plexus becomes more convoluted and, under the stereoscopic dissecting microscope, appears to be tightly spiralled. Third, the subepithelial vascular plexus appears to be dilated and congested. Fourth, obvious indications of mucosal and submucosal hemorrhage are present, as manifested by leakage of injection compound (Figs. 9 and 10).

The observed architectural changes can be correlated with several of the known actions of endotoxin in the microvasculature. The shortening of the villi and the coiling, or folding, of their

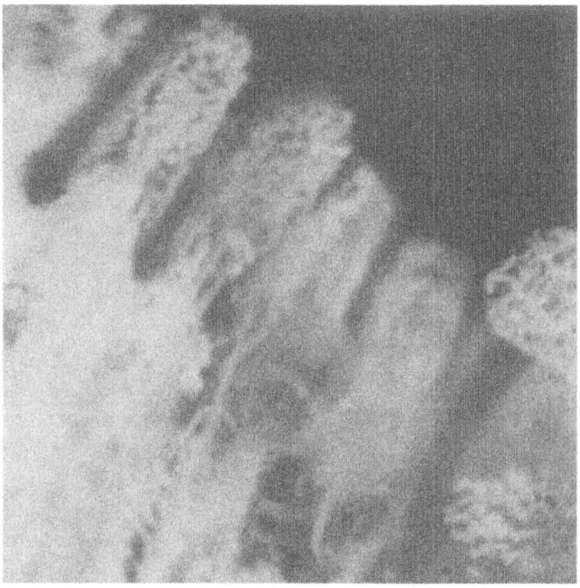

FIG. 9. Cross-section of canine mucosa 4 hours after administration of endotoxin. Microscopic detail shows shortening of villi, folding of the subepithelial plexus and, at the base of the villi, extravasation of rubber from the core vessels. Magnification X72.

small vessels might result from the demonstrated constrictor action of endotoxin on vascular smooth muscle (4,10). Contraction of the smooth muscle component of the lamina propria could also be responsible. However, no available evidence suggests such an action of endotoxin. Another consideration relates to the probable elasticity of the villi and the possibility that during hypotension the elastic recoil of the structure causes the shortening and coiling.

Figure 8 suggests the subepithelial vascular plexus to be both dilated and congested. Such an observation would agree both with the detrimental effect of the intestinal arteriovenous reflex described by Johnson (7) and with the late venous constriction and arteriolar dilation during endotoxemia reported by Meyer and Visscher (10). Figures 9 and 10 demonstrate the presence of mucosal and submucosal hemorrhage in endotoxin shock. The intra-arterial hemorrhage suggested by Palmerio (11) might be represented by the extravasation of rubber from the core vessels of the villi shown in Figure 9.

When canine intestines are also examined histopathologically,

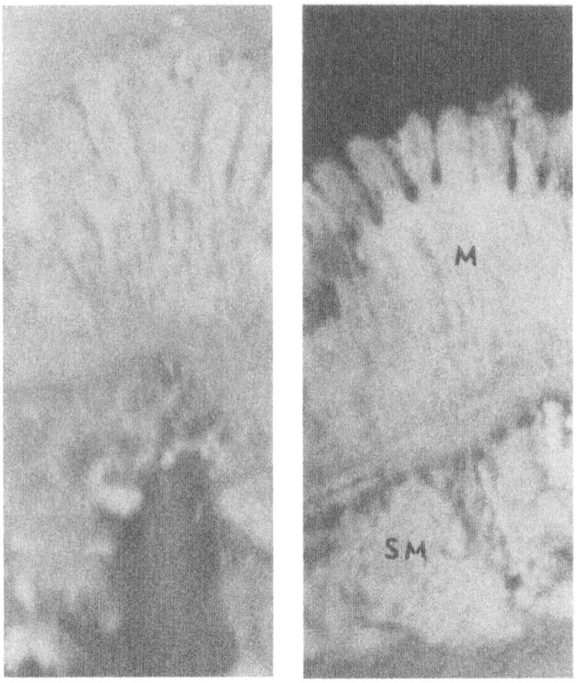

FIG. 10. Cross-section of canine jejunum (X22.5). Left, normal vascular architecture; right, 4 hours after the intravenous injection of a lethal dose of endotoxin. The microscopic appearance reveals villus shortening and both mucosal (M) and submucosal (SM) rubber extravasation, suggesting hemorrhage.

the expected tissue changes are verified, including submucosal hemorrhage, edema of the muscularis, mucosal inflammation with lymphocytic infiltration, and epithelial degeneration of the villi.

Baboon Intestinal Mucosa

When the mesenteric vascular beds of baboons are injected with silicone rubber in a similar manner after exposure to a lethal dose of endotoxin, the gross morphology of the baboon mucosa remains unaltered in the presence of endotoxemia, as does the microvascular architecture of these tissues. The only architectural alteration suggested by microscopic examination is a possible mild dilation of the subepithelial plexus (Fig. 11). These tissues, when subjected to histopathological study, are unremarkable.

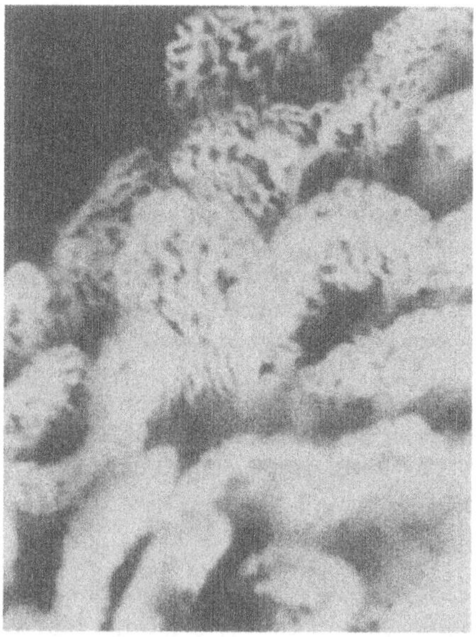

FIG. 11. High magnification of baboon villi (X55). The subepithelial plexus appears to be moderately dilated. There are no other changes from the control vascular patterns.

GENERAL INTERPRETATION

The difference in the microvascular response to endotoxin between the dog and baboon, as described above, suggests a mechanism that might account for their opposite mesenteric circulatory responses to endotoxin. In the dog the villi are shortened, and both the core and subepithelial vessels are coiled or folded upon themselves. By implication, then, these changes would indicate a significant increase in the resistance of blood flow through the microvasculature of the mucosa. The observed dilation and congestion of the subepithelial plexus further suggests an increased vascular resistance. In contrast, these changes are absent in monkeys. The subepithelial plexus may actually be slightly dilated, so that no active increase in resistance to blood flow occurs. One should note, however, that the present studies reveal only the morphological differences between the two species and do not explain why mesenteric blood flow in the baboon is unchanged by hypotension. The distinct difference between the species in terms of normal architecture may be functionally related to the different mesenteric vascular responses to endotoxin. Supporting this possibility is the observation that both rats (18) and rabbits (19) suffer severe mesenteric ischemia in endotoxin shock and, as pointed out earlier, their microvascular architecture resembles that in the dog.

These observations also suggest that endotoxin might have a direct constrictor effect on the intestinal microvasculature of the dog. Such an action has been reported elsewhere (4,10), and recent work from our laboratory supports its validity (unpublished data). Dogs were administered a low dose of endotoxin through either the inferior vena cava, portal vein, or superior mesenteric artery, and mesenteric blood flow was monitored for 5 1/2 hours. When endotoxin was delivered through the vena cava or portal vein, the animals exhibited prolonged hypotension and mesenteric ischemia. However, when endotoxin was delivered via the superior mesenteric artery, mesenteric ischemia occurred without a change in blood pressure. Thus, endotoxin would appear to have exerted a direct constrictor effect on the mesenteric vasculature.

SUMMARY

The silicone-rubber injection technique was used to characterize the microvascular architecture of canine and baboon intestinal mucosa. The specimens revealed a basic anatomical difference in the vasculature of the two species. In the dog, both arterioles and venules in the core of the villus serve the subepithelial vascular plexus. The baboon, on the other hand, has a single central villus vein, and the arterial supply is distributed to the base of the mucosa. The subepithelial plexus is derived directly from the cryptic plexus of the mucosa. After a lethal dose of endotoxin, the canine villi shorten, the microvasculature is coiled upon itself, the subepithelial plexus is congested, and mucosal and submucosal hemorrhage becomes apparent. None of these changes occurs in the baboon when an equivalent dose of endotoxin is administered. The data indicate a direct, morphological difference between the species in their response to endotoxin; moreover, they suggest a mechanism to explain the increase of mesenteric vascular resistance that is typical of the canine shock model and absent in the primate model.

REFERENCES

1. Bond, R.F., E.S. Manley, and H.D. Green. Cutaneous and skeletal muscle vascular responses to hemorrhage and irreversible shock. Am. J. Physiol. 212:488-497, 1967.

2. Branemark, P.I. Rheological aspects of low flow states. In: *Microcirculation as Related to Shock*, edited by D. Shepro and G.P. Fulton. New York: Academic Press, 1968, pp. 161-180.

3. Brobmann, G.F., H.B. Ulano, L.B. Hinshaw, and E.D. Jacobson. Mesenteric vascular responses to endotoxin in the monkey and dog. Am. J. Physiol. 219:1464-1467, 1970.

4. Delaunay, A., P. Boquet, and L. Lebrun. Le mode d'action des endotoxines bactériennes. IV. Les troubles vaso-moteurs chèz les animaux intoxiques et leurs conséquences. J. Physiol., (Paris) 40:89-110, 1948.

5. Gilbert, R.P. Mechanisms of the hemodynamic effects of endotoxin. Physiol. Rev. 40:245-279, 1960.

6. Green, H.D. Physiology of peripheral circulation in shock. Fed. Proc. (Suppl. 9) 20:61-68, 1961.

7. Johnson, P.C. The splanchnic microcirculation in shock and hypotension. In: *Microcirculation as Related to Shock*, edited by D. Shepro and G.P. Fulton. New York: Academic Press, 1968, pp. 3-22.

8. Lillehei, R.C., J.K. Longerbeam, and J.C. Rosenberg. The nature of irreversible shock: Its relation to intestinal changes. In: *Shock: Pathogenesis and Therapy*, edited by K.D. Bock. Berlin: Springer-Verlag, 1962, pp. 106-129.

9. Mall, F.P. Die blut und lymphwege in dunndarm des hundes. Abh. d. Mat. - phys. el. d. Konig. sachs. Gesell. d. Wiss. 14:153-200, 1887.

10. Meyer, M.W., and M.B. Visscher. Partial analysis of segmental resistances in intestinal vessels after endotoxin. Am. J. Physiol. 202:913-918, 1962.

11. Palmerio, C., S.C. Ming, E. Frank, and J. Fine. The role of the sympathetic nervous sytem in the generalized Shwartzman reaction. J. Exptl. Med. 115:609-615, 1962.

12. Reynolds, D.G., J. Brim, and J.E. McClain. Silicone-rubber technique for microvascular studies. Lab. Manage. 6:24, 1968.

13. Reynolds, D.G., J. Brim, and T.W. Sheehy. The vascular architecture of the small intestinal mucosa of the monkey *(Macaca mulatta)*. Anat. Rec. 159:211-218, 1967.

14. Rothe, C.F., and E.E. Selkurt. Cardiac and peripheral failure in hemorrhagic shock in the dog. Am. J. Physiol. 207: 203-214, 1964.

15. Sobin, S.S., W.G. Frasher, and H.M. Tremer. Vasa vasorum of

the pulmonary artery of the rabbit. Circ. Res. 11:257-263, 1962.

16. Sobin, S.S. Vascular injection methods. Methods Med. Res. 11:233-238, 1965.

17. Swan, K.G., R.W. Barton, and D.G. Reynolds. Mesenteric hemodynamics during endotoxemia in the baboon. Gastroenterology, in press.

18. White, F.N., G. Ross, L. Barajas, and E.D. Jacobson. Hemodynamics of endotoxin shock in the rat and the effect of phenoxybenzamine. Proc. Soc. Exptl. Biol. Med. 122:1025-1029, 1966.

19. Zweifach, B.W., and K. Fronek. Effect of anesthesia on lethal response to endotoxin in rabbits. Fed. Proc. 30:373, 1971.

ROLE OF VASOPRESSIN AND ANGIOTENSIN IN RESPONSE OF SPLANCHNIC RESISTANCE VESSELS TO HEMORRHAGE

J. Robert McNeill, Ph.D.[1]

Department of Physiology and Biophysics, University of Oklahoma Medical Center, Oklahoma City, Oklahoma

After hemorrhage, total hepatic flow decreases approximately in proportion to the decrease in cardiac output. This is associated with a slight increase in splanchnic vascular resistance (2,10,15). However, this response is the net result of marked vasoconstriction of the intestinal and splenic resistance vessels and vasodilatation of the hepatic arterial resistance vessels (2,12,14,15,18,20,29). Although these responses of the splanchnic resistance vessels to hemorrhage are well established, the mechanisms have not been investigated until recently.

INTESTINAL VASOCONSTRICTION

Intestinal vasoconstriction following hemorrhage has generally been assumed to be mediated by the sympathetic nerves. In the normovolemic cat, however, stimulation of the sympathetic nerves and infusions of norepinephrine do not cause sustained vasoconstriction, and autoregulatory escape occurs (6,7). Epinephrine infusions cause intestinal vasodilatation (11,24). When intestinal flow is reduced by partial occlusion of the superior mesenteric artery, the response to sympathetic nerve stimulation becomes impaired (7). On the basis of these reports, it would be surprising if the innervation to the intestine or adrenal medullary secretions were the main factors causing intestinal vasoconstriction after hemorrhage. Other vasoconstrictor factors may contribute. Renin is released from the kidneys and large amounts of angiotensin have

[1]Present address: Department of Pharmacology, University of Saskatchewan, Saskatoon, Saskatchewan, Canada.

been found in the blood after hemorrhage (17,22,27). Similarly, large amounts of vasopressin have been found in the blood after hemorrhage (1,3,23,31). Both vasopressin and angiotensin are potent vasoconstrictors and, unlike norepinephrine, can cause sustained intestinal vasoconstriction (4,6).

The role of the sympathetic nerves and of vasopressin secretion and angiotensin formation in the mechanism of the intestinal vasoconstriction after hemorrhage was studied in anesthetized cats with all organ systems intact and in cats after intestinal denervation, adrenalectomy, nephrectomy, and hypophysectomy in various combinations. The methods have been described in detail elsewhere (20).

Cats were anesthetized by intraperitoneal injection of sodium pentobarbital (30 mg/kg). A noncannulating electromagnetic flowmeter probe and, downstream from this, a micrometer-controlled arterial clamp were placed around the superior mesenteric artery. In each experiment, the relationship of superior mesenteric arterial flow to arterial pressure was investigated by graded clamping of the superior mesenteric artery, and a pressure-flow curve was obtained. Then, rapid hemorrhage was induced by withdrawing blood from a femoral artery at a rate of 15±1.1 ml/min/kg until the arterial pressure had dropped to 50 mm Hg. A little more blood was then removed to maintain this pressure for 1 minute. Thereafter, no more blood was removed and arterial pressure was allowed to recover. In some experiments, slow hemorrhage was induced by removing blood for 25 minutes at the rate of 0.6 ml/min/kg.

Simple comparison of the changes in intestinal vascular resistance before and after hemorrhage is not the best method to assess the role of extrinsic vasoconstrictor factors (9). Although changes in calculated resistance may be due to extrinsic influences acting on the vascular smooth muscle elements, they may also be due to local adjustments in response to changes in arterial pressure. Arterial pressure decreases after hemorrhage, and the pressure-flow curve for the intestinal vascular bed is not linear. We have therefore compared the actual flows after hemorrhage with the flows expected from the changes in arterial pressure. These latter flows were determined from the pressure-flow curves and are described as the passive flows. The actual flows are expressed as percentages of the passive flows. Thus the extent of deviation from 100% represents the extent to which flows were altered by extrinsic influences.

The blood volumes removed and the arterial pressures and flows before and after hemorrhage in the various groups of animals are listed in Table 1. The flow response to extrinsic factors was calculated for the various groups of animals, described below

TABLE 1

PRESSURES, FLOWS, AND VASCULAR RESISTANCE IN DIFFERENT GROUPS OF CATS SUBJECTED TO RAPID HEMORRHAGE

	Group 1[a]	Group 2[b]	Group 3[c]	Group 4[d]	Group 5[e]
Blood vol. removed (ml/kg)	20±2.4	10±1.0	19±1.5	17±1.7	11±1.0
Arterial pressure (mm Hg)					
Prehemorrhage	122±3.8	102±5.4	118±3.0	118±5.4	110±5.4
2 min after hemorrhage	51±0.6	50±1.8	52±1.4	52±1.1	51±0.4
60 min after hemorrhage	96±6.5	76±8.0	91±7.5	85±6.2	73±8.3
Mesenteric flow (ml/min/kg)					
Prehemorrhage	43±2.7	47±2.9	34±4.2	48±3.4	36±5.4
2 min after hemorrhage	13±2.0	19±2.4	9±0.9	16±1.4	16±2.0
60 min after hemorrhage	17±1.6	27±3.5	12±1.2	15±1.9	18±3.5
Vascular resistance (% of prehemorrhage level, 60 min after hemorrhage)	200	130	220	204	132

Values are means ±SE.

[a]Five cats with intact organ systems.

[b]Six cats subjected to intestinal denervation, adrenalectomy, nephrectomy, and hypophysectomy.

[c]Six cats subjected to intestinal denervation, adrenalectomy, and nephrectomy.

[d]Three cats subjected to intestinal denervation, adrenalectomy, and hypophysectomy.

[e]Four cats subjected to nephrectomy and hypophysectomy.

(Courtesy of Am. J. Physiol. 219:1343, 1970.)

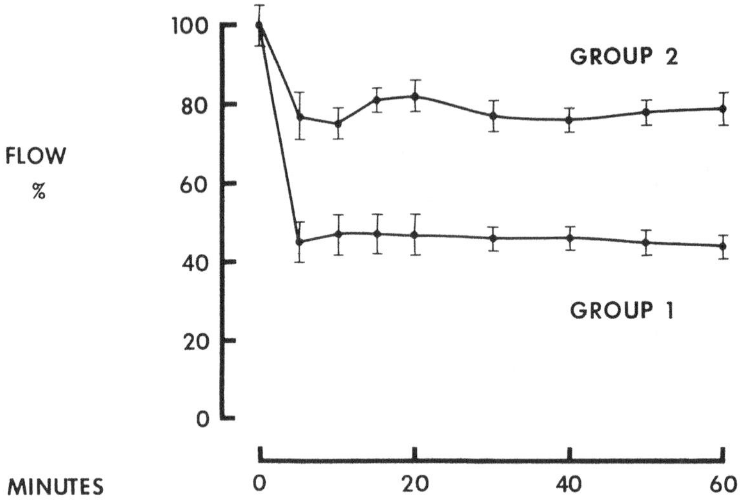

FIG. 1. The means ±SE of the superior mesenteric flows after rapid hemorrhage, expressed as percentages of the passive flows expected from the changes in arterial pressure. Group 1, intact cats; Group 2, cats after denervation, adrenalectomy, nephrectomy, and hypophysectomy. (Courtesy of Am. J. Physiol. 219:1344, 1970.)

(see also Figs. 1,2, and 3).

Group 1: Cats with intact organ systems. In five cats in which the intestinal nerves, adrenals, kidneys, and pituitary were all left intact, vasoconstriction developed within 5 minutes after hemorrhage and was well maintained for the next 55 minutes (Fig. 1, lower curve).

Group 2: Cats subjected to intestinal denervation, adrenalectomy, nephrectomy, and hypophysectomy. The flow response to hemorrhage in six cats is shown in Figure 1 (upper curve). The values were significantly different from those of Group 1 cats ($P < 0.005$, unpaired t-test). Thus, intestinal vasoconstriction was greatly reduced by denervation, adrenalectomy, nephrectomy, and hypophysectomy.

In this group of cats, the arterial pressure was reduced to 50 mm Hg by the removal of a smaller volume of blood than in Group 1 (Table 1). This seemed most likely to be a consequence of the inability of these animals to undergo vasoconstriction after hemorrhage. However, an alternative explanation could not be excluded: the smaller vasoconstriction might be due to the smaller reduction in blood volume, even though arterial pressure decreased to a

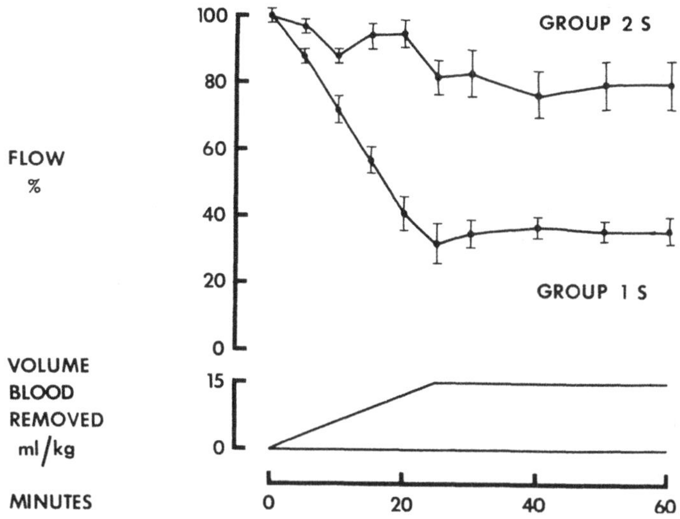

FIG. 2. The means ±SE of the superior mesenteric flows during and after slow hemorrhage, expressed as percentages of the passive flows expected from the changes in arterial pressure. Group 1S, intact cats; Group 2S, cats after denervation, adrenalectomy, nephrectomy, and hypophysectomy. (Courtesy of Am. J. Physiol. 219: 1345, 1970.)

similar extent. To exclude this second possibility, in additional experiments similar blood volumes were removed slowly and continously.

Group 1S and 2S: Slow hemorrhage. In four cats with intact intestinal innervation, adrenals, kidneys, and pituitary, blood was removed at the rate of 0.6 ml/min/kg for 25 minutes (Group 1S). Vasoconstriction was similar to that following rapid hemorrhage (Fig. 2).

In seven cats, the intestines were denervated and the adrenal glands, kidneys, and pituitary were removed before the animals were bled at the same rate, *i.e.*, 0.6 ml/min/kg for 25 minutes (Group 2S). Vasoconstriction (Fig. 2, Group 2S) was significantly less ($P < 0.001$) than in the cats with intact organ systems (Group 1S). Arterial pressure fell more in group 2S than in group 1S cats. Thus, when identical slow hemorrhages were induced in the two groups, the arterial pressure fell more and vasoconstriction was less in the group in which the intestine was denervated and the adrenals, kidneys, and pituitary were removed. These experiments suggest that, in Group 2, the smaller volume of blood

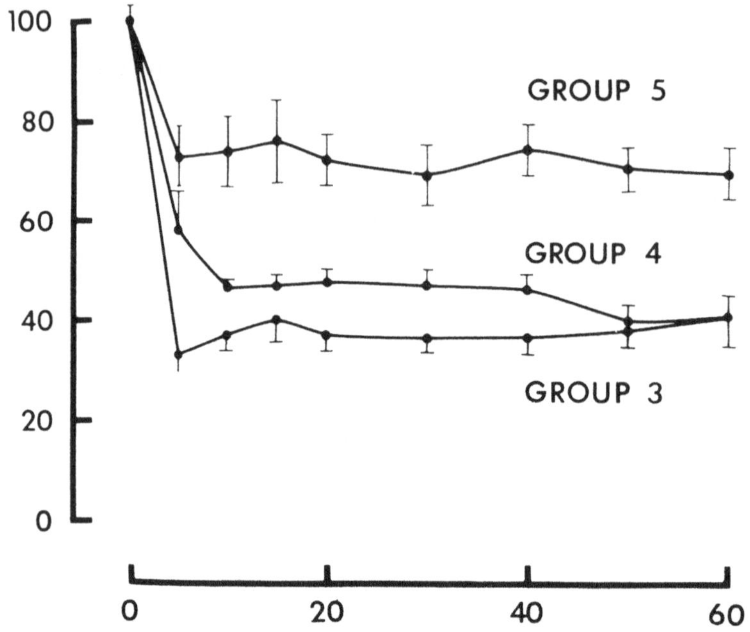

FIG. 3. The means ±SE of the superior mesenteric flows after rapid hemorrhage, expressed as percentages of the passive flows expected from the changes in arterial pressure. Group 3, intestinal denervation, adrenalectomy, and nephrectomy; Group 4, intestinal denervation, adrenalectomy, and hypophysectomy; Group 5, nephrectomy and hypophysectomy. (Courtesy of Am. J. Physiol. 219: 1345, 1970.)

removed acutely to reduce arterial pressure to 50 mm Hg was a consequence of, and not the cause of, the lesser vasoconstriction.

Thus, intestinal vasoconstriction after hemorrhage was significantly reduced by denervation of the intestine and removal of the adrenals, kidneys, and pituitary. The results were the same (a) whether a given degree of hypotension was produced or similar volumes of blood were removed and (b) whether the hemorrhage was rapid or slow. Further experiments were designed to investigate the role of each factor in the over-all response.

Group 3: Cats subjected to intestinal denervation, adrenalectomy, and nephrectomy. The flow response to hemorrhage of six cats in this group is shown in Figure 3 (Group 3). The values did not differ significantly from those for Group 1 cats ($P > 0.1$). Thus, the response to hemorrhage was not reduced by denervation, adrenalectomy, and nephrectomy, and the presence of the pituitary alone was sufficient to ensure a maximal response to hemorrhage.

Group 4: Cats subjected to intestinal denervation, adrenalectomy, and hypophysectomy. The flow response to hemorrhage of three cats in this group is shown in Figure 3 (Group 4). The values did not differ significantly from those of Group 1 cats ($P > 0.5$). Thus, the response to hemorrhage was not reduced by intestinal denervation, adrenalectomy, and hypophysectomy, and the presence of the kidneys alone was sufficient to ensure a maximal response to this stimulus.

Group 5: Cats subjected to nephrectomy and hypophysectomy. The flow response to hemorrhage of four cats in this group is shown in Figure 3 (Group 5). The values differ significantly from those of Group 1 ($P < 0.01$) but not from those of Group 2 ($P > 0.1$). Thus, the small remaining vasoconstriction in animals subjected to denervation, adrenalectomy, nephrectomy, and hypophysectomy (Group 2) was unmodified by the presence of the nerves and adrenal glands.

Hemorrhage after phenoxybenzamine. In two cats with intact innervation, adrenals, kidneys, and pituitary, phenoxybenzamine (5 mg/kg) was administered intravenously, followed by 5% dextran (Rheomacrodex diluted with 0.9% NaCl, 10 mg/kg). One hour later, blood was removed at the rate of 0.6 ml/min/kg for 25 minutes. In two more cats, the dose of phenoxybenzamine was increased to 10 mg/kg. Since the responses in all four cats were very similar, the data were pooled. The mean arterial pressure before hemorrhage was 110±6.9 mm Hg, and the mean superior mesenteric arterial flow was 34±3.4 ml/min/kg. The arterial pressure dropped to 73±7.8 mm Hg during blood removal and recovered to 88±13 mm Hg over the next 35 minutes. The vasoconstrictor response was calculated, with the results shown in Figure 4. The responses did not differ significantly ($P > 0.1$) from those in cats not receiving phenoxybenzamine (Group 1S, Fig. 2). Before and after phenoxybenzamine administration, norepinephrine (0.2-2.0 μg) was injected into the superior mesenteric artery. After phenoxybenzamine, the vasoconstrictor response was abolished or converted to a small vasodilatation. Stimulation of the intestinal nerves at the end of the experiments produced a small increase or no change in superior mesenteric arterial flow.

Discussion

Experiments were designed to investigate the mechanism of the intestinal vasoconstriction following hemorrhage. The sympathetic nerves have usually been assumed to be the most important factor in the mechanism of vasoconstriction after hemorrhage, but circulating vasoactive factors may also contribute. The roles of these factors were investigated by removing the major sources of

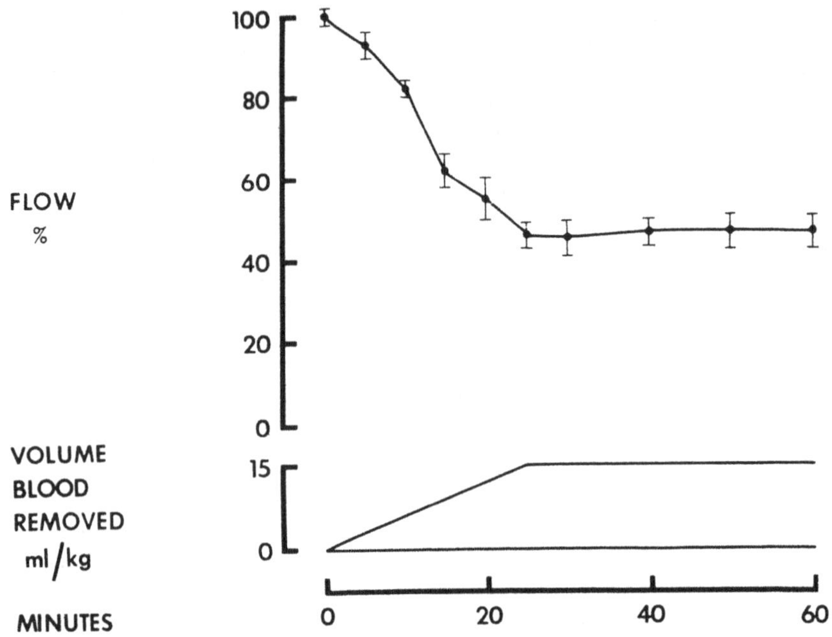

FIG. 4. The means ±SE of the superior mesenteric flows during and after slow hemorrhage, expressed as percentages of the passive flows expected from the changes in arterial pressure. Cats with intact organ systems, 1 hour after administration of phenoxybenzamine (5 or 10 mg/kg). (Courtesy of Am. J. Physiol. 219:1346, 1970.)

these agents and by intestinal denervation. The results do not prove that the effects of hypophysectomy and nephrectomy were due solely to the absence of circulating vasopressin and angiotensin. However, since the concentrations of these agents in the blood increase markedly after hemorrhage, the results have been interpreted accordingly.

In most experiments, hemorrhage was standardized by inducing a controlled degree of hypotension. Under these conditions, the degree of intestinal vasoconstriction and the volume of blood removed in order to produce a given degree of hypotension are both indications of the integrity of the complex mechanisms by which the animal compensates for hemorrhage. To show that the responses did not depend on the different volumes of blood removed, similar volumes were removed in some animals.

The results of all these experiments were consistent. After intestinal denervation and removal of the adrenals, kidneys, and pituitary, the intestinal vasoconstriction was significantly reduced. In addition, the blood volume removed to produce a given degree of hypotension was reduced.

After denervation, adrenalectomy, and nephrectomy, the intestinal vasoconstriction did not differ significantly from the response in the control animals. This suggested either that vasopressin was the sole vasoconstrictor factor or that several overlapping and simultaneous mechanisms were involved. Further experiments in which other combinations of the factors were selectively excluded showed clearly that either vasopressin secretion alone or angiotensin production alone caused responses similar to those produced when both factors acted simultaneously in the presence of the adrenals and intestinal innervation.

The responses in the cats after nephrectomy and hypophysectomy are of particular interest. Since stimulation of the sympathetic nerves and infusions of norepinephrine do not cause sustained vasoconstriction, and autoregulatory escape occurs, and since epinephrine infusions cause intestinal vasodilatation, it is perhaps not surprising that the innèrvation and adrenal medullary secretions played no significant part in the vasoconstriction of the intestinal resistance vessels after hemorrhage or that the response was unchanged after administration of phenoxybenzamine.

SPLENIC VASOCONSTRICTION

The mechanism of the splenic vasoconstriction was studied in a manner similar to that described for the intestinal vascular bed. However, it had been shown previously that splenic denervation together with the removal of the adrenals and kidneys significantly reduced, but did not abolish, the splenic vasoconstriction after hemorrhage (14). Since denervation and adrenalectomy alone had no effect, the conclusion was drawn that angiotensin formation subsequent to renin release from the kidneys caused part of the splenic vasoconstriction (14). However, a significant vasoconstriction still remained. Thus, experiments were designed to determine whether hypophysectomy in addition to denervation, adrenalectomy, and nephrectomy would abolish the splenic vasoconstriction. It was also of interest to demonstrate whether the sympathetic nerves and adrenal glands could affect splenic flow after hemorrhage. Therefore, experiments were carried out to determine whether the splenic nerves and adrenals would cause splenic vasoconstriction when the renal and pituitary factors were absent.

The methods have been described in more detail elsewhere (29). Splenic arterial flow was measured with a noncannulating electromagnetic flowmeter probe. Hemorrhage consisted of removing blood (15 ml/kg) at a constant rate for 20 minutes. Prior to hemorrhage, a pressure-flow curve was obtained, and the actual flows after hemorrhage were expressed as percentages of the passive flows expected from the changes in arterial pressure as calculated from the pressure-flow curve.

Group 1: Cats with intact organ systems. In three cats, the splenic nerves, adrenals, kidneys, and pituitary were all left intact. Splenic vasoconstriction developed during the period of blood removal, and the vasoconstriction was well maintained (Fig. 5, Group 1).

Group 2: Cats subjected to splenic denervation, adrenalectomy, nephrectomy, and hypophysectomy. The flow response to hemorrhage in four cats is shown in Figure 5 (Group 2). The values did not differ significantly from pre-hemorrhage control values. It was concluded that all extrinsic factors had been removed. Thus, hypophysectomy in addition to splenic denervation, adrenalectomy, and nephrectomy completely abolished the splenic vasoconstriction.

Group 3: Cats subjected to nephrectomy and hypophysectomy. The flow response to hemorrhage in four cats is shown in Figure 5 (Group 3). The values for this group were significantly different ($P < 0.05$) both from those obtained in cats with intact organ systems (Group 1) and from those obtained when cats were subjected to denervation, adrenalectomy, nephrectomy, and hypophysectomy (Group 2). Thus, in contrast to the intestinal bed, the sympathetic nerves and secretions from the adrenal glands were capable of causing splenic vasoconstriction.

Discussion

It had been previously shown that endogenous angiotensin formation caused part of the splenic vasoconstriction after hemorrhage (see above). The present results show that removal of the pituitary, in addition to denervation, adrenalectomy, and nephrectomy, completely abolished the vasoconstriction. Thus, in addition to angiotensin, vasopressin also appears to play an important role in this response.

After nephrectomy and hypophysectomy, significant splenic vasoconstriction occurred. Thus, in contrast to the intestinal vascular bed, the sympathetic nerves and the adrenal medullary secretions are capable of causing splenic vasoconstriction, although significantly less than when the kidneys and pituitary are also intact. In the intestinal vascular bed, autoregulatory

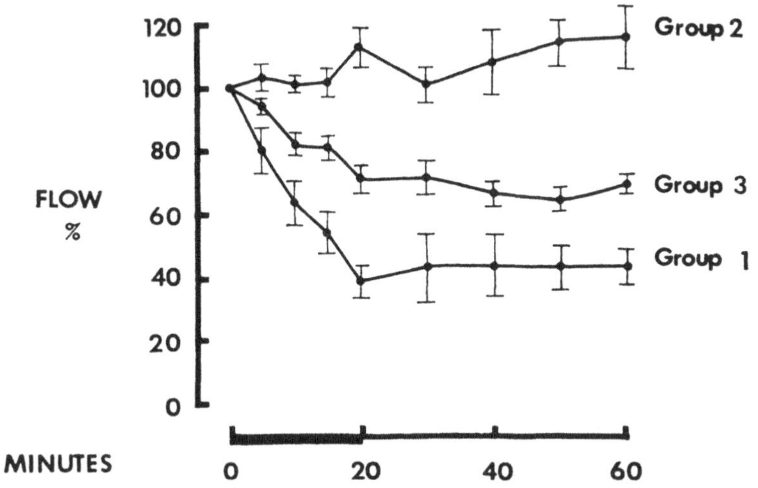

FIG. 5. Means ±SE of splenic flows after hemorrhage, expressed as percentages of passive flows expected from changes in arterial pressure. Group 1, sham-operated cats with all organ systems intact; Group 2, cats with splenic denervation, adrenalectomy, nephrectomy, and hypophysectomy; Group 3, cats with nephrectomy and hypophysectomy. Blood was removed during period shown by bar at bottom. (Courtesy of Am. J. Physiol. 220:838, 1971.)

escape occurs in response to stimulation of the sympathetic nerves and to infusions of norepinephrine (6,7), whereas in the spleen the extent of autoregulatory escape is much smaller (13). Also, the splenic flow response to stimulation of the sympathetic nerves is well maintained during periods of reduced blood flow (13), but in the intestinal vascular bed the flow response is impaired (7). These findings are consistent with the hypothesis that the sympathetic innervation is involved in the vasoconstriction after hemorrhage in the spleen but not in the intestine.

INFUSIONS OF VASOPRESSIN AND ANGIOTENSIN

In contrast to the intestinal and splenic vasoconstriction after hemorrhage, the hepatic arterial resistance vessels dilate. If vasopressin and angiotensin play important roles in the splanchnic response to hemorrhage, then intravenous infusions of these agents in amounts likely to be found in blood after hemorrhage should cause a similar response. Therefore, the responses of the intestinal, splenic, and hepatic arterial resistance vessels were compared during intravenous infusions of vasopressin and angiotensin.

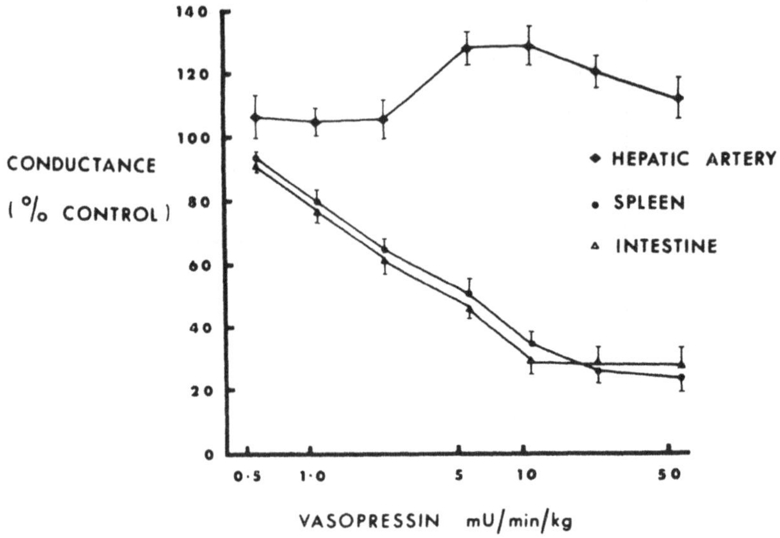

FIG. 6. Dose-response curves to vasopressin infusions for resistance vessels of hepatic arterial, splenic, and intestinal vascular beds. Each curve represents means ±SE of responses in five to seven cats. (Courtesy of Am. J. Physiol. 218:1705, 1970.)

The methods used have been described in detail elsewhere (4). In one series of animals, hepatic arterial flow was measured with a noncannulating electromagnetic flowmeter probe. In a second series, superior mesenteric artery flow was recorded. In a third series, splenic arterial flow was recorded. At each dose level, infusions were continued for 6 minutes, by which time the flow was steady at its new level. The conductance to flow was calculated 1 minute before and at the 5-minute mark during each infusion. The conductance during the infusion was expressed as a percentage of that before infusion began.

Infusions of vasopressin caused marked vasoconstriction of the intestinal and splenic vascular beds, and the decrease in conductance at each dose level was very similar in the two beds (Fig. 6). In contrast, vasopressin caused an increase in conductance of the hepatic arterial bed.

Infusions of angiotensin caused a decrease in conductance in all three vascular beds, but the vasoconstriction of the hepatic arterial bed was significantly less than that which occurred in the intestinal and splenic beds (Fig. 7).

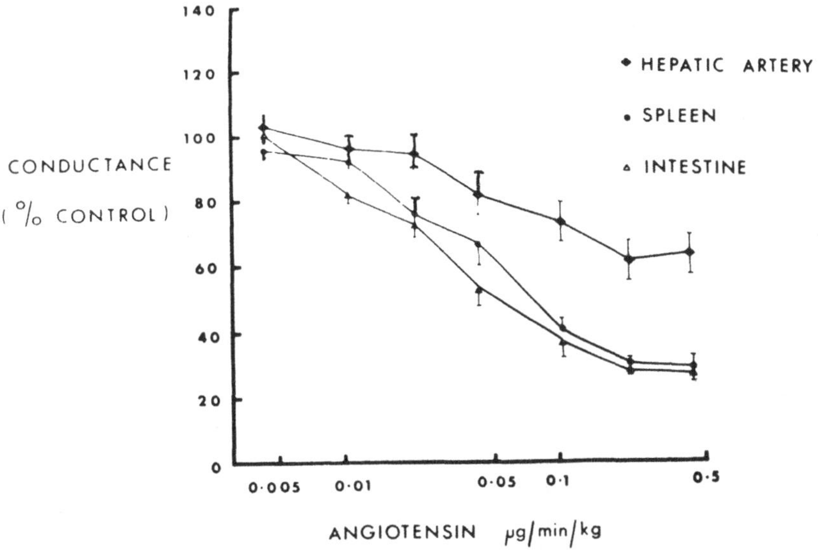

FIG. 7. Dose-response curves to angiotensin infusions for resistance vessels of hepatic arterial, splenic, and intestinal vascular beds. Each curve represents means ±SE of responses in five to seven cats. (Courtesy of Am. J. Physiol. 218:1705, 1970.)

Discussion

Intravenous infusions of vasopressin caused marked intestinal and splenic vasoconstriction and hepatic arterial vasodilatation. In these experiments, infusions of vasopressin from 0.5 to 10 mU/min/kg body weight would be expected to produce blood levels similar to those reported to occur after hemorrhage in the cat (1,3,23) and in the dog(31). Intravenous infusions of angiotensin caused vasoconstriction of the splenic and intestinal vascular beds and weak vasoconstriction of the hepatic arterial bed. The blood levels of angiotensin after hemorrhage have not been studied in the cat, but the blood levels produced by our infusions would not be unlike those reported to occur in the dog (17,22,27).

Since intra-arterial administration of either vasopressin or angiotensin causes hepatic arterial vasoconstriction (19,26,28), it seems likely that the effects of these agents on the hepatic arterial bed during hemorrhage and during intravenous administration must be counteracted by some vasodilator mechanism which opposes the direct action of these agents. The existence of such a mechanism is established. Splenic and intestinal vasoconstriction resulted in a decreased portal venous flow and this, in turn, caused a relaxation of the hepatic arteriolar smooth muscle. This mechanism was difficult to elicit in experiments where the basal tone of the hepatic arterioles was already reduced, for example, by arterial long-circuits or in isolated perfusions of the liver (5,8,30). However, in experiments where these technical procedures were avoided, a decrease in portal vein flow caused a marked hepatic arterial vasodilatation (21,25). As Hanson and Johnson pointed out (16), the data are best explained on the basis of a myogenic response of the hepatic arteriolar smooth muscle to changes in sinusoidal pressure.

It seems likely, therefore, that no fundamental differences exist among the responses of the intestinal, splenic, and hepatic arterial resistance vessels to vasopressin and angiotensin. However, in the hepatic arterial bed, the vasoconstrictor actions of these drugs are counteracted by a myogenic vasodilatation secondary to the decrease in portal vein flow. In our experiments, the net result was a vasodilatation with vasopressin and a weak vasoconstriction with angiotensin. However, hepatic arterial flow was measured after the splenic vessels had been ligated and the spleen removed (4). Thus portal vein flow was already partly reduced, and it seems likely that the effectiveness of the vasodilator mechanism in antagonizing the direct constrictor effects of vasopressin and angiotensin is greater in the intact animal than in the present experiments.

In summary, the over-all response of the splanchnic resistance vessels to hemorrhage can now be described. After hemorrhage, portal vein flow decreases due to marked intestinal and splenic vasoconstriction. Vasopressin secretion from the pituitary gland and angiotensin formation subsequent to renin release from the kidneys appear to play major roles in the mechanism of the intestinal and splenic vasoconstriction. The sympathetic nerves and adrenal medullary secretions may also play a role in the mechanism of the splenic vasoconstriction, but they appear to be unimportant in the mechanism of the intestinal vasoconstriction. In contrast to the marked vasoconstriction of the intestinal and splenic vascular beds, the hepatic arterial resistance vessels dilate. This vasodilatation probably reflects a myogenic relaxation of the hepatic arteriolar smooth muscle as a response to the decrease in portal vein flow. The hepatic arterial vasodilatation may be important in maintaining the oxygen supply to the liver. Under conditions where portal flow decreases, a smaller increase in hepatic arterial flow would be sufficient to maintain the oxygen supply to the liver.

SUMMARY

The mechanism of the response of the splanchnic resistance vessels to hemorrhage was investigated in cats anesthetized with pentobarbital. After acute intestinal denervation, adrenalectomy, nephrectomy, and hypophysectomy, intestinal vasoconstriction after hemorrhage was greatly reduced. When either the kidneys or pituitary was left intact, the vasoconstriction did not differ significantly from that when all organs were intact. In the absence of the kidneys and pituitary, the intestinal nerves and adrenal glands did not contribute to the small residual response. The intestinal vasoconstriction after hemorrhage was unaltered by phenoxybenzamine. After splenic denervation, adrenalectomy, nephrectomy, and hypophysectomy, the posthemorrhagic splenic vasoconstriction was completely abolished. In the absence of the kidneys and pituitary, the splenic nerves and adrenal glands caused a significant vasoconstriction, but the response was reduced from that which occurred when all the organs were intact. The data suggest that vasopressin secretion and angiotensin formation play major roles in the intestinal and splenic vasoconstriction following hemorrhage. The sympathetic nerves and adrenal medullary secretions may also contribute to splenic vasoconstriction, but they appear not to be important in the intestinal vasoconstriction. The responses of the intestinal, splenic, and hepatic arterial resistance vessels to intravenous infusions of vasopressin and angiotensin were consistent with the postulated roles for these peptides in the splanchnic response to hemorrhage.

REFERENCES

1. Beleslin, D., G.W. Bisset, J. Haldar, and R.L. Polak. The release of vasopressin without oxytocin in response to hemorrhage. Proc. Roy. Soc., London, S.B. 166:443, 1967.

2. Chien, S. Role of the sympathetic nervous system in hemorrhage. Physiol. Rev. 47:214, 1967.

3. Clark, B.J., and M. Rocha e Silva, Jr. An afferent pathway for the selective release of vasopressin in response to carotid occlusion and hemorrhage in the cat. J. Physiol. 191:529, 1967.

4. Cohen, M.M., D.S. Sitar, J.R. McNeill, and C.V. Greenway. Vasopressin and angiotensin on resistance vessels of spleen, intestine, and liver. Am. J. Physiol. 218:1704, 1970.

5. Condon, R.E., L.M. Nyhus, N.D. Chapman, and H.N. Harkins. Portal vein and hepatic artery interactions: Studied in the

isolated, perfused liver. Gastroenterology 43:547, 1962.

6. Dresel, P.E., and I. Wallentin. Effects of sympathetic vasoconstrictor fibres, noradrenaline, and vasopressin on the intestinal vascular resistance during constant blood flow or blood pressure. Acta. physiol. scandinav. 66:427, 1966.

7. Folkow, B., D.H. Lewis, O. Lundgren, S. Mellander, and I. Wallentin. The effect of graded vasoconstrictor fibre stimulation on the intestinal resistance and capacitance vessels. Acta physiol. scandinav. 61:445-457, 1964.

8. Green, H.D., L.S. Hall, J. Sexton, and C.P. Deal. Autonomic vasomotor responses in the canine hepatic arterial and venous beds. Am. J. Physiol. 196:196, 1959.

9. Green, H.D., C.E. Rapela, and M.C. Conrad. Resistance (conductance) and capacitance phenomena in terminal vascular beds. In: *Handbook of Physiology*, Section 2, edited by W.F. Hamilton and P. Dow. Baltimore: Williams & Wilkins, 1963, vol. 2, pp. 935-960.

10. Greenway, C.V., and A.E. Lawson. The effect of haemorrhage on venous return and regional blood flow in the anesthetized cat. J. Physiol. 184:856-871, 1966.

11. Greenway, C.V., and A.E. Lawson. Effect of adrenaline and propranolol on the superior mesenteric artery blood flow. Can. J. Physiol. Pharmacol. 46:906-908, 1968.

12. Greenway, C.V., A.E. Lawson, and R.D. Stark. The effect of hemorrhage on hepatic artery and portal vein flows in the anesthetized cat. J. Physiol. 193:375, 1967.

13. Greenway, C.V., A.E. Lawson, and R.D. Stark. Vascular responses of the spleen to nerve stimulation during normal and reduced blood flow. J. Physiol. 194:241, 1968.

14. Greenway, C.V., and R.D. Stark. Vascular responses of the spleen to rapid hemorrhage in the anesthetized cat. J. Physiol. 204:169, 1969.

15. Greenway, C.V., and R.D. Stark. Hepatic vascular bed. Physiol. Rev. 51:23, 1971.

16. Hanson, K.M., and P.C. Johnson. Local control of hepatic arterial and portal venous flow in the dog. Am. J. Physiol. 211:712, 1966.

17. Hodge, R.L., R.D. Lowe, and J.R. Vane. The effects of alteration of blood volume on the concentration of circulating angiotensin an anesthetized dogs. J. Physiol. 185: 613, 1966.

18. Lillehei, R.C., J.K. Longerbeam, and J.C. Rosenberg. The nature of irreversible shock: Its relationship to intestinal changes. In: *Shock, Pathogenesis and Therapy: An International Symposium* (Ciba), edited by K.D. Bock. Berlin: Springer-Verlag, 1962.

19. Mahfouz, M., and G. Aida. Pharmacodynamics of intrahepatic circulation in shock. Surgery 61:755, 1967.

20. McNeill, J.R., R.D. Stark, and C.V. Greenway. Intestinal vasoconstriction after hemorrhage: Roles of vasopressin and angiotensin. Am. J. Physiol. 219:1342, 1970.

21. Price, J.B., R.C. Britton, L.M. Peterson, J.W. Reilly, and A.B. Vorhees. The validity of chronic blood flow measurements obtained by the electromagnetic flowmeter. J. Surg. Res. 5:313, 1965.

22. Regoli, D., and J.R. Vane. The continuous estimation of angiotensin formed in the circulation of the dog. J. Physiol. 183:513, 1966.

23. Rocha e Silva, Jr., M., and M. Rosenberg. The release of vasopressin in response to hemorrhage and its role in the mechanism of blood pressure regulation. J. Physiol. 202: 535-557, 1969.

24. Ross, G. Effects of epinephrine and norepinephrine on the mesenteric circulation of the cat. Am. J. Physiol. 212: 1037, 1967.

25. Schenk, W.G., J.C. McDonald, K. McDonald, and T. Drapanas. Direct measurement of hepatic blood flow in surgical patients, with related observations on hepatic flow dynamics in experimental animals. Ann. Surg. 156:463, 1962.

26. Scholtholt, J., and T. Shiraishi. The action of acetylcholine, bradykinin and angiotensin on the liver blood flow of the anesthetized dog and on the pressure in the ligated ductus choledochus. Pflugers Archiv. 300:189, 1968.

27. Scornik, O.A., and A.C. Paladini. Angiotensin blood levels in haemorrhagic hypotension and other related conditions. Am. J. Physiol. 206:553, 1964.

28. Shoemaker, C.P. A study of hepatic hemodynamics in the dog. Circ. Res. 15:216, 1964.

29. Stark, R.D., J.R. McNeill, and C.V. Greenway. Sympathetic and hypophyseal roles in the splenic response to hemorrhage. Am. J. Physiol. 220:837-840, 1971.

30. Takeuchi, J., T. Kitagawa, T. Kubo, I. Murai, and T. Tone. Autoregulation of hepatic circulation. Japan Heart J. 7: 168, 1966.

31. Weinstein, H., R.M. Berne, and H. Sachs. Vasopressin in blood: Effect of hemorrhage. Endocrinology 66:712, 1960.

PLATELET, HEMODYNAMIC, AND RESPIRATORY CHANGES IN SHOCK, SEPSIS, AND TRAUMA

Robert F. Wilson, M.D., and Herbert J. Robb, M.D.

Department of Surgery, School of Medicine, Wayne State University, Detroit, Michigan

Increasing experimental and clinical evidence suggests that platelet aggregates play an important role in the hemodynamic and respiratory changes occurring in shock, sepsis, and trauma. The purpose of this paper is to present some experimental and clinical data from the Wayne State University School of Medicine supporting this view.

Using high-resolution cinephotomicrography, studies of the microcirculation in the bowel, mesentery, skeletal muscle, and lungs of rabbits were performed under a variety of circumstances. Hypovolemia by itself caused contraction of arterioles and venules, producing some stasis but not complete occlusion of flow. When norepinephrine was given, severe spasm of the vessels occurred, producing complete obstruction to the blood flow (3). Platelet and red cell aggregates formed during the hypovolemic period and tended to remain in the local area. With readministration of the blood and raising of the blood pressure, the aggregates moved and became lodged at narrowed areas and bifurcations or embolized to the liver or lungs (1).

Direct trauma caused platelet aggregates to form (4). The aggregates were much firmer than red cell aggregates and did not break apart as they traveled in the microcirculation (5). The platelet aggregates embolized and tended to occlude the microcirculation at areas of bifurcation or narrowing. Aggregates from the bowel and mesentery lodged in the liver, while those from skeletal muscle embolized to the lung (1).

In anaphylactic shock, a pronounced aggregation of platelets was associated with marked drops in platelet counts from 450,000/mm^3 to 40,000±20,000/mm^3 within 5 minutes. Concurrent cinemicrophotographic examination of the lung demonstrated a shower of platelet emboli in the pulmonary capillaries within 5 minutes after antigen injection (2). At the same time, venous pressure rose, the arterial pressure fell, the heart slowed, the right side of the heart distended, and a heart block developed (6). Either death occurred rapidly, or the animal survived. When the animal survived, the platelet counts would progressively rise during the next 1 1/2 hours.

Endotoxin tended to cause similar, but less severe, changes than those seen in acute anaphylaxis. None of the animals died in the immediate postendotoxin period, and the hemodynamic changes and platelet count would gradually improve. However, 6, 8, or 10 hours later, a second phase of endotoxin shock seemed to occur. In this phase, the platelet aggregates again formed and embolized to the lung. The arterial pressure and platelet counts fell relentlessly until the animals died several hours later (6).

In a prospective study of patients admitted to Detroit General Hospital for trauma and/or shock, over half of them had a reduced platelet count. The more severe the trauma and shock, the greater the thrombocytopenia. Surprisingly, even uncomplicated extremity fractures were associated with a decreased platelet count in 23 of 50 such patients studied (8). Although the initial fibrinogen levels were usually normal, they rose progressively until they were two to three times normal within 6-8 days. An alveolar-arterial oxygen difference (A-aDO_2) of 40 mm Hg or more while the patient breathes room air is generally considered indicative of significant pulmonary change. It was found in 28% of patients studied within 48 hours of admission and in 35% during the second 48 hours. The patients with the lowest platelet counts were most apt to have increased A-aDO_2. This tendency for the patients with a reduced platelet count to have an increased A-aDO_2 of 40 mm Hg or more was statistically significant ($P < 0.05$) during the first 48 hours. During the second 48 hours, the correlation was not significant ($P < 0.2$).

Experimental extremity fractures in dogs have shown similar results, with an abrupt drop in platelet and fibrinogen levels followed by a slow rise of the platelet count to normal over several days and a rapid increase in fibrinogen to above-normal levels within a few days (7). The role of platelets in clinical shock, sepsis, and trauma is less clear. Patients with shock associated with massive transfusions often have greatly reduced platelet counts. Of 31 patients with prospective coagulation studies during and after massive transfusions of 10 or more units of blood in 24 hours, 25 had platelet counts less than 200,000/mm^3 and six had platelet counts less than 50,000/mm^3. Of the six patients with severe thrombocytopenia, four had excessive oozing, five were in shock, and five died (9).

The platelet count in shock is determined primarily by the severity and duration of the shock and the number of transfusions the patient has received. Of 13 patients who developed platelet counts of less than 50,000/mm^3, 11 (85%) died; of 28 with platelet counts of 50,000-99,000/mm^3, 18 (64%) died; and of 63 with higher platelet counts, only 32 (51%) died. The patients with the lowest platelet counts were also most apt to have a significant acidosis. Of 19 patients with an arterial pH of less than 7.30, 15 (79%) had platelet counts below 100,000/mm^3. In contrast, of 85 patients with a higher pH, only 26 (31%) had less than 100,000 platelets/mm^3. The patients with the lowest platelet counts were also most apt to have other coagulation abnormalities.

REFERENCES

1. Robb, H.J. Microembolism in the pathophysiology of shock. Angiology 16:405, 1965.

2. Robb, H.J. Observations on the dynamics of microembolism during experimental anaphylaxis. Ann. Allergy 24:78, 1967.

3. Robb, J.H., D.E. Ingham, and H.M. Nelson. Observations in vascular dynamics during hemorrhagic shock and its therapy. Am. J. Surg. 95:659, 1958.

4. Robb, H.J., and L.F. Jacobson. Microvascular responses to trauma. J. Trauma 3:407, 1963.

5. Robb, H.J., and C.M. Jobs. Distortion and dynamics of cellular elements in the microcirculation. Angiology 19:602, 1968.

6. Robb, H.J., R.R. Margules, and C.M. Jobs. Role of pulmonary microembolism in the hemodynamics of endotoxin shock. Ann. Surg., in press.

7. Mammen, E. Unpublished data.

8. McCarthy, B., E. Mammen, L.P. LeBlanc, and R.F. Wilson. Subclinical fat embolism: A prospective study of 50 patients with extremity fractures. J. Trauma, in press.

9. Wilson, R.F., E. Mammen, and A.J. Walt. Eight years of experience with massive blood transfusions. J. Trauma 11:275, 1971.

DISCUSSION

DR. I. M. SMITH *(Iowa City, Iowa):* You mentioned, Dr. Wilson, that the albumin disappears rapidly in a model of septic shock. In mice with staphylococci, we find this happens very rapidly—1 hour. Do you know from your labeling where this goes? And the second question, in relation to your biochemical changes, can you tell us what happens to glucose and inorganic phosphorus?

DR. WILSON: We don't really know where the infused albumin goes. Since only a small amount of it comes out in the urine, we assume that it is moving into the interstitial space through capillaries which have an increased permeability. This increased capillary permeability, especially in our septic patients, creates many problems with our studies and treatment. We like to get some estimate of the relative hypovolemia and cardiac function in each patient by noting the changes in central venous pressure and cardiac index before and after fluid loads. Sometimes rather large fluid loads cause relatively little change in the blood pressure, central venous pressure, or cardiac index, even though the patient may gain considerable weight and become quite edematous. Obviously, such patients require more colloids and blood and less crystalloids.

Of the factors which affect the glucose levels in our patients, the most important appear to be the amount of glucose given to the patient and the extent of his sepsis. We see many patients who have had surgery for generalized peritonitis, and one of the main problems we have is to decide, in those who are recovering poorly, whether or not an abscess is developing. It is becoming increasingly apparent that clinical evidence of these abscesses tends to come rather late, when treatment is much less effective. Our laboratory tests, however, are much more sensitive and can be of considerable help. If there is no other significant source of sepsis, and the patient has increasing physiologic shunting in the lung, increasing cardiac output, decreasing total peripheral resistance, and increasing blood glucose levels when receiving 150-250 g of glucose per day, the patient is probably developing an intra-abdominal abscess which needs surgical drainage. Regardless of what else you do and what drugs you give for peritonitis, if a large abscess is left undrained, the patient will probably die. The incidence of undrained abscesses is very difficult to find when reviewing the literature for survival data on septic shock due to peritonitis, but it is probably the main determinant of life or death.

We have paid no special attention to phosphorous levels so far.

DR. W. C. SHOEMAKER, *Panel Moderator (New York, N.Y.):* A very well-stated position. The primary problem is infection, and unless you can deal with that, you're in bad shape. The rest of the manipulations are supportive and do not have definite implications, the mechanisms being precisely those of infection.

I should like to attempt to summarize one or two ideas in closing.

The problem in shock is a perfusion defect but, like so many things, it's easier to say that a perfusion problem exists than it is to measure it. As Mark Twain said about the weather: Everybody talks about it but nobody does anything about it. The perfusion defect precedes the development of cellular alterations in cell death. After that event, nothing that you can do to flow makes much difference. The perfusion defect is not necessarily low flow, but it may well be uneven flow. And with the uneven flow, there may be inefficient oxygen transport. From the standpoint of therapy, therefore, one can look at a number of different parameters. Not the least of these is arterial pressure, volume, flow, and, if you will, changes in oxygen transport as reflecting this perfusion defect. What I mean to presume is that, if you can change the oxygen consumption under certain specific conditions, you presume that this will change perfusion. Optimally, you want to improve all of these, especially the oxygen consumption of the patient who may have critical problems of sustaining cell integrity.

DR. M. H. WEIL *(Los Angeles, Calif.)*: I think the issue that was raised by Dr. Duff is pertinent, and I want to underscore something that Dr. Emerson said. We assembled here with great enthusiasm, about 7 years ago, to perform under controlled conditions experiments to confirm what we had individually claimed in our home laboratories was effective treatment for experimental animals. You've been reminded of the results today, that we couldn't really come up with regimens that were unequivocally effective. Now, Dr. Duff asked that we not speak in broad terms with regard to our patients and how well they do. We can perhaps raise a somewhat persuasive argument, since we are going on to 1,100 patients in an attempt to objectively study some of these issues, and we've used some rather forceful objective methods to try to understand which of the hemodynamic and metabolic measurements are primary. Dr. Duff is entirely correct when he says that, for the untreated patient, the arterial blood pH and, for the treated patient, the arterial or central venous lactate concentrations do give you a measure of the input into your system. Furthermore, I think that, unless we classify and then stage the disease category that we're talking about, we mix up ventilatory with other complications and then put them into our total disease category. Finally, if we try to do a cluster analysis of the etiological types of shock and then try to find out whether the very same parameters, save acidosis, actually cross-cut in terms of cardiac output, arterial blood pressure, peripheral resistance, and blood volume, we are going to be very disappointed when we look at large volumes of data. This is a brief way of putting in a plea, Mr. Chairman, that we mustn't take the license of walking from the refinement of our experimental laboratories to the bedsides of our patients and try to overgeneralize by lumping together conditions of varying etiology, varying severities, multiple complications. When we do this, we tend to come up with either a panacea or a disappointment.

DR. SHOEMAKER: Very well stated. And there couldn't have been a better summary of this complex problem.

SESSION II

SHOCK AND METABOLISM

Panel Moderator:

Louis R. M. Del Guercio, M.D.
Department of Surgery
Saint Barnabas Medical Center
Livingston, New Jersey

SESSION II: INTRODUCTORY REMARKS

Louis R. M. Del Guercio, M.D., *Panel Moderator*

Department of Surgery, Saint Barnabas Medical Center,
Livingston, New Jersey

In this session of the symposium, we are getting down to fundamental issues—what happens in the cells. Metabolism, however, applies not only to the cell but to specific organs, so we will not limit ourselves to cellular metabolism. In the backs of our minds, however, lurks the fact that thus far we have learned about the cell and its function primarily from autolytic "washout" products; we have failed to uncover what is happening in real time, as far as the cell is concerned (*i.e.,* the kinetics of exchange and the kinetics of oxygen consumption). Drs. Chance at the University of Pennsylvania and Roughton in England have been some of the pioneers in this area, trying to develop systems for analyzing cellular function on a real-time basis without the need for measuring "washout" products alone. We are perfectly aware that perfusion must be adequate, not only to get nutrients and oxygen into the cell but to remove the lactate and other autolytic and enzyme products which are indicators of cellular function.

The panel is composed of physiologists, biochemists, surgeons, and internists. The field of shock being what it is, however, I think that one's original discipline makes no difference. I might even predict that the day will come when there is a Department of Shock in each medical school, which will probably represent the only truly interdisciplinary concept in most medical schools. To me, the most stimulating aspect of working in shock is the fact that you never know who is what, from the standpoint of their original field.

IMMUNOCHEMICAL AND PHYSIOLOGIC INSULIN LACK DURING LETHAL *E. coli* SEPTICEMIA IN THE SUBHUMAN PRIMATE[1]

Philip E. Cryer, M.D., Clifford M. Herman, M.D., Jonas Sode, M.D., Arnold G. Coran, M.D., and David Horwitz, M.D., Ph.D.[2]

Department of Clinical Medical Sciences, Naval Medical Research Institute, and the Medical Service, Naval Hospital; National Naval Medical Center, Bethesda, Maryland, and the Bureau of Medicine and Surgery, Navy Department

Depressed insulin secretion is a feature of severe stress, and it is usually, though not invariably, associated with hypotension. Absolute hypoinsulinemia develops during experimental hemorrhagic hypotension (5,18) and experimental gram-negative septicemia (7) in the baboon. In man, investigators have observed relative hypoinsulinemia after combat trauma (4) and impaired serum insulin responses to intravenous glucose or tolbutamide after acute myocardial infarction (1,2,6,23). After cranial trauma, the serum insulin response to intravenous glucose may be impaired (14).

We have studied the mechanisms and physiologic consequences of septicemic hypoinsulinemia (7-9), as well as the relationship between depressed insulin secretion and the duration of survival (10), in unanesthetized adult male baboons subjected to lethal *Escherichia coli* septicemia.

MATERIALS AND METHODS

The septicemic baboon model used in this laboratory has been described elsewhere (7). All experiments were performed on adult male baboons (*Papio doguera*) after an overnight fast. Since the

[1]Research Task No. M4305. 05-3056 AGG2.

[2]Teaching and Research Scholar, American College of Physicians.

adrenergic modulation of insulin secretion could theoretically be altered by anesthesia, all animals were studied in the unanesthetized state with baseline observations begun at least 4 hours after tranquilization with 1.0 mg/kg of 1-(1-phenylcyclohexyl) piperidine hydrochloride (Sernylan) intramuscularly. At no time between *E. coli* injection and ultimate loss of consciousness did the animals suffer overt pain.

The Dunwald strain B15:0125 of *E. coli*, kindly provided from the laboratory of Dr. Lerner B. Hinshaw, Oklahoma City, Oklahoma, was used in all studies. Two dosage regimens were used. In most studies, each baboon was given approximately 10^{11} *E. coli* organisms per kilogram of body weight. This dose was invariably lethal. The median survival time among 30 baboons given this dose was just under 2 hours. In the final studies, a dose of less than 5×10^{10} organisms per kilogram was given. Survival among six animals given this dose ranged from 2.1 to 24.3 hours, although fluid infusion may well have contributed to the longer survival of this group of animals.

Immunoreactive insulin was measured in arterial samples by radioimmunoassay using dextran-coated charcoal to separate antibody-bound insulin from unbound insulin (13). Porcine insulin standards were used; dilution of a baboon serum containing a high concentration of measured insulin produced appropriate changes in the insulin concentration, documenting adequate cross-reactivity between baboon insulin and porcine insulin with respect to the antiserum used. Arterial serum glucose was measured by the ferricyanide method with a Technicon AutoAnalyzer, as was the serum urea nitrogen, sodium, chloride, carbon dioxide, and potassium. Blood lactate was determined enzymatically (22) and serum free fatty acids were measured by a colorimetric technique (16). Serum creatinine was measured by the AutoAnalyzer technique.

RESULTS

Figure 1 depicts serum glucose and insulin concentrations in five control baboons given saline alone, in five *E. coli*-injected baboons, and in seven baboons injected with *E. coli* during phentolamine-induced alpha-adrenergic blockade (9). In contrast to saline-injected control animals, the animals injected with *E. coli* showed a rapid drop in the serum insulin concentration (with a serum half-time approximating the serum half-time of insulin in man), mirrored by a rise in the serum glucose concentration. Additional studies demonstrated absence of the normal serum insulin response to intravenous administration of glucose during septicemia and a twofold prolongation of the serum half-time of exogenous regular insulin injected intravenously during septicemia (8).

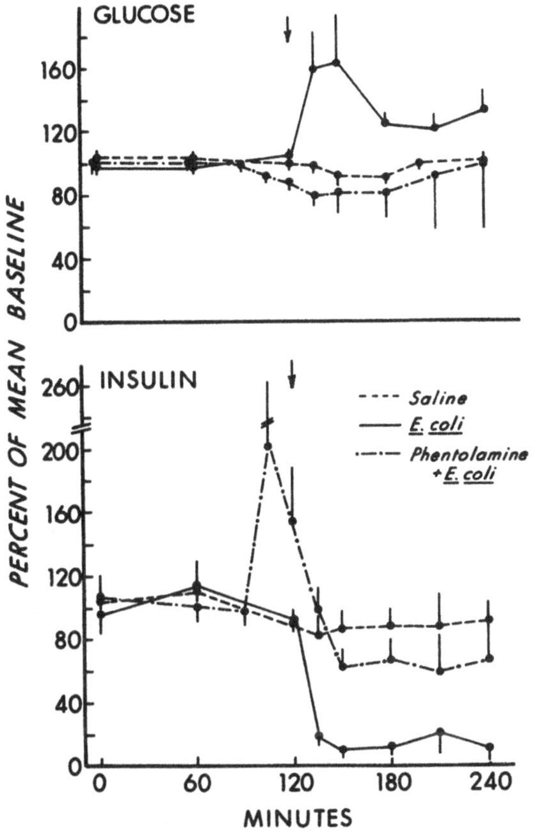

FIG. 1. The mean (±SE) serum insulin and glucose concentrations in baboons during baseline observations and after injection (arrows) of saline (five animals), approximately 10^{11} *E. coli* organisms per kilogram body weight (five animals), and similar doses of *E. coli* during phentolamine-induced alpha-adrenergic blockade (seven animals). In the latter group, 5.0 mg of phentolamine was injected intravenously and an intravenous infusion of phentolamine, 25 μg/minute, was begun at 90 minutes and continued throughout the experiment.

Alpha-adrenergic blockade was produced by the rapid intravenous injection of 5.0 mg of phentolamine (Regitine) and then sustained infusion of this drug at a rate of 25 μg/minute throughout the remainder of the experiment. Phentolamine was begun 30 minutes before *E. coli* injection. It produced an increase in the serum insulin concentration in four baboons with baseline glucose concentrations above 100 mg/100 ml; the three animals with baseline concentrations lower than this showed no rise in the serum insulin concentration. Thus, insulin release during alpha-adrenergic blockade occurred only in hyperglycemic animals (11). Preliminary studies in nonsepticemic phentolamine-infused baboons documented the adequacy of alpha-adrenergic blockade. In the absence of phentolamine, the intravenous injection of 2.5 μg/kg of epinephrine produced the expected depression of the serum insulin concentration, whereas during phentolamine infusion the serum insulin concentration increased after injection of the same dose of epinephrine (9).

In contrast to the rapid development of hypoinsulinemia and hyperglycemia after *E. coli* injection in baboons not given phentolamine, the serum insulin concentration was not significantly lower than control values and the serum glucose concentration was not higher than control values after *E. coli* injection during phentolamine-induced alpha-adrenergic blockade (Fig. 1). Thus, alpha-adrenergic blockade prevented septicemic hypoinsulinemia and septicemic hyperglycemia. In additional studies, the injection of exogenous regular insulin (0.2 units/kg) (8) and the release of endogenous insulin (after the rapid intravenous injection of 5.0 mg of phentolamine) (9) 20 minutes after *E. coli* injection were shown to abort the developing septicemic hyperglycemia. Two examples of the latter phenomenon are shown in Table 1.

The relationship between the degree of depression of insulin secretion and the survival time of *E. coli* septicemic baboons was examined in six animals injected with a smaller dose of *E. coli* (3.0×10^{10} to 4.2×10^{10} organisms/kg) and infused with 2.5% albumin in saline at rates of 12 ml/kg/hour for the first 6 hours, 6 ml/kg/hour the second 6 hours, and 3 ml/kg/hour thereafter. The infusions were begun 20 minutes after *E. coli* injection. The degree of suppression of insulin secretion in these septicemic baboons was variable; *i.e.*, only three of six developed definite hypoinsulinemia with serum insulin concentrations less than 60% of baseline throughout septicemia. The duration of survival of these six animals ranged from 2.1 to 24.3 hours and correlated significantly with the serum immunoreactive insulin levels, expressed as a percent of the mean of two baseline observations for each animal, determined at 30 minutes ($r = 0.896$; $P < 0.02$), 45 minutes ($r = 0.962$; $P < 0.01$)(Fig. 2), and 60 minutes ($r = 0.900$; $P < 0.02$) after *E. coli* injection (10). In contrast, the survival time did not correlate significantly with the initial hematocrit, body weight, or *E. coli* dose, or with the early changes in blood lactate, mean arterial pressure, or arterial pH. The three hypoinsulinemic septicemic baboons survived a mean (±SE) of 3.0 ± 0.5 hours, significantly less than the euinsulinemic animals (16.4 ± 3.9 hours, $P < 0.05$). The mean survival time for the six septicemic baboons was 9.7 ± 3.5 hours.

TABLE 1

EFFECT OF *E. coli* INJECTION AND RAPID PHENTOLAMINE INJECTION UPON SERUM GLUCOSE AND INSULIN CONCENTRATIONS IN BABOONS DURING SEPTICEMIA

Time (minutes)	Baboon 1 Glucose (mg/100 ml)	Baboon 1 Insulin (μU/ml)	Baboon 2 Glucose (mg/100 ml)	Baboon 2 Insulin (μU/ml)
0	122	8.5	122	10.2
60	116	11.0	112	10.0
120[a]	108	10.5	104	10.0
135	111	<5.0	146	6.8
140[b]	154	<5.0	148	5.2
145	165	8.5	128	5.8
150	150	9.2	150	7.8
155	132	8.5	140	8.0
165	114	9.2	132	10.5
180	126	11.2	140	10.6

[a]*E. coli* injection was administered immediately after 120-minute sample.

[b]Phentolamine, 5.0 mg, was administered intravenously immediately after 140-minute sample.

An additional five septicemic baboons were given infusions of similar volumes of 2.5% albumin in saline containing regular insulin (Ileitin, 10 units/liter), glucose (100 g/liter), and potassium chloride (80 mEq/liter) after an intravenous injection of 0.2 units/kg of regular insulin 20 minutes after *E. coli* injection. Despite evidence of metabolic effectiveness of the infused insulin (75% suppression of the serum free fatty acid concentration and prevention of the rise in serum urea nitrogen despite an increment in the serum creatinine), the mean over-all duration of survival was 9.8 ± 1.5 hours, virtually identical to that of the septicemic

TABLE 2

EFFECT OF INSULIN-GLUCOSE-POTASSIUM INFUSION ON SURVIVAL TIME IN SEPTICEMIC BABOONS

	Baboons treated with 5×10^{10} *E. coli* organisms/kg		
	Control[a]	Insulin-glucose-potassium infused[b]	Statistical significance
Total no. baboons	6	5	
Mean survival±SE (hours)	9.7±3.5	9.8±1.5	NS
Hypoinsulinemic baboons[c]	3/6	4/5	
Mean survival±SE (hours)	3.0±0.5	9.4±1.9	$P<0.05$

[a]Infused with 2.5% albumin in saline.

[b]Infused with comparable volumes of 2.5% albumin in saline, containing regular insulin (10 units/liter), glucose (100 g/liter), and potassium chloride (80 mEq/liter).

[c]Serum insulin concentration less than 60% of baseline throughout septicemia in the control group and before insulin infusion in the insulin-glucose-potassium infused group.

baboons not given insulin, glucose, and potassium chloride (Table 2). However, the four septicemic baboons which were hypoinsulinemic before infusion of insulin, glucose, and potassium chloride did survive longer (9.4 ± 1.9 hours) than the three hypoinsulinemic septicemic animals not infused with this combination (3.0 ± 0.5 hours), as shown in Table 2.

DISCUSSION

The hypoinsulinemia associated with lethal *E. coli* septicemia is due to depressed insulin secretion rather than to expansion of the insulin distribution space or acceleration of the insulin degradation rate. This is apparent from several observations, including the rapid drop in serum insulin during septicemia (with a half-time approximating the serum half-time of insulin in man) (7), the failure of intravenously injected glucose to elicit a serum insulin response during septicemia (8), and the prolongation, rather than shortening, of the serum half-time of regular insulin injected intravenously during septicemia (8).

Stress-initiated inhibition of insulin secretion is mediated through alpha-adrenergic mechanisms. Porte and co-workers have demonstrated that the infusion of epinephrine (19) or norepinephrine (20) inhibits insulin secretion in man and that this inhibition is prevented by alpha-adrenergic blockade (21). The demonstration that phentolamine-induced alpha-adrenergic blockade prevented the development of septicemic hypoinsulinemia in the baboon (Fig. 1) is consistent with the concept of alpha-adrenergic mediation of the depressed insulin secretion associated with this lethal stress.

Stress-initiated inhibition of insulin secretion appears to be a relatively high-threshold phenomenon. The unanesthetized baboons used in these studies were clearly stressed in the baseline state, as reflected in their elevated urinary catecholamine excretion and serum cortisol concentrations before *E. coli* injection (7). Nonetheless, similarly prepared nonsepticemic animals not only have readily measurable baseline serum insulin levels, they are also able to respond with a threefold rise in the serum insulin concentration after intravenous administration of glucose (8). Furthermore, although hypoinsulinemia was a common feature of rapidly lethal septicemia in baboons given approximately 10^{11} *E. coli* organisms per kilogram, definite suppression of insulin secretion occurred in only three of six septicemic baboons given a smaller, but still lethal, dose of *E. coli*.

The demonstration of immunochemical hypoinsulinemia during lethal *E. coli* septicemia does not, in itself, establish that the septicemic animal is physiologically insulin-deficient. However, considerable evidence is available that septicemic hypoinsulinemia is a major determinant of septicemic hyperglycemia and, therefore, that the depressed immunoreactive insulin levels associated with septicemia are physiologically reflected. First, the drop in the serum insulin concentration is temporally related to the rise in the serum glucose concentration (7) during septicemia. Second, the measured rise in serum glucose concentration during septicemia correlates significantly with the measured decrease in serum insulin concentration (7). Third, as illustrated in Figure 1, the prevention of septicemic hypoinsulinemia by phentolamine-induced alpha-adrenergic blockade also prevents the development of septicemic hyperglycemia (9).

These observations are consistent with the interpretation that septicemic hypoinsulinemia mediates septicemic hyperglycemia. They do not exclude the possibility that depressed pancreatic insulin secretion and increased hepatic glucose release are common, though independent, responses to sympathetic activation of alpha-adrenergic mechanisms. However, the ability of exogenous insulin injected during septicemia (8) and of endogenous insulin released by phentolamine injection (9) during septicemia (Table 1) to abort the developing hyperglycemia indicates that septicemic hyperglycemia is not an obligatory response to factors other than insulin lack.

The degree of depression of insulin secretion early in lethal *E. coli* septicemia is inversely related to the survival time of the septicemic animal (10). In six animals given less than 5×10^{10} *E. coli* organisms per kilogram, the serum insulin concentration, measured at 30, 45 (Fig. 2), and 60 minutes after *E. coli* injection and expressed as a percent of the mean of two baseline observations for each animal, was significantly correlated with the duration of survival. Indeed, the serum insulin concentration, relative to baseline, was a highly sensitive prognostic indicator since significant relationships between the duration of survival and the blood lactate concentration, mean arterial pressure, or arterial pH, all expressed relative to baseline, were not achieved in this small group of animals.

The statistical correlation between serum insulin levels and survival from *E. coli* septicemia does not establish a pathogenetic link between these two variables. Insulin modulates hepatic glucose release (17,12) as well as peripheral glucose uptake. Insulin-deficient states are typified by accelerated hepatic glucose production and diminished peripheral glucose utilization by insulin-sensitive tissues (3,15). Accordingly, the depression of insulin secretion and physiologic insulin lack associated with severe gram-negative septicemia may be viewed as an adaptive metabolic response to life-threatening stress which involves the provision of glucose to the underperfused central nervous system as well as the mobilization of other metabolic fuels such as fatty acids and amino acids. Conceivably, however, prolonged insulin lack in the periphery may contribute to the cardiovascular decompensation which generally precedes the death of the septicemic animal.

With the latter possibility in mind, five septicemic baboons were infused with fluids containing insulin, glucose, and potassium, and the duration of their survival was compared with that of six animals given similar doses of *E. coli* and infused with similar volumes of fluid not containing insulin, glucose, and potassium. Despite documented hyperinsulinemia and evidence of metabolic

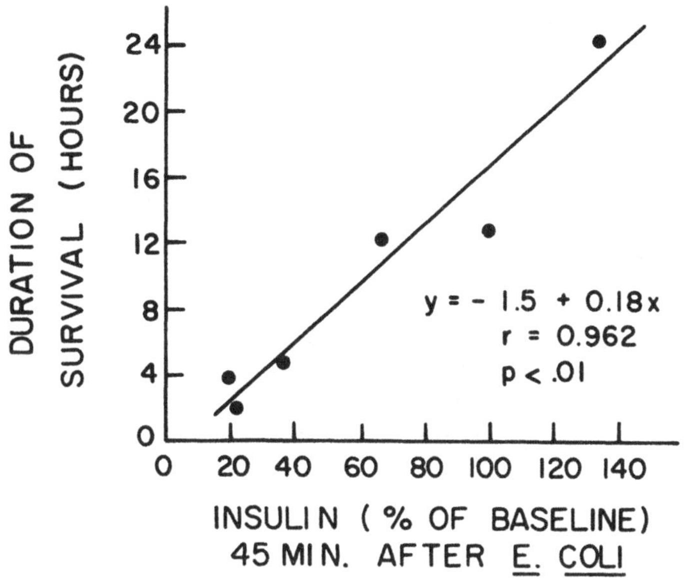

FIG. 2 Relationship between the serum insulin concentration, expressed as a percent of the mean of two baseline observations for each animal, at 45 minutes after the injection of less than 5×10^{10} *E. coli* organisms per kilogram, and the duration of survival of six septicemic baboons.

effectiveness of the infused insulin (lowered free fatty acid and urea nitrogen levels), the over-all mean survival of the two groups of animals was virtually identical (Table 2). These observations do not support the pharmacologic use of insulin in the treatment of shock states. Interestingly, however, only three of six control animals became hypoinsulinemic during septicemia, and the mean survival time of these hypoinsulinemic animals was significantly shorter than that of the four initially hypoinsulinemic septicemic animals infused with insulin, glucose, and potassium (Table 2). The mean (±SE) duration of survival of hypoinsulinemic septicemic controls, infused with albumin in saline only, was 3.0 ± 0.5 hours, whereas that of initially hypoinsulinemic septicemic animals infused with insulin, glucose, and potassium in albumin in saline was 9.4 ± 1.9 hours. Thus, the provision of insulin, along with glucose and potassium, to hypoinsulinemic septicemic baboons may have been beneficial.

SUMMARY

In these experiments, alpha-adrenergic inhibition of insulin secretion was a common feature of lethal *E. coli* septicemia in baboons injected with approximately 10^{11} *E. coli* organisms per kilogram. Only three of six baboons given less than 5 x 10^{10} *E. coli* organisms per kilogram became hypoinsulinemic. The survival time of these six septicemic baboons ranged from 2.1 to 24.3 hours. The duration of survival correlated significantly with the serum insulin concentration, expressed as a percent of the mean baseline concentration for each animal, measured at 30, 45, and 60 minutes after *E. coli* injection. The inclusion of metabolically effective doses of regular insulin, along with glucose and potassium, in the intravenous fluids of five additional septicemic baboons did not prolong the over-all mean duration of survival beyond that of the group of six septicemic animals not given insulin. However, the mean (±SE) duration of survival of the four initially hypoinsulinemic baboons infused with glucose, insulin, and potassium was 9.4 ± 1.9 hours, significantly longer than that of the three hypoinsulinemic septicemic animals not infused with insulin, glucose, and potassium (3.0 ± 0.5 hours).

ACKNOWLEDGMENTS

The authors are grateful to Mrs. R. Chestnut for technical assistance in the performance of these studies. The procedures were supported by several Navy corpsmen, including P. Vangeloff, W. Hawker, R. Dostalek, F. Kizis, J. Shoulders, J. Strohman, W. Volker, R. Rearly, J. Roulston, A. Chester, W. Mayfield, F. Chisholm, E. Thompson, M. Martinson, and R. West, under the direction of HMC J. Horton, USN, and Mr. J. Ewell. Logistical support was provided by HMC J. Magee, USN (Ret).

NOTE

The opinions or assertions contained herein are the private ones of the authors and are not to be construed as official or reflecting the views of the Navy Department or the Naval service at large.

The experiments reported herein were conducted according to the principles enunciated in "Guide for Laboratory Animal Facilities and Care", prepared by the Committee on the Guide for Laboratory Animal Resources, National Academy of Sciences-National Research Council.

REFERENCES

1. Allison, S.P., M.J. Chamberlain, and P. Hinton. Intravenous

glucose tolerance, insulin, glucose and free fatty acid levels after myocardial infarction. Brit. Med. J. 4:776-778, 1969.

2. Allison, S.P., S.K. Prowse, and M.J. Chamberlain. Failure of insulin response to glucose load during operation and after myocardial infarction. Lancet 1:478-481, 1967.

3. Cahill, G.F., Jr. Starvation in man. New Engl. J. Med. 282:668-675, 1970.

4. Carey, L.C., B.D. Lowery, and C.Y. Cloutier. Blood sugar and insulin response of humans in shock. Ann. Surg. 172: 342-350, 1970.

5. Cerchio, G.M., G.S. Moss, P.A. Popovich, E. Butler, and D.C. Siegel. Serum insulin and growth hormone response to hemorrhagic shock. Endocrinology 88:138-143, 1971.

6. Ceremuzynski, L., J. Kuch, L. Markiewicz, J. Lawecki, and J. Taton. Patterns of endocrine reactivity in patients with recent myocardial infarction. Brit. Heart J. 32: 603-610, 1970.

7. Cryer, P.E., C.M. Herman, and J. Sode. Carbohydrate metabolism in the baboon subjected to gram-negative (*E. coli*) septicemia. I. Hyperglycemia with depressed plasma insulin concentrations. Ann. Surg. 174:91-100, 1971.

8. Cryer, P.E., C.M. Herman, and J. Sode. Carbohydrate metabolism in the baboon subjected to gram-negative (*E. coli*) septicemia. II. Depressed insulin secretion with glucose intolerance and sensitivity to exogenous insulin. In: *Current Topics in Surgical Research,* edited by D.B. Skinner and P.A. Ebert. New York: Academic Press, 1971, Vol. II, pp. 117-125.

9. Cryer, P.E., C.M. Herman, and J. Sode. Alpha-adrenergic inhibition of insulin secretion during lethal *E. coli* septicemia in the baboon. In preparation (abstracted in: Clin. Res. 19:456, 1971).

10. Cryer, P.E., A. Coran, J. Sode, C.M. Herman, and D. Horwitz. Gram-negative septicemia in the subhuman primate: Inverse relationship between the depression of insulin secretion and the duration of survival. In preparation.

11. Cryer, P.E., C.M. Herman, and J. Sode. Insulin release during alpha-adrenergic receptor blockade: Primacy of the glycemic stimulus. Endocrinology 89:918-920, 1971.

12. Felig, P., and J. Wahren. Influence of endogenous insulin secretion on splanchnic glucose and amino acid metabolism in man. J. Clin. Invest. 50:1702-1711, 1971.

13. Herbert, V.K., K. Lay, C.W. Gottlieb, and S.J. Bleicher. Coated charcoal immunoassay of insulin. J. Clin. Endocrinol. 25:1375-1384, 1965.

14. King, L.R., H.C. Knowles, R.L. McLaurin, and H.P. Lewis. Glucose tolerance and plasma insulin in cranial trauma. Ann. Surg. 173:337-343, 1971.

15. Levine, R., and D.E. Haft. Carbohydrate homeostasis. New Engl. J. Med. 283:175-183, 237-246, 1970.

16. MacKenzie, R.D., T.R. Blohm, E.M. Auxier, and A.C. Luther. Rapid colorimetric micromethod for free fatty acids. J. Lipid Res. 8:589-597, 1967.

17. Madison, L.L. Role of insulin in the hepatic handling of glucose. Arch. Intern. Med. 123:284-292, 1969.

18. Moss, G.S., G.M. Cerchio, D.C. Siegel, P.A. Popovich, and E. Butler. Serum insulin response in hemorrhagic shock in baboons. Surgery 68:34-39, 1970.

19. Porte, D., Jr., A.L. Graber, T. Kuzuya, and R.H. Williams: The effect of epinephrine on immunoreactive insulin levels in man. J. Clin. Invest. 45:228-236, 1966.

20. Porte, D., Jr., and R.H. Williams. Inhibition of insulin release by norepinephrine in man. Science 152:1248-1250, 1966.

21. Porte, D., Jr. A receptor mechanism for the inhibition of insulin release by epinephrine in man. J. Clin. Invest. 46:86-94, 1967.

22. Rosenberg, J.C., and B.F. Rush. An enzymatic-spectrophotometric determination of pyruvic and lactic acid in blood. Clin. Chem. 12:299-307, 1966.

23. Taylor, S.H., C. Saxton, P.A. Majid, J.R.W. Dykes, P. Ghosh, and J.B. Stoker. Insulin secretion following myocardial infarction. Lancet 2:1373-1377, 1969.

WHAT MECHANISMS INFLUENCE OXYGEN TRANSPORT AND OXYGEN TISSUE DELIVERY IN ENDOTOXIC AND HEMORRHAGIC SHOCK?

Frank E. Gump, M.D.

Department of Surgery, College of Physicians and Surgeons, Columbia University, New York, New York

Oxygen is the most flow-limited of all substances carried by the blood. Fully one fourth of the arterial oxygen is removed during the course of a single transit through the normal resting body. Under such circumstances, it is obvious that proper tissue oxygenation is uniquely dependent on an adequate circulation. The ability to transport oxygen to the tissues is critical for survival, and its importance is reflected in the extensive animal research in this area. Unfortunately, human studies are much more limited, and our understanding of the adjustments that take place in clinical shock remains fragmentary.

The circulatory and metabolic adjustments seen in shock associated with a decreased cardiac output are far better defined than those in septic hypotension with a normal or increased cardiac output. Cournand's pioneering hemodynamic studies in shock patients stressed a decrease in cardiac output associated with peripheral vasoconstriction. Oxygen consumption was maintained in the presence of decreased blood flow by above-normal oxygen extraction (4). Although a similar increase in oxygen extraction has been described in experimental shock, one should recognize that, despite increased oxygen extraction, animal shock studies have consistently stressed the presence of abnormally low oxygen consumption values. Blood flow is greatly decreased in the usual hemorrhagic shock preparation, and since oxygen delivery to the tissues represents the product of blood flow and arterial oxygen content, less oxygen is delivered to the tissues. When cardiac output is reduced to such an extent, increased extraction can no longer maintain normal levels of tissue oxygenation. This has led to the concept of "oxygen debt", which can be calculated by assuming that tissue requirements, as judged by prehemorrhage oxygen consumption, remain unchanged during the shock period.

A similar debt has been suspected in clinical shock, but the limits have not been well defined. Physiologists have demonstrated an oxygen debt during exercise associated with both aerobic and anaerobic metabolism. Their studies resemble the usual experimental shock protocol: a control period, an exercise period, and a period of recovery. In the clinical situation, shock may start just as abruptly, but the duration as well as the variations in treatment and recovery create complex patterns. It is important to appreciate that oxygen debt in the exercising subject exists in the presence of oxygen consumption far above basal levels. Conceivably, the entire debt is incurred by striated muscle and oxygen delivery to vital organs remains normal. The oxygen debt in experimental shock reflects an oxygen consumption that has fallen below basal levels; however, a similar situation has been difficult to document clinically. Cournand's study included four patients with hemorrhagic shock, none of whom had depressed levels of oxygen consumption. Shock patients with skeletal trauma or abdominal injury actually had moderate increases in oxygen consumption. After further studies, Cournand reported that even in patients who had lost up to 40% of their blood volume, oxygen consumption did not decrease below predicted basal levels.

The literature indicates that oxygen consumption measurements are being made with greater frequency. Kho and Shoemaker studied seven patients with hemorrhagic shock whose mean arterial pressure was 65 mm Hg (12). Although oxygen consumption was normal in these patients, cardiac output was also close to normal. Conversely, nine patients reported by Duff and his associates (8) had cardiac indices below 2.5 liters/minutes/m^2. An unquestionable decrease in oxygen consumption was seen in only one patient (86 ml/minute/m^2) who had a blood pressure of 35/30 mm Hg and a cardiac index of 1.2 liters/minute/m^2. This patient died, and may well have been studied in a terminal state. Border's studies also confirm that oxygen consumption in conscious man appears to be maintained near normal until it falls rapidly near death (2). Admittedly, very few patients in severe hemorrhagic shock have been studied prior to any resuscitative measures. A recent report by Shoemaker and his associates (15) represents one of these exceptions. In patients whose shock was due to rapid blood loss, the cardiac index fell to 2 liters/minute/m^2 and oxygen extraction rose. Although the authors reported a decrease in calculated oxygen consumption, the fall was minimal and the final values remained within the normal range. While experimental studies contrast oxygen consumption during shock to control levels in the same animal, as a rule clinical measurements must be evaluated in terms of the predicted normal value. Since the normal range is quite broad, an appreciable change in oxygen consumption must take place before it can be recognized with certainty.

Despite the fact that the heart has been shown to be affected by hypoxia (5), Downing demonstrated that myocardial contractility did not decrease in animals with marked hypoxemia unless the pH was less than 7.1 (7). In the patients reported by Shoemaker, decreased transport of oxygen appeared to have no deleterious effect on myocardial function, judged by the finding that most patients were functioning on a normal or augmented ventricular function curve. Thus, hemodynamic adjustments and increased oxygen extraction appear to maintain oxygen consumption near normal levels in clinical hemorrhagic shock. The oxygen debt of limited duration seen in experimental shock or exercise is less obvious over the longer time span affecting the injured patient.

However, certain questions remain unanswered at this time. Calculations of oxygen debt assume that oxygen requirements are unchanged from basal or control levels during the period of hemorrhage. Similarly, in clinical studies of hemorrhagic shock, oxygen consumption has been reported to be in the predicted normal range. Possibly oxygen requirements are increased at this time so that the observed "normal" levels of oxygen consumption constitute inadequate tissue oxygenation. Sequential measurements in our unit have often shown oxygen consumption to be above normal after resuscitation; this may reflect the fact that previously elevated oxygen requirements were not satisfied during the hypotensive period. A similar increase in oxygen consumption after resuscitation was observed in Shoemaker's patients.

Elevated blood lactate levels also suggest that oxygen requirements are not being met during hemorrhagic shock. However, some question exists about the significance of increased circulating lactate in these patients, except for extremely high levels and plasma levels that remain elevated after appropriate therapy. Redistribution of blood flow designed to preserve cerebral and myocardial circulation may lead to hypoxia in less critical vascular beds, with resulting increases in lactic acid. Furthermore, measurable lactate production has been demonstrated in well-perfused resting striated muscle (1). Obviously, the ideal indicator of tissue oxygenation has yet to be discovered. Tolerance to hypoxia varies in different organs, and regional rather than whole-body oxygen uptake may have to be examined in order to advance our knowledge in this area.

The previous section dealt with oxygen transport and consumption in hemorrhagic shock associated with a decreased cardiac output. The situation is far more complex in septic shock, which is often associated with a normal or increased cardiac output. Although much effort has gone into the study of septic shock in laboratory animals, the resulting data are less directly applicable to man than those obtained in hypovolemic shock. Marked species differences are apparent in responses to endotoxin, and the characteristic low-flow state that follows the administration of pure endotoxin is not ordinarily evident in the patient with sepsis. The hemodynamic alterations in clinical sepsis and septic shock have been extensively studied since 1964, when Clowes first described raised circulatory requirements in these patients (3). Since then, the term "hyperdynamic circulation" has come into usage, and the combination of increased cardiac output and decreased peripheral resistance has been repeatedly documented. However, the mechanisms of oxygen delivery and consumption in these patients remain controversial. In 1966, Border, Gallo, and Schenk studied a group of critically ill patients with high cardiac outputs and commented on the decreased arteriovenous (AV) oxygen tension (2). Systemic arteriovenous shunting was postulated as an explanation for their findings. Similar reports by Hopkins (11), Del Guercio (6), and their associates discussed the possible significance of AV shunts in septic shock, while the work of Siegel, Greenspan, and Del Guercio (14) suggested that AV shunting might explain the low oxygen consumption seen in some septic shock patients. At this time, certain questions remain to be clarified. Little doubt exists that mixed venous oxygen tension is increased in many of these patients, and, as a result, AV oxygen differences are decreased. The effect on whole-body oxygen consumption is less certain.

The increase in cardiac output as well as the fact that arterial oxygen content is usually well maintained insures increased oxygen delivery to the tissues. Therefore, oxygen consumption may not actually fall below the normal range, despite the decreased AV difference. When oxygen uptake is measured directly, as opposed to a calculated value, oxygen consumption usually falls within the normal range. This is not entirely reassuring, since the tissue requirements for oxygen during septic shock are unknown. Lactic acid levels have been recorded, as was the case in hemorrhagic shock, in an effort to evaluate tissue oxygen supply. Duff and his associates demonstrated a significant inverse correlation between total arterial blood lactate and oxygen consumption, as measured by analysis of expired air (8). However, blood lactate levels have been shown to increase dramatically with hyperventilation despite the presence of normal amounts of oxygen. Similar increases in blood lactate have been seen with glucose or epinephrine infusions, once again in the absence of hypoxia. The source of the increased circulating lactate remains unidentified and the relationship between lactate release and actual hypoxic cellular damage uncertain. A better indicator of tissue hypoxia would obviously be valuable, but at this time lactic acid determination is still the most widely used index of the adequacy of tissue oxygenation.

Oxygen consumption values in septic shock are probably not as low as suspected from the early work utilizing calculated figures, since values derived from analysis of expired air usually fall within the predicted normal range. While it is certainly possible that these patients have supranormal requirements, this has not been proven. The normal oxygen consumption values seen in sepsis and septic shock contrast sharply with the far greater increases in blood flow. The combination of large increases in flow and a decreased peripheral resistance, as well as the evidence of flow going to nonmetabolizing (or non-oxygenextracting) areas, led to the suggestion that AV shunts were involved. Anatomic demonstration of such channels has never been convincing, and alternative explanations have been sought. It is worthwhile remembering that blood flow can vary independently of oxygen consumption in both normal and pathologic states. The ability to increase cutaneous blood flow is important in heat exchange and bears no relationship to the metabolic needs of the skin. Similarly, renal blood flow is large because of decreased renal vascular resistance related to the requirements for clearing the blood of waste products rather than renal oxygen requirements. Changes in blood viscosity due to anemia will affect flow far more than oxygen consumption; in fact, anemia represents the original hyperdynamic state, since it was recognized to increase heart action even before cardiac output could be measured. Increased cardiac output is the primary response to moderate anemia, and the decreased oxygen content of both arterial and venous blood results in a narrowed AV difference. Increased oxygen extraction (increased AV oxygen difference) is usually not a factor in surgical anemia since it does not become manifest until hemoglobin levels fall below 7 g. Oxygen consumption is unchanged in moderate anemia, and the final result—*i.e.*, increased blood flow, narrowed AV oxygen difference, and decreased peripheral resistance—resembles that seen in sepsis. However, shunting need not be invoked to explain these findings. We recently studied 23 patients who developed septic intraperitoneal complications after operation or injury (10). All patients were febrile and some were hypotensive, but none could be considered to be in shock at the time of the study. The mean increase in cardiac index in this group was +36% while oxygen consumption increased far less (+15%). The mean AV oxygen difference was slightly decreased, and at first glance the results appeared to resemble those of previously reported studies in which this constellation of findings was ascribed to arteriovenous shunting. However, the mixed venous (from a pulmonary artery catheter) oxygen saturation remained very close to 70% in all patients, provided that no arterial desaturation had occurred. Under these circumstances, the AV oxygen difference depends on hemoglobin concentration, which determines blood oxygen content. Simple calculations will show that AV oxygen difference decreases as hemoglobin levels fall. Thus, the increased cardiac outputs recorded in our study can be explained by a combination of anemia and increased metabolic requirements. While this study demonstrates that decreased hemoglobin levels produce a circulatory picture indistinguishable from that often ascribed to multiple arteriovenous shunts, it certainly does not rule out the possibility of extensive nonnutritional blood flow in patients with more severe sepsis or septic shock. For instance, patients with severe burns have cardiac output values far in excess of tissue oxygen requirements, even when allowances are made for decreased hemoglobin levels. Evidently the extent and nature of the septic process is an important factor in oxygen transport and uptake by the tissues.

The contribution of increased cutaneous blood flow to the increased cardiac output seen in sepsis cannot readily be quantitated. Febrile patients have increased skin blood flow, and since little oxygen is extracted from this blood, some narrowing of the whole-body AV oxygen difference will result. If patients with hyperthyroidism can be taken as a guide, increased circulatory requirements for heat dissipation exist in the presence of hypermetabolism, even without an increase in body temperature. Significant sepsis is usually associated with an increased metabolic rate so that the need for heat transport plays a role in the circulatory response.

While anemia and increased cutaneous blood flow needed for heat exchange contribute to the hyperdynamic state, it is also true that typical hyperdynamic changes can exist in afebrile patients with normal hemoglobin values. We recently reported a series of measurements in eight patients with severe third-degree burns (9). The burned patients were compared with other febrile surgical patients, and hemoglobin values and temperature elevations in both groups were comparable. Despite this fact, blood flow tended to be higher at any level of oxygen consumption in the burned patients, indicating the presence of flow through tissues that failed to extract oxygen. Whether this flow was through arteriovenous channels or simply vasodilatation was unclear, but normal lactate levels suggested that cellular oxygenation was maintained.

Recently attention has been directed to shifts in the oxyhemoglobin dissociation curve as an explanation for decreased oxygen extraction septic states. Miller and his associates have reported low levels of 2,3-diphosphoglycerate (2,3-DPG) in clinical septic shock and have postulated that this contributed to poor tissue oxygenation (13). Unfortunately, dissociation curves represent *in vitro* measurements made at a set pH of 7.4, and this is equally true when the curve is characterized by its P_{50} value. The over-all *in vivo* effect of the many factors known to influence oxyhemoglobin dissociation remains speculative. The metabolic upset associated with septic shock may inhibit the synthesis of 2,3-DPG while the increased oxygen requirements associated with sepsis would be expected to stimulate an increase in 2,3-DPG levels. The result of these forces is unclear, but in a recent study we have attempted to plot *in vivo* dissociation curves by measuring the pO_2 and saturation of venous blood drawn from multiple sites in the body as well as arterial and venous blood obtained while varying the concentration of oxygen in the inspired air. This makes it possible to obtain a reasonable range of values that can be used to plot an *in vivo* dissociation curve. Preliminary studies in four patients suggest that the *in vivo* curve is not displaced in sepsis and septic shock despite abnormally low 2,3-DPG levels. At this point further studies are needed. Apparently, there are important factors in addition to 2,3-DPG levels influencing the oxyhemoglobin dissociation curve.

If oxyhemoglobin dissociation curve shifts are really not responsible for the decreased oxygen extraction in septic states, alternate explanations should be investigated. Since oxygen transport is inevitably increased because of increased blood flow, decreased oxygen extraction is not necessarily associated with inadequate tissue oxygenation. More extensive clinical measurements of oxygen consumption are needed, although, as noted previously, interpretation will always be difficult. Lactic acid levels have been discussed previously, and might be more valuable if the vascular bed (or beds) responsible for the release of lactate could be identified. A similar regional, as opposed to whole-body, approach to the adequacy of tissue oxygenation might utilize tissue pO_2 or lymph pO_2 measurements. Finally, it may be necessary to look beyond oxygen consumption to individual metabolic events. We have recently found a defect in ^{14}C glucose oxidation to $^{14}CO_2$ and H_2O during the reinfusion period after hemorrhagic shock, even though oxygen consumption had returned to baseline levels.

SUMMARY

Oxygen transport is well maintained in septic shock with normal or increased cardiac output. Decreased oxygen extraction from circulating blood was originally thought to be associated with decreased levels of oxygen consumption. However, most direct (as opposed to calculated) measurements are within the normal range. Since the tissue requirements for oxygen are unknown in these patients, hypoxia may still exist. Efforts have been made to document this by measuring circulating lactate. The results are somewhat inconclusive, but might be improved if regional studies of oxygen consumption and lactate production could be performed in conjunction with whole-body measurements.

REFERENCES

1. Andres, R., G. Cader, and K.L. Zierler. The quantitatively minor role of carbohydrate in oxidative metabolism by skeletal muscle in intact man in the basal state. J. Clin. Invest. 35:671-687, 1956.

2. Border, J.R., E. Gallo, and W.G. Schenk, Jr. Systemic arteriovenous shunts in patients under severe stress: A common cause of high output cardiac failure. Surgery 60:225-231, 1966.

3. Clowes, G.H.A., Jr., M. Vucinic, and M.G. Weidner. Circulatory and metabolic alterations associated with survival or death in peritonitis. Ann. Surg. 163:866-885, 1966.

4. Cournand, A., M.D. Riley, S.E. Bradley, E.S. Breed, R.P. Noble, H.D. Lauson, M.I. Gregerson, and D.W. Richards. Studies of the circulation in clinical shock. Surgery 13:964-995, 1943.

5. Crowell, J.W. In: *Shock and Hypotension: Pathogenesis and Treatment,* edited by L.C. Mills and J.H. Moyer. New York: Grune and Stratton, 1965, pp. 605-608.

6. Del Guercio, L.R., J.D. Cohn, M. Greenspan, N.R. Geins, and G. Kornitzer. Pulmonary and systemic arteriovenous shunting in clinical septic shock. In: *Third International Conference on Hyperbaric Medicine,* edited by I.W. Brown, Jr., and B.G. Cox. Washington, D.C.: National Academy of Sciences-National Research Council, 1966, pp. 337-342.

7. Downing, S.E., N.S. Talner, and T.H. Gardner. Influences of hypoxia and acidemia on left ventricular function. Am. J. Physiol. 210:1327-1334, 1966.

8. Duff, J.H., A.C. Groves, A.P.H. McLean, R. LaPointe, and L.D. Maclean. Defective oxygen consumption in septic shock. Surg. Gynecol. Obstet. 128:1051-1060, 1969.

9. Gump, F.E., J.B. Price, Jr., and J.M. Kinney. Blood flow and oxygen consumption in patients with severe burns. Surg. Gynecol. Obstet. 130:23-28, 1970.

10. Gump, F.E., J.B. Price, Jr., and J.M. Kinney. The relationship

of blood flow and oxygen consumption in surgical infections. Current Topics Surg. Res. 2:385-394, 1970.

11. Hopkins, R.W., G. Sabaga, I. Penn, and F.A. Simeon. Hemodynamic aspects of hemorrhagic and septic shock. JAMA 191: 731-735, 1965.

12. Kho, L.K., and W.C. Shoemaker. Evaluation of therapy in clinical shock by cardiorespiratory measurements. Surg. Gynecol. Obstet. 127:81-88, 1968.

13. Miller, L.D., F.A. Oski, J.F. Diaco, H.J. Sugarman, A.J. Gottlieb, and M. Delivoria. The affinity of hemoglobin for oxygen: Its control as well as *in vivo* significance. Surgery 68:187-195, 1970.

14. Siegel, J.H., M. Greenspan, and L.R.M. Del Guercio. Abnormal vascular tone, defective oxygen transport and myocardial failure in human septic shock. Ann. Surg. 165:504-517, 1967.

15. Vladeck, B.C., R. Bassin, A.E. Kark, and W.C. Shoemaker. Rapid and slow hemorrhage in man. Ann. Surg. 173:331-336, 1971.

OXYHEMOGLOBIN DISSOCIATION CURVE IN HEMORRHAGIC AND SEPTIC SHOCK

C.R. Valeri, CDR, MC, USNR[1], and C.J. Kopriva, LCDR, MC, USNR[2]

Naval Blood Research Laboratory, Chelsea, Massachusetts

Blood flow through the microcirculation, hemoglobin concentration, and affinity of hemoglobin for oxygen all affect tissue pO_2 tension. In patients with hemorrhagic or septic shock, the adaptive responses for maintaining adequate partial pressure of oxygen in tissue (pO_2, measured in mm Hg) are mediated by mechanisms that maintain blood flow to vital organs, while they usually decrease blood flow to the nonvital organs (skin, gastrointestinal tract, and the extremities) (13,15,23,33). There are usually simultaneous changes that lead to facilitation of oxygen release from hemoglobin (2-4,6,7,24,32,34).

This paper presents data obtained (a) from combat casualties with severe musculoskeletal injuries, with or without severe sepsis, after massive transfusion of stored blood, (b) from chronically ill patients with anemic hypoxia, with or without sepsis, after transfusion of stored blood, and (c) from a patient in septic shock. The role of the oxyhemoglobin dissociation curve during acute impairment of oxygen delivery to tissue is also discussed.

---

[1]Officer-in-Charge, Naval Blood Research Laboratory, Chelsea, Massachusetts.

[2]Naval Medical Research Institute, National Naval Medical Center, Bethesda, Maryland.

MATERIALS AND METHODS

Hemorrhagic Shock With or Without Sepsis

Each of 23 combat casualties with severe musculoskeletal injuries received at least 12 units of whole blood. Some of the blood had been stored in acid-citrate-dextrose (500 ml of whole blood collected in 75 ml of ACD, National Institutes of Health, Formula A) for at least 14 days after collection, hereafter referred to in this report as "stored blood". Some of it was transfused within 24 hours of collection, hereafter referred to as "fresh blood". Most of the stored blood had been collected in the United States and air-shipped to South Vietnam, whereas all of the fresh blood was collected in South Vietnam. Peripheral venous blood samples were obtained from each patient during or immediately after operation for multiple traumatic injuries. The first sample of blood was obtained immediately after 12 or more units of blood had been given; the time of this initial sampling is referred to as "zero hour". Additional samples were obtained 12,48, and 120 hours after the initial sample. In many cases, the first blood sample was obtained while the patient was still under general anesthesia. Administration of 12 units of blood took from 4 to 8 hours. Most of the patients were febrile (99-102° F) during the study period. During the study, four of the patients with traumatic injuries developed severe sepsis characterized by positive blood cultures, grossly infected wounds, and a fever of at least 103° F. None of the other 19 patients with traumatic injuries developed severe sepsis, cardio-pulmonary insufficiency, or renal insufficiency. It was often necessary to transfuse both ACD-stored and fresh blood between the sampling periods because of postoperative bleeding (Fig. 1).

Routine intensive clinical treatment, including administration of fluid, antibiotics, and oxygen and respiratory care, was carried out as required.

The mean corpuscular hemoglobin concentration (MCHC, %) was derived from the microhematocrit and the hemoglobin concentration, as measured by the cyanmethemoglobin method. Venous blood pH was measured with a pH-gas analyzer (Instrumentation Laboratories) at 37° C.

Control subjects for this study were 16 healthy Marines on duty in South Vietnam. They smoked from zero to as many as four packages of cigarettes a day.

Immediately after collection, 2 ml of heparinated whole blood was deproteinized with 4 ml of cold 6% perchloric acid. The mix-

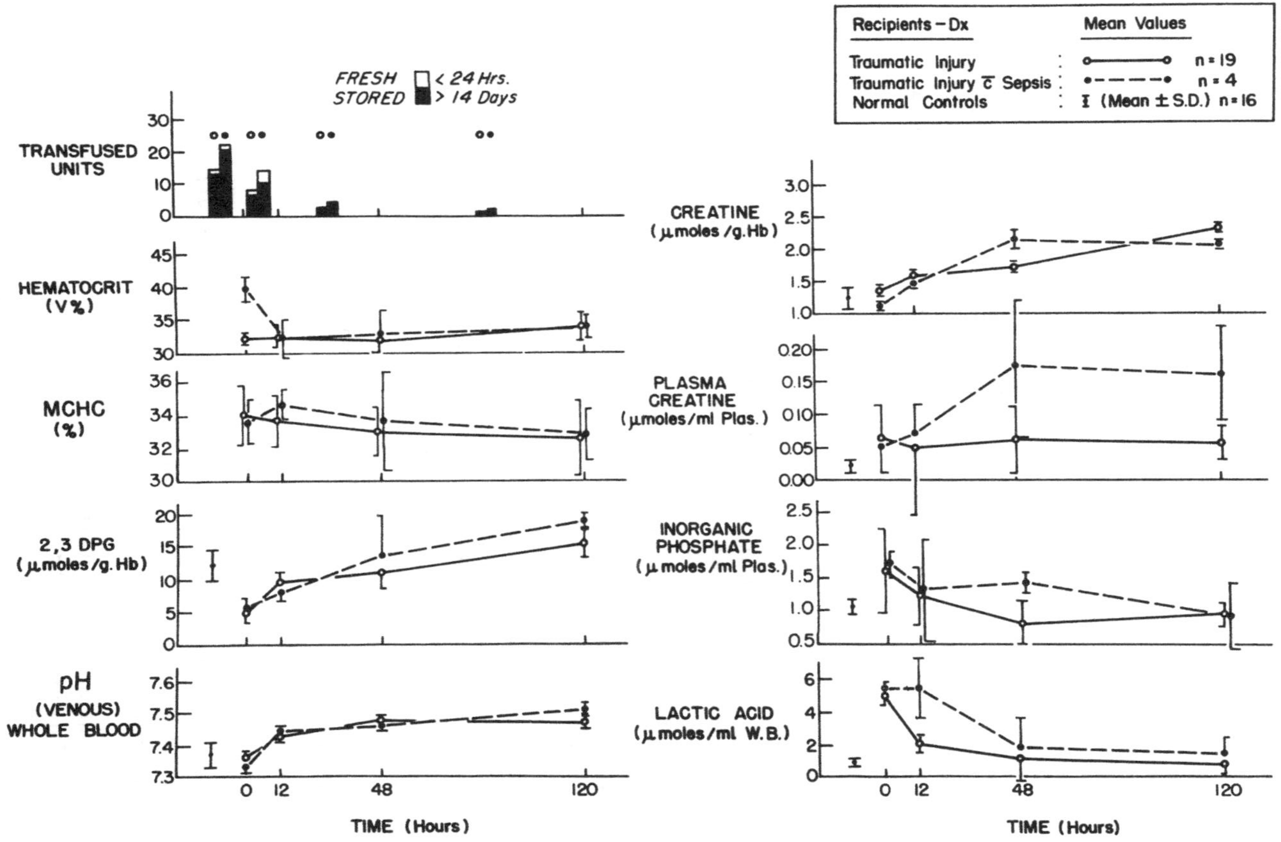

FIG. 1. Hematologic and biochemical measurements in venous blood after massive transfusion of fresh and stored liquid blood to acutely injured casualties with or without severe sepsis.

ture was agitated and centrifuged, and the supernatant solution was neutralized with potassium hydroxide. Another sample of whole blood was then centrifuged, and 2 ml of plasma was deproteinized with 4 ml of perchloric acid solution and neutralized as described above. The extracts were stored at about -20° C for up to 1 year. The 2,3-diphosphoglycerate (2,3-DPG) in the extracts was measured in duplicate as previously described (37). Since 2,3-DPG exists predominantly in the red cells, the level of 2,3-DPG is reported as μmoles per gram of hemoglobin. Creatine was measured spectrophotometrically in both the plasma and whole blood extracts. Since plasma creatine was present, the whole blood extract was corrected for the plasma fraction; creatine is reported in μmoles per gram of cellular hemoglobin and μmoles per milliliter of plasma. Whole blood lactate (μmoles per milliliter of whole blood) was measured spectrophotometrically using enzymatic kits (Calbiochem). Plasma phosphorus was measured by the Fiske and Subbarow method (17).

Anemic Hypoxia With or Without Sepsis

Two male patients requiring blood transfusions were studied at the Boston Naval Hospital, Chelsea, Massachusetts. At the time of study, one patient had carcinoma of the colon with intra-abdominal abscess, septicemia, and fever. The other patient was comatose from a brain contusion and had gastrointestinal bleeding without sepsis. They had been bedridden for at least 2 weeks. Chromium-51 was used to measure the red cell volume of each patient, and the red cell hemoglobin mass was calculated from the red cell volume (milliliters) multiplied by the MCHC (%, grams of hemoglobin per 100 ml of red cells) as previously described (35,37). The theoretical red cell hemoglobin mass was estimated from the product of the body surface area, the factor 1091, and the MCHC of 33%.

The red cell mass deficit was corrected by transfusion, usually within 3 hours, of four units of washed, liquid ACD-stored red cells. The red cell volume was measured again 3 to 4 days after transfusion. Before and immediately after the transfusion, and 4, 8, and 24 hours after transfusion, oxygen consumption was measured directly for at least 15 minutes with a basal metabolic rate indicator (Hartmann and Braun) by measurements of the expired oxygen content and flow rates.

Cardiac outputs were measured directly by the indocyanine green dye technique usually before and immediately after transfusion, and 4, 8, and 24 hours after transfusion. Cardiac output was determined by the standard indicator dilution curve, as described by Del Guercio *et al.* (16).

For preserved blood, whole blood (450 ml) was collected from each healthy volunteer into 67.5 ml of acid-citrate-dextrose (ACD, National Institutes of Health, Formula A). Eight units of whole blood were stored at 4° C up to 21 days.

Four units of stored blood were transfused to each patient at one time. Each unit was washed by an automated programmed wash cycle with 2,000 ml of phosphate-buffered glucose-saline solution. The final hematocrit value of the pooled units was approximately 40%, and the pH of the supernatant of the washed red cells was 6.8-6.9. The units were transfused usually within 4 hours of washing. The red cell survival was measured by an automated differential agglutination procedure (35).

Measurements were taken as follows. Arterial and mixed venous blood samples from the pulmonary artery were obtained in heparinated syringes. Whole blood pH, pO_2, and pCO_2 were measured at 37° C in a pH-gas analyzer. Oxygen and carbon dioxide content (vol%) were measured in duplicate by the Van Slyke procedure (26).

The patient's whole blood prior to transfusion, and the blood samples obtained after transfusion, were assayed for 2,3-DPG (μmoles/g hemoglobin) and creatine (μmoles/g hemoglobin).

The oxyhemoglobin dissociation curve was measured at 37° C by the method of Bellingham and Huehn (5), using a diluted washed red cell suspension in 0.9% sodium chloride and 0.108 g% disodium phosphate buffered to pH 7.2. The amount of carboxyhemoglobin in the blood samples was measured spectrophotometrically with a Model 182 Co-oximeter (Instrumentation Laboratories).

Septic Shock

A 50-year-old female, patient A.M., died in septic shock which was characterized by fever, hypotension, positive blood cultures, a bleeding diathesis, and renal insufficiency. The patient developed a perinephric abscess after operation for removal of a pheochromocytoma. Red cell 2,3-DPG levels, arterial blood pH, and P_{50} values of the oxyhemoglobin dissociation curve were measured on the 6 days before her death.

RESULTS

Patients with traumatic injuries who developed sepsis received more blood (mean of 21.5 units with a standard deviation of ±5.3) prior to the initial blood sample (t = 3.566; degrees of freedom, or df = 21; P<0.002) than those without sepsis (mean of

16.0 ±SD of 5.0 units) (Fig. 1) (20). Both groups received the same number of fresh units of blood (t = 0.460, df= 21, P>0.5). At the 12-, 48-, and 120-hour periods, both groups received the same number of units.

At 12, 48, and 120 hours post-transfusion there were no significant differences in the following measurements: hematocrit, MCHC, red cell 2,3-DPG and creatine levels, peripheral venous blood pH, and plasma inorganic phosphorus.

At the 12-hour period there was a significant difference in the blood lactic acid level (t = 3.458, df = 20, P<0.003) between the patients with sepsis (mean of 5.5 μmoles/ml whole blood ±1.6) and those without (mean of 2.1 μmoles/ml whole blood±1.5); however, there were no significant differences at the 48- and 120-hour periods. At the 48-hour period, the plasma creatine level was significantly increased in the patients with sepsis (mean of 0.18 μmoles/ml plasma ± 0.10) compared to those without (mean of 0.06 μmoles/ml plasma ± 0.05) (t = 3.377, df = 16, P<0.004); at 120 hours a similar difference was noted (t = 3.54, df= 6, P <0.01).

Three of the four patients with sepsis died, and two of the 19 patients without sepsis died.

Patient R.V., with anemia and sepsis, had an increased arteriovenous difference in oxygen content and a normal oxygen consumption (Fig. 2). The red cell 2,3-DPG level was elevated to 18.0 μmoles/g hemoglobin (normal 12.0±1.2 μmoles/g), and the P_{50} value of the oxyhemoglobin dissociation curve was 32 mm Hg (normal 27±1.0 mm Hg). The red cell creatine level was elevated to 4.0 μmoles/g hemoglobin (normal 1.2±0.6 μmoles/g). After transfusion of preserved red cells with low 2,3-DPG levels (1.3 μmoles/g hemoglobin) and high affinity for oxygen (P_{50} value of 22 mm Hg), restoration *in vivo* of the red cell 2,3-DPG level and the P_{50} value occurred. During the 24-hour post-transfusion period, the arterial pH ranged from 7.40 to 7.45, pO_2 ranged from 85 to 90 mm Hg, and the pCO_2 ranged from 38 to 42 mm Hg. Although the patient received four units of washed red cells, the red cell mass 3 days after the transfusion was similar to the pretransfusion level. Five days after transfusion the red cell level of 2,3-DPG was 22 μmoles/g hemoglobin, the P_{50} value was 35 mm Hg, and the red cell creatine level was 4.5 μmoles/g hemoglobin. The patient's clinical condition did not improve after transfusion.

Patient M.F., with anemia without sepsis, had normal arteriovenous difference in oxygen content, normal cardiac output, and normal oxygen consumption (Fig. 3). Prior to the transfusion, red cell levels of 2,3-DPG (13.5 μmoles/g hemoglobin) and creatine

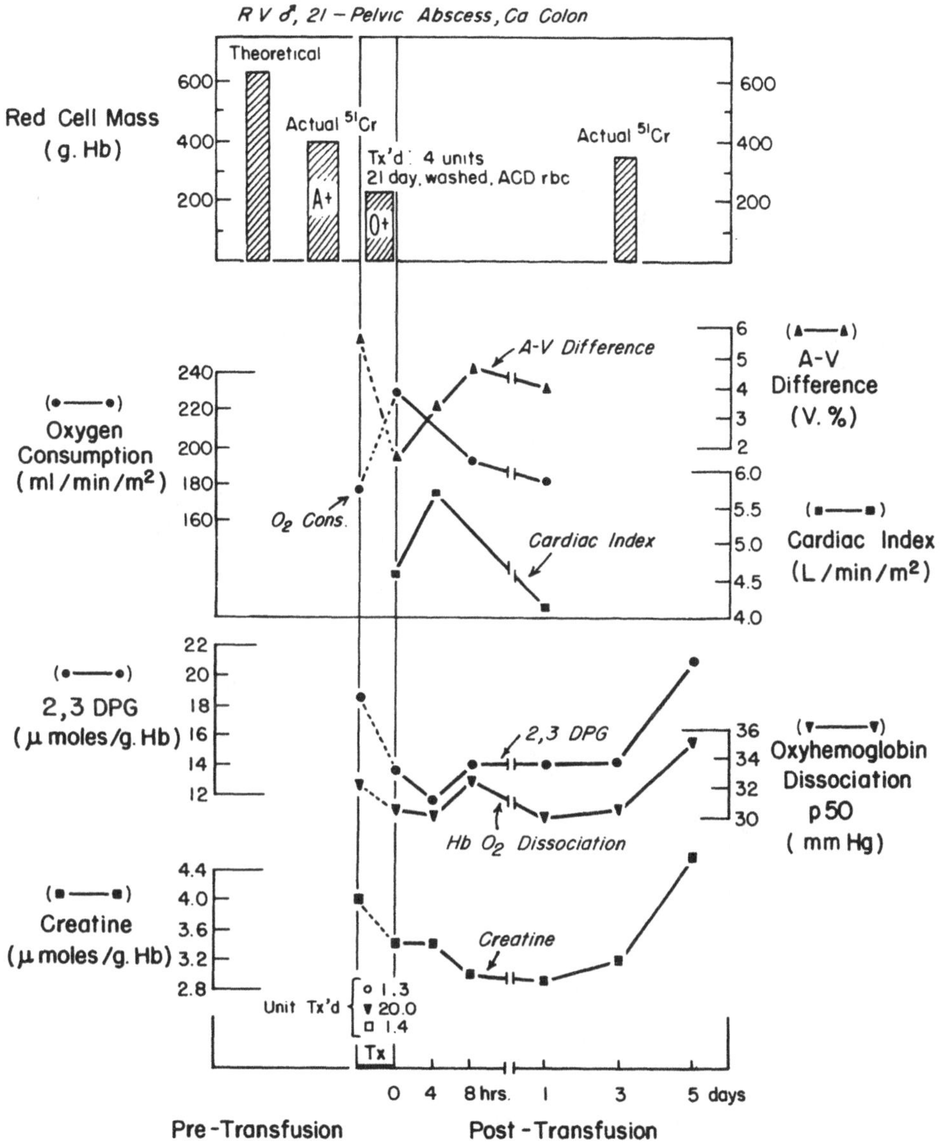

FIG. 2. Cardiac index, oxygen consumption, and arteriovenous difference in oxygen content before and after transfusion of four units of washed stored red cells, P_{50} values and red cell levels of 2,3-DPG, and creatine levels in patient R.V. with anemic hypoxia and severe sepsis.

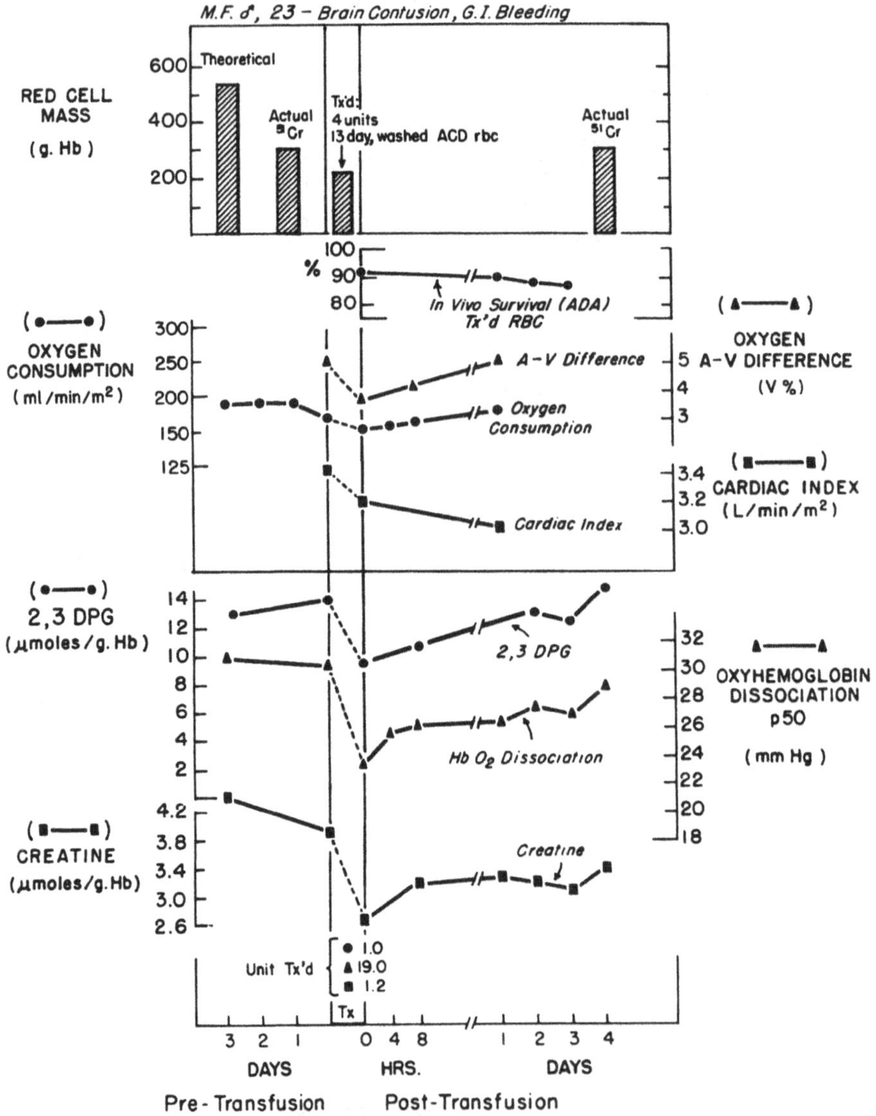

FIG. 3. Cardiac index, oxygen consumption, and arteriovenous difference in oxygen content before and after transfusion of four units of washed stored red cells, P_{50} values and red cell levels of 2,3-DPG, and creatine in a patient with anemic hypoxia without sepsis.

(3.9 μmoles/g hemoglobin) were elevated, and the P_{50} value of the oxyhemoglobin dissociation curve was 31 mm Hg. After the transfusion of four units of washed red cells with low 2,3-DPG level and high affinity for oxygen, restoration *in vivo* of the red cell 2,3-DPG levels and the P_{50} values of the oxyhemoglobin dissociation curve were similar to values noted in patient R.V. with anemia and sepsis. The 24-hour survival value of the preserved red cells was 90%. However, because gastrointestinal bleeding continued throughout the post-transfusion period, the patient's red cell mass 4 days after transfusion was similar to the pretransfusion value. Red cell levels of 2,3-DPG and creatine and P_{50} values of the oxyhemoglobin dissociation curve were still elevated on the fourth day after transfusion.

In patient A.M. with septic shock, the arterial blood pH was elevated throughout the 6-day period of study, ranging from 7.40 to 7.53. Her temperature was elevated to 103° F. The patient developed oliguria and underwent dialysis for acute renal insufficiency. The red cell 2,3-DPG level ranged from 14 to 24 μmoles/g hemoglobin throughout the study. The P_{50} value of the oxyhemoglobin dissociation curve was increased, ranging from 30 to 32 mm Hg. Figure 4 shows the effects of the elevated arterial pH and the elevated red cell level of 2,3-DPG on the P_{50} value of the oxyhemoglobin dissociation curve. When the 2,3-DPG level was about 14 μmoles/g hemoglobin and the arterial pH was about 7.48, the P_{50} value of the *in vitro* oxyhemoglobin dissociation curve was about 32 mm Hg. When the red cell 2,3-DPG level was 22 μmoles/g hemoglobin and the arterial pH was about 7.53, the P_{50} value of the *in vitro* oxyhemoglobin dissociation curve was about 30 mm Hg.

DISCUSSION

Several investigators have reported a relation between the oxyhemoglobin dissociation curve and the levels of the organic phosphate compounds, 2,3-diphosphoglycerate and adenosine triphosphate (1,8,12,14). This study demonstrates that restoration *in vivo* of red cells depleted of 2,3-DPG correlates temporally with restoration *in vivo* of the oxyhemoglobin dissociation curve; these findings are in accord with previous reports (9,36,38).

The biochemical and hematologic changes in peripheral blood that occurred in patients with acute severe traumatic injuries after resuscitation indicated rapid increases in red cell 2,3-DPG levels during the 120-hour post-transfusion period. Red cells stored in acid-citrate-dextrose (ACD) for longer than 14 days at 4° C have low 2,3-DPG levels and high affinity for oxygen (1,12, 34,38). After the rapid infusion of at least 12 units of stored blood, the circulating red cells had low red cell 2,3-DPG levels

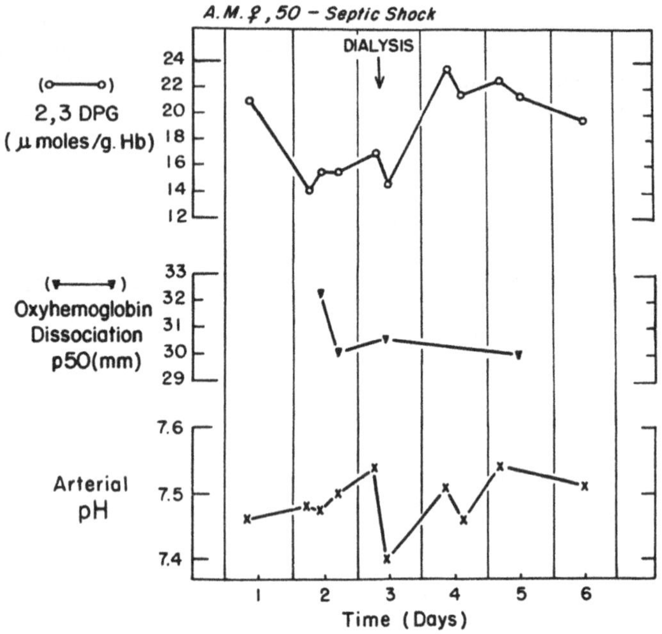

FIG. 4. Arterial blood pH, red cell 2,3-DPG levels, and P_{50} values of the oxyhemoglobin dissociation curve in a patient with septic shock.

---

and high affinity for oxygen. Restoration *in vivo* of the 2,3-DPG level was the same in the four patients with traumatic injuries who had developed severe sepsis as it was in the 19 patients with traumatic injuries without severe sepsis. Restoration of the red cell level of 2,3-DPG was associated with an increase in the venous blood pH (Fig. 1); an increase in blood pH occurred mainly during the initial 12 hours, whereas the red cell 2,3-DPG level progressively increased for 120 hours.

Although a relation between the P_{50} value of the oxyhemoglobin dissociation curve and the level of red cell 2,3-DPG has been established, the mechanism for the change in the intraerythrocyte 2,3-DPG level *in vivo* is not completely understood. Astrup has reported that red cell pH is the main determinant of the intra-erythrocytic concentration of 2,3-DPG and that this relationship, through its effect on the oxyhemoglobin dissociation curve, forms a feedback control system for maintaining normal oxygen release from hemoglobin (3,4). Systemic alkalosis in the patients with traumatic injuries (Fig. 1) may have represented the effect of massive blood replacement and hyperventilation response to anemia, arterial hypoxemia, and fever (10,18,22,25). Alkalosis is an excellent stimulus for increasing red cell glycolysis and red cell 2,3-DPG level (18,29,31). Systemic alkalosis and elevated plasma inorganic phosphate levels (Fig. 1) provide environmental conditions for rapid restoration of the red cell 2,3-DPG level. The increased 2,3-DPG level observed 5 days after the initial sample was similar to the observations of Proctor and his collaborators (28). It reflected an attempt by circulating red cells to compensate for an impairment in supply of oxygen to tissue by facilitating the release of oxygen from red cells. The only biochemical difference in the peripheral blood of patients with traumatic injuries between those with and those without sepsis was at the 48- and 120-hour periods: the plasma creatine level was elevated in the four patients who developed severe sepsis. The increase in the red cell creatine level throughout the study period was similar in patients with severe sepsis and those without. Figures 1, 2, and 3 show a relation between the red cell levels of 2,3-DPG and creatine. An increase in the red cell 2,3-DPG level is usually associated with a parallel increase in the level of red cell creatine (37). The red cell 2,3-DPG level affects the affinity of the red cells for oxygen, whereas the role of red cell creatine remains obscure.

Some investigators have suggested that restoration of the preserved red cell 2,3-DPG level may be impaired in patients with sepsis (34); our study, however, does not support this view. Two of our patients with red cell mass deficits received washed stored red cells which had low 2,3-DPG levels and high affinity for oxygen; in both cases, the presence of severe sepsis did not impair restoration of either the 2,3-DPG level or the P_{50} value of the oxyhemoglobin dissociation curve. There was no significant increase in the red cell mass 4 days after transfusion in either of the patients. At the end of the study, red cell 2,3-DPG and creatine levels and P_{50} values of the oxyhemoglobin dissociation curves were elevated. These findings indicate that in response to tissue hypoxia, the peripheral red cells facilitated oxygen delivery to tissue by increasing the 2,3-DPG level and decreasing the affinity of the red cells for oxygen (37).

In some patients in septic shock who have increased cardiac output, a relation has been suggested between the decreased arteriovenous difference in oxygen content and increased affinity for oxygen by red cells secondary to decreased 2,3-DPG (24). Our patient with septic shock had elevated levels of red cell 2,3-DPG and arterial blood alkalosis, and the red cells had decreased affinity for oxygen. Our data and the data of other investigators suggest that the decreased arteriovenous difference in oxygen content during septic shock is probably due to arteriovenous shunting in the peripheral tissue (15,33).

The oxyhemoglobin dissociation curve of intact red cells that contain normal adult hemoglobin (hemoglobin A) is affected by (a) temperature and the red cell concentrations of hydrogen, sodium, potassium, chloride, and bicarbonate ions, (b) red cell levels of CO_2, 2,3-DPG, ATP, and reduced glutathione, (c) the MCHC, and (d) the amount of carboxyhemoglobin and methemoglobin in the red cells (2-9, 11,12,14,19,21,30,32).

Bellingham, Detter, and Lenfant (7) have reported on the regulatory mechanisms of hemoglobin's oxygen affinity in acidosis and alkalosis. They studied the effect of induced acidosis and alkalosis on the oxyhemoglobin dissociation curve in normal men. Their studies defined, in addition to the effects of blood pH, temperature, red cell 2,3-DPG level, and whole blood base excess (BE) on the oxyhemoglobin dissociation curve, the role of the MCHC.

Bellingham and his associates have also reported the role of hemoglobin's affinity for oxygen and red cell 2,3-DPG in the management of diabetic ketoacidosis (6). They described the interaction of blood pH with red cell 2,3-DPG on the P_{50} value of the oxyhemoglobin dissociation curve *in vivo*. Because the response of red cell 2,3-DPG to changes in blood pH is slow in contrast to the immediate pH (Bohr) effect on the P_{50} value of the oxyhemoglobin dissociation curve, rapid correction of blood pH in diabetic ketoacidosis causes an increased affinity for oxygen which impairs tissue oxygen availability.

The *in vivo* conditions affecting the hemoglobin-oxygen interaction in clinical conditions of hemorrhagic and septic shock are defined in the Bellingham, Detter, and Lenfant equation (7):

$$\log P_{50}\ (\textit{in vivo}) = \log [\ 26.6 + 0.5\ (\text{MCHC}-33) + 0.69\ (\text{DPG}-14.5)] + 0.0013\text{BE} + 0.48\ (\text{pH}-7.4) + 0.024\ (\text{T}-37)$$

Increased temperature, decreased pH, and increased MCHC are immediate changes that occur which facilitate oxygen delivery to tissue, while the change in red cell 2,3-DPG is delayed, occurring usually 4 to 12 hours after the change in blood pH. When pH is increased or decreased there is usually a parallel increase or decrease in the red cell 2,3-DPG level (3,4,6,7,19,29,31).

Herman and his associates (data to be published) have bled baboons 40% of their blood volume and then rapidly infused them with a volume of sodium chloride in an amount three times that of the hemorrhage at 50 ml/minute. They reported a significant decrease in the red cell affinity for oxygen and a significant increase in red cell 2,3-DPG level within 24 hours after the red cell volume depletion. Their studies demonstrated the compensatory role of the oxyhemoglobin dissociation curve in the baboons when oxygen supply to tissue was impaired by acute blood loss.

The ability of the peripheral red cell to monitor tissue demands for oxygen and to appropriately decrease the hemoglobin affinity for oxygen is one example of a compensatory mechanism for maintaining adequate tissue oxygen tension. Animals that have adapted to high altitude have been shown to better tolerate shock of certain causes (hemorrhage, tourniquet, burns, and endotoxin) than animals at sea level (39). This tolerance may be partly due to the position of the oxyhemoglobin dissociation curve. If animals that have oxyhemoglobin dissociation curve displaced to the right can be protected against endotoxin and hemorrhagic shock, then attention should be directed toward treatment of hemorrhagic and endotoxin shock with pharmacological agents which facilitate oxygen release from hemoglobin. Horejsi has reported that, when blood supplemented with reduced glutathione (GSH) was administered to dogs that had been subjected to experimental hemorrhagic shock, the survival improved (21). He also reported that a GSH concentration of 40 mg% produced significant shifts to the right in the oxyhemoglobin dissociation curve both *in vitro* and *in vivo*. A complete explanation of the beneficial effects of GSH-supplemented blood is still lacking. Pollock and his associates have reported the *in vivo* effect of inosine-pyruvate-phosphate (IPP) in decreasing the red cells' affinity for oxygen in baboons (27). Six hours after administration of the IPP solution, a significant increase in red cell 2,3-DPG level and a significant decrease in red cell affinity for oxygen occurred. The 2,3-DPG level remained elevated for 24 hours and then gradually returned to normal within 4 days. The concept of pharmacologic therapy in facilitating oxygen delivery from hemoglobin during acute periods of tissue hypoxia should be explored.

SUMMARY

After massive transfusions of fresh and stored blood to acutely injured casualties, hematologic and biochemical measurements in the peripheral venous blood showed that red cell 2,3-DPG levels in patients with musculoskeletal injuries were similar whether or not severe sepsis was present. In patients with traumatic injuries and severe sepsis, a significant increase in plasma creatine was observed at the 48- and 120-hour periods.

When preserved red cells with low red cell 2,3-DPG levels and high affinity for oxygen were transfused to patients with anemic hypoxia, there was no difference in restoration of the red cell 2,3-DPG level or the P_{50} value of the oxyhemoglobin dissociation curve whether or not sepsis was present.

A patient in septic shock had an increased red cell 2,3-DPG level, arterial alkalosis, and decreased red cell affinity for oxygen.

In patients in hemorrhagic or septic shock, red cell affinity for oxygen *in vivo* is affected by whole blood pH, body temperature, red cell 2,3-DPG level, mean corpuscular hemoglobin concentration, and whole blood base excess.

NOTE

The opinions or assertions contained herein are those of the authors, and are not to be construed as official or reflecting the views of the Navy Department or Naval Service at large.

REFERENCES

1. Akerblom, O., C.H. deVerdier, L. Garby, and C. Högman. Restoration of defective oxygen transport function of stored red blood cells by addition of inosine. Scand. J. Clin. Lab. Invest. 21:245-248, 1968.

2. Astrup, P., K. Engel, J.W. Severinghaus, and E. Munson. The influence of temperature and pH on the dissociation curve of oxyhemoglobin of human blood. Scand. J. Clin. Lab. Invest. 17:515-523, 1965.

3. Astrup, P. Red cell pH and oxygen affinity of hemoglobin. New Engl. J. Med. 283:202-204, 1970.

4. Astrup, P. Dependence of oxyhemoglobin dissociation and intraerythrocytic 2,3-DPG on acid-base status of blood. II. Clinical and experimental studies. In: *Red Cell Metabolism and Function*, edited by G.J. Brewer, Advan. Exptl. Med. Biol. 6:67-79, 1970.

5. Bellingham, A.J., and E.R. Huehns. Compensation in haemolytic anemias caused by abnormal hemoglobins. Nature 218: 618-622, 1969.

6. Bellingham, A.J., J.C. Detter, and C. Lenfant. The role of hemoglobin affinity for oxygen and red-cell 2,3-diphosphoglycerate in the management of diabetic ketoacidosis. Trans. Assoc. Am. Physicians 83:113-120, 1970.

7. Bellingham, A.J., J.C. Detter, and C. Lenfant: Regulatory mechanisms of hemoglobin oxygen affinity in acidosis and

and alkalosis. J. Clin. Invest. 50:700-706, 1971.

8. Benesch, R., and R.E. Benesch. The effect of organic phosphates from the human erythrocyte on the allosteric properties of hemoglobin. Biochem. Biophys. Res. Commun. 26:162-167, 1967.

9. Beutler, E., and L. Wood. The *in vivo* regeneration of red cell 2,3-diphosphoglyceric acid (DPG) after transfusion of stored blood. J. Lab. Clin. Med. 74:300-304, 1969.

10. Blumgart, H.L., and M.D. Altschule. Clinical significance of cardiac and respiratory adjustments in chronic anemia. Blood 3:329-348, 1948.

11. Bohr, C., K. Hasselbalch, and A. Krogh. Ueber einen in biologischer Beziehung wichtigen Einfluss, den die Kohlen säurespannung des Blutes auf dessen Sauerstoffbindung übt. Skand. Arch. Physiol. 16:402-412, 1904.

12. Bunn, H.F., M.H. May, W.F. Kocholaty, and C.E. Shields. Hemoglobin function of stored blood. J. Clin. Invest. 48: 311-321, 1969.

13. Carey, J.S., P.A. Mohr, R.S. Brown, and W.C. Shoemaker. Cardiovascular function in hemorrhage, trauma and sepsis: Determinants of cardiac output and cardiac work. Ann. Surg. 170:910-921, 1969.

14. Chanutin, A., and R.R. Curnish. Effect of organic and inorganic phosphates on the oxygen equilibrium of human erythrocytes. Arch. Biochem. 121:96-102, 1967.

15. Cohn, J.D., M. Greenspan, C.R. Goldstein, A.L. Gudwin, J.H. Siegel, and L.R.M. Del Guercio. Arteriovenous shunting in high cardiac output shock syndromes. Surg. Gynecol. Obstet. 127:282-288, 1968.

16. Del Guercio, L.R.M., R.P. Coomaraswamy, and D. State. Cardiac output and other hemodynamic variables during external cardiac massage in man. New Engl. J. Med. 269:1398-1404, 1963.

17. Fiske, C.H., and Y. Subbarow. The colorimetric determination of phosphorus. J. Biol. Chem. 66:375-400, 1925.

18. George, W.F., W.D. George, Jr., J.P. Smith, F.T. Gordon, E.E. Baird, and G.C. Mills. Changes in serum calcium, serum phosphate, and red cell phosphate during hyperventilation. New Engl. J. Med. 270:726-728, 1964.

19. Guest, C.M., and S. Rapoport. Role of acid-soluble phosphorus compounds in red blood cells in experimental rickets, renal insufficiency, pyloric obstruction, gastroenteritis, ammonium chloride acidosis, and diabetic acidosis. Am. J. Dis. Child. 58:1072-1089, 1939.

20. Hays, W.L. *Statistics for Psychologists*. New York: Holt, Rinehart & Winston, 1963.

21. Horejsi, J. Effect of glutathione and some other substances on the oxygen dissociation curve of hemoglobin and experimental therapy of hemorrhagic shock with solutions enriched with glutathione. In: *Red Cell Metabolism and Function*, edited by G.J. Brewer, Advan. Exptl. Med. Biol. 6:9-20, 1970.

22. Litwin, M.S., L.L. Smith, and F.D. Moore. Metabolic alkalosis following massive transfusion. Surgery 45:805-813, 1959.

23. MacLean, L.D., W.G. Mulligan, A.P.H. McLean, and J.H. Duff. Patterns of septic shock in man: A detailed study of 56 patients. Ann. Surg. 166:543-562, 1967.

24. Miller, L.D., F.A. Oski, J.F. Diaco, H.J. Sugerman, A.J. Gottlieb, D. Davidson, and M. Delivoria-Papadopoulos. The affinity of hemoglobin for oxygen: Its control and *in vivo* significance. Surgery 68:187-195, 1970.

25. Oski, F.A., A.J. Gottlieb, M. Delivoria-Papadopoulos, and W.W. Miller. Red-cell 2,3-diphosphoglycerate levels in subjects with chronic hypoxemia. New Engl. J. Med. 280:1165-1166, 1969.

26. Peters, J.P., and D.D. Van Slyke. *Quantitative Clinical Chemistry Methods*. Baltimore: Williams & Wilkins, 1932, vol. 2, pp. 229-442.

27. Pollock, T.W., H.J. Sugerman, F.A. Oski, E.F. Rosato, and L.D. Miller. *In vivo* effect of inosine, pyruvate, and phosphate (IPP) on oxygen-hemoglobin affinity. Fed. Proc. 30: Abstract #1965, 1971.

28. Proctor, H.J., J.C. Parker, and G. Johnson, Jr. Alterations in erythrocyte 2,3-diphosphoglycerate in postoperative patients. Ann. Surg. 173:357-362, 1971.

29. Rapoport, S. Regulation of concentration of DPG and ATP in red blood cells. Forsvarsmedicin 5:168-174, 1969.

30. Rooth, G., H. Sommerkamp, and H. Bartels. The influence of

base excess and cation concentration in the red cells on the position of the oxygen dissociation curve. Clin. Sci. 23: 1-4, 1962.

31. Rörth, M. Dependence of oxyhemoglobin dissociation and intra-erythrocytic 2,3-DPG on acid-base status of blood. I. *In vitro* studies on reduced and oxygenated blood. In: *Red Cell Metabolism and Function*, edited by G.J. Brewer, Advan. Exptl. Med. Biol. 6:57-65, 1970.

32. Severinghaus, J.W. Blood gas calculator. J. Appl. Physiol. 21:1108-1116, 1966.

33. Siegel, J.H., M. Greenspan, and L.R.M. Del Guercio. Abnormal vascular tone, defective oxygen transport and myocardial failure in human septic shock. Ann. Surg. 165:504-517, 1967.

34. Sugerman, H.J., D.T. Davidson, S. Vibul, M. Delivoria-Papadopoulos, L.D. Miller, and F.A. Oski. The basis of defective oxygen delivery from stored blood. Surg. Gynecol. Obstet. 131:733-741, 1970.

35. Valeri, C.R. Viability and function of preserved red cells. New Engl. J. Med. 284:81-88, 1971.

36. Valeri, C.R., and N.M. Hirsch. Restoration *in vivo* of erythrocyte adenosine triphosphoglycerate, potassium ion, and sodium ion concentrations following the transfusion of acid-citrate-dextrose-stored human red blood cells. J. Lab. Clin. Med. 73:722-733, 1969.

37. Valeri, C.R., and N.L. Fortier. Red cell 2,3-diphosphoglycerate and creatine levels in patients with red cell mass deficits or with cardiopulmonary insufficiency. New Engl. J. Med. 281:1452-1455, 1969.

38. Valtis, D.J., and A.C. Kennedy. Defective gas transport function of stored red blood cells. Lancet 1:119-125, 1954.

39. Zapata-Ortiz, V., R. Castro de la Mata, E. Fernandez, L. Batalla, and A. Geu. Experimental hemorrhagic shock in animals adapted to high altitudes. Acta Physiol. Latinoam. 17:194-199, 1967.

EFFECTS OF ENDOTOXIN AND *E. coli* SHOCK ON THE METABOLISM OF LIPIDS AND CARBOHYDRATE[1]

David L. Horwitz, LCDR, MC, USNR[2]

Naval Medical Research Institute, Bethesda, Maryland,
Bureau of Medicine and Surgery, Navy Department

Many investigators have shown that injection of endotoxin of gram-negative bacilli or infection with various bacteria causes hyperlipidemia in experimental animals (4,5,8,11,13,17). In one of the few clinical studies in this area, Gallin *et al.* have shown that in gram-negative infections a significant hyperlipidemia occurs that is related to elevated concentrations of phospholipids, free fatty acids, and triglycerides (6). They further reported an initial rise in free fatty acids 2 hours after *Escherichia coli* injection in rabbits; at 24 hours after injection fatty acid values had reverted toward normal, whereas triglycerides were rising. It is important to investigate how these alterations in blood lipids may be related to changes in the mechanism of energy production in cells. In particular, does it represent a normal and beneficial adaptation to a particular type of stress or, rather, a pathological and detrimental condition requiring correction?

NORMAL FATTY ACID METABOLISM

The current state of knowledge concerning fatty acid metabolism is summarized in Figures 1 and 2. Figure 1 depicts how ingested fat is transported from the gut almost entirely as chylomicrons. (Medium-chain triglycerides are an exception to this, but not of physiological significance.) Although the exact mechanism of chylomicron metabolism is controversial, apparently at least

---

[1]Research Task No. M4305.05.3007BGGO.

[2]Current adress: Department of Medicine, University of Chicago, Chicago, Illinois.

some chylomicron triglycerides are taken up by the adipose tissue and are either stored or released into the blood as free fatty acids, loosely bound to albumin. These may be metabolized by heart or skeletal muscle as an energy source, or re-esterified by the liver to triglycerides and released as very-low-density lipoproteins (VLDL, or pre-beta lipoproteins). Metabolism of VLDL is under active investigation, but at least some of it appears to release triglyceride to adipose tissue in the presence of glucose and insulin.

Figure 2 diagrams adipose tissue metabolism in more detail. Chylomicron triglycerides are acted on by lipoprotein lipase, either on or near the cell membrane, to release fatty acids. Glucose enters the cell under control of insulin and is metabolized either by the Embden-Meyerhoff glycolytic pathway or the pentose-phosphate shunt to produce both acetyl-CoA and NADPH, both of which form *de novo* fatty acids. The fatty acid pool may be stored as triglycerides or released to the blood. Stored triglycerides may be released by action of an intracellular lipase which seems to be activated by cyclic AMP (16). Epinephrine stimulates this lipolysis through beta receptors, while insulin inhibits it, probably by blocking the action of cyclic AMP.

BIOCHEMICAL OBSERVATIONS IN ENDOTOXEMIA

To help elucidate the pathogenesis of observed blood lipid changes in sepsis, measurements of blood free fatty acid and total lipid levels were made in an acute fatal endotoxic shock model. The study, which consisted of rapid intravenous injection of *E.*

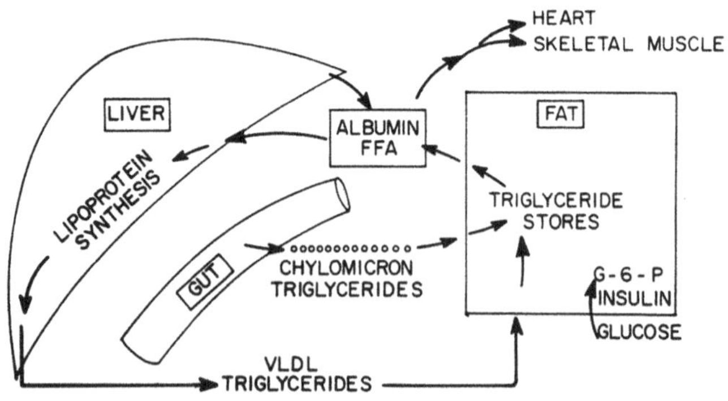

FIG. 1. Schematic illustration of triglyceride and free fatty acid (FFA) transport between gut, liver, and adipose tissue.

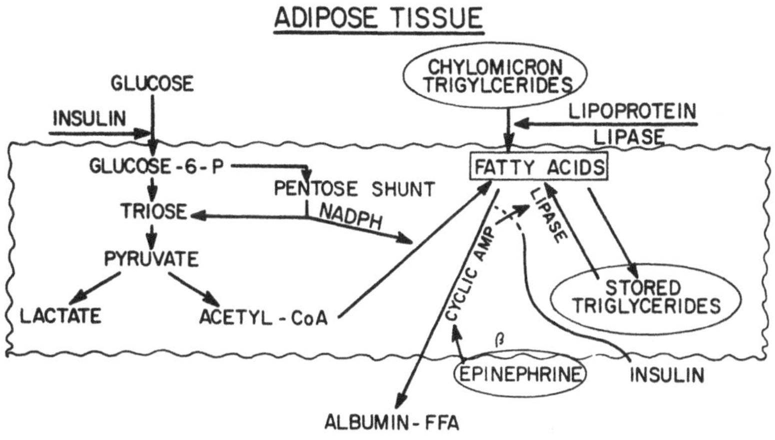

FIG. 2. Diagrammatic summary of carbohydrate and lipid metabolism in adipose tissue, and sites of regulation by insulin and epinephrine.

---

coli endotoxin (5 mg/kg, Difco) into five conscious baboons, will be reported in detail elsewhere. The data are summarized in Figure 3. Free fatty acids were significantly elevated within 30 minutes of endotoxin injection, while total serum lipids had not changed significantly even after 2 hours. In interpreting the data in Figure 3, one should note that insufficient animals survived to 3 hours to calculate significant changes at that point. Free fatty acids were expressed as percent of baseline free fatty acid levels which appear to be related to varying levels of anesthesia and adrenergic stimulation (Coran and Horwitz, manuscript in preparation). We found similar free fatty acid and total lipid changes in baboons subjected to live *E. coli* septicemia.

Previous work in our laboratory has indicated that the early phase of septic shock is manifest by hyperglycemia and hypoinsulinemia (2). The mechanism seems to be alpha-adrenergic inhibition of insulin release, with resultant hyperglycemia (Cryer, manuscript in preparation). Hyperglycemia and hypoinsulinemia occur within an hour after *E. coli* infusion. These data are not completely in accord with those of Guenter *et al.*, who found that the catecholamine response in rhesus monkeys infused with live *E. coli* or endotoxin was delayed until the second hour of hypotension(9). However, they measured catecholamines in mixed arterial blood, while the pancreatic beta cells are probably much more sensitive to small local increases in catecholamine level.

Gilette *et al.* have observed that goats receiving a lethal

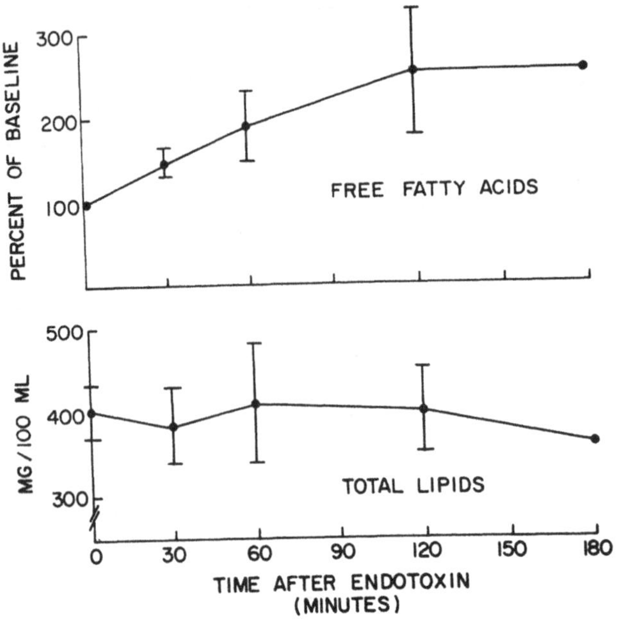

FIG. 3. Response of serum free fatty acids and total lipids to injection of *E. coli* endotoxin in the conscious baboon.

dose of *E. coli* endotoxin show increases in blood non-protein nitrogen, urea, creatine, and creatinine (7). While nitrogen metabolism has not been studied as extensively in septic shock as in traumatic and other types of shocks, this evidence would suggest increased protein catabolism and possibly gluconeogenesis in sepsis. Data concerning this are scanty and conflicting. in all types of shock, however (3). Increased gluconeogenesis would be quite compatible with the hyperglycemic, hypoinsulinemic state seen in early sepsis, and, indeed, would at least partly explain the hyperglycemia.

POSSIBLE PATHOPHYSIOLOGIC EFFECTS OF BIOCHEMICAL ABNORMALITIES

To satisfactorily treat septic shock, we must establish whether the observed elevation of fatty acids, hyperglycemia, and hypo-insulinemia are beneficial or detrimental to the organism, *i.e.*, whether they represent an appropriate response to stress or a pathological effect of sepsis which can further derange metabolic functions. Unfortunately, we still lack sufficient information to precisely define the mechanisms of cellular energy production in sepsis, so we must base our conclusions on indirect evidence.

One clear experimental approach is to attempt pharmacological reversal of observed biochemical abnormalities. In the studies of Cryer *et al.*, this was done in baboons receiving lethal doses of live *E. coli* by infusion of a glucose-insulin-potassium mixture (1). This study suggested an improved survival in animals so treated. Hence, we might conclude that cell survival is diminished, rather than lengthened, by the hyperglycemic or hypoinsulinemic condition. Naturally, more studies must be done, preferably on the cellular level with endotoxin-treated cells or tissues, before firm conclusions can be drawn.

More is known, however, about the cellular effects of elevated free fatty acids. Free fatty acids potentially offer a plentiful source of metabolic substrate to cells. However, insulin deficiency may interfere with free fatty acid utilization by muscle cells. Even in those tissues where insulin probably does not affect free fatty acid entry (such as liver), fatty acid oxidation cannot proceed under the hypoxic conditions obtained in shock. Thus, it is doubtful whether the elevation of free fatty acids is beneficial.

Moreover, substantial data indicate the harmful effects of free fatty acids. Soloff has shown that cardiac arrhythmias are provoked by injection of long-chain saturated fatty acids (18). Meester and Sekhar have shown the effect of free fatty acids on potentiating platelet aggregation (14). This could contribute to the coagulation problems observed in sepsis. Hageman factor activation may also be initiated by free fatty acids (12). Other reported adverse effects of free fatty acids are inflammatory lesions of pulmonary tissue (15) and depression of myocardial contractility under hypoxic conditions (10).

SUMMARY

Data are too fragmentary to permit a precise definition of the roles of glucose and lipids in metabolism during shock. The basic pathogenesis can be outlined, however, if certain initial steps are hypothesized. These include epinephrine release and diminished microcirculation. Unfortunately, the mechanisms by which endotoxin or bacteria produce these responses are not yet known. Epinephrine release then leads to hypoinsulinemia. As shown in Figure 2, hypoinsulinemia prevents glucose uptake and fatty acid synthesis in adipose tissue, while epinephrine promotes lipolysis. The blocking effect of insulin on lipolysis is also lost.

While the elevated free fatty acids and glucose represent a

theoretical substrate for cellular energy production, these probably cannot be metabolized efficiently without insulin or adequate oxygen. Furthermore, the potential toxic effects of elevated free fatty acids are likely to negate their possible benefits as an energy source.

NOTE

The opinions or assertions contained herein are the private ones of the authors and are not to be construed as official or reflecting the views of the Navy Department or the Naval service at large.

The experiments reported herein were conducted according to the principles set forth in "Guide for Laboratory Animal Facilities and Care", prepared by the Committee on the Guide for Laboratory Animal Resources, National Academy of Sciences-National Research Council.

REFERENCES

1. Cryer, P.E., A.G. Coran, J. Sode, C.M. Herman, and D.L. Horwitz. Gram-negative septicemia in the subhuman primate: Inverse relationship between the depression of insulin secretion and the duration of survival. In preparation.

2. Cryer, P.E., C.M. Herman, and J. Sode. Carbohydrate metabolism in the baboon subjected to gram-negative (*E. coli*) septicemia. I. Hyperglycemia with depressed plasma insulin concentrations. Ann. Surg. 174:91-100, 1971.

3. Cuthbertson, D., and W.J. Tilstone. Metabolism during the postinjury period. Advan. Clin. Chem. 12:1-55, 1969.

4. Farshtchi, D., and V.J. Lewis. Effects of three bacterial infections on serum lipids in rabbits. J. Bacteriol. 95: 1615-1621, 1968.

5. Foldvari, P., and P. Kertai. Changes in the serum lipid fractions of cholest cholesterol-fed and control rabbits induced by *Salmonella typhi* endotoxin. J. Atheroscler. Res. 7:714-717, 1967.

6. Gallin, J.I., D. Kaye, and W.M. O'Leary. Serum lipids in infection. New Engl. J. Med. 281:1081-1086, 1969.

7. Gillette, R.W., A.R. Mansberger, C.E. Johnston, and G.J.

Kookootsedes. A new preparation for the study of experimental shock in massive wounds. V. Changes in some serum electrolytes and nitrogenous fraction values. Surgery 43: 747-757, 1958.

8. Graves, A.C., J.H. Duff, A.P.H. McLean, and L.D. MacLean. Hyperlipidemia and pulmonary fat embolism in dogs with *E. coli* bacteremia. Surgery 68:656-661, 1970.

9. Guenter, C.A., V. Fiorica, and L.B. Hinshaw. Cardiorespiratory and metabolic responses to live *E. coli* and endotoxin in the monkey. J. Appl. Physiol. 26:780-786, 1969.

10. Henderson, A.H., A.S. Most, W.W. Parley, R. Garlin, and E.H. Sonnenblick. Depression of myocardial contractility in rats by free fatty acids during hypoxia. Circ. Res. 26:439-449, 1970.

11. Hirsch, R.L., D.G. MacKay, R.I. Travers, and R.K. Skraly. Hyperlipidemia, fatty liver, and bromsulfalein retention in rabbits injected intravenously with bacterial endotoxins. J. Lipid Res. 5:563-568, 1964.

12. Hook, J.C., W.E. Connor, J.W. Eckstein, and E.D. Warner. Fatty acid induced thrombosis and death: Mechanisms and prevention. J. Lab. Clin. Med. 63:791-800, 1964.

13. LeQuire, V.S., J.D. Hutcherson, R.L. Hamilton, and M.E. Gray. The effects of bacterial endotoxin on lipid metabolism. I. The responses of serum lipids of rabbits to single and repeated injections of Shear's polysaccharide. J. Exptl. Med. 110:293-309, 1959.

14. Meester, W.D., and N.C. Sekhar. The effect of epinephrine-induced elevation of plasma-free fatty acids on platelet aggregation in man. Blood 34:537-538, 1969.

15. Pomerontz, M., and B. Eiseman. Experimental shock lung model. J. Trauma 8:782-787, 1968.

16. Rizack, M.A. Hormone-sensitive lipolytic activity of adipose tissue. In: *Adipose Tissue*, Handbook of Physiology. Washington, D.C.: American Physiological Society, 1965, pp. 309-311.

17. Seifter, J., and D.H. Baeder. Relation of endocrines and clearing factor inhibitors to hyperlipemia in fasted animals. Proc. Soc. Exptl. Biol. Med. 93:63-67, 1956.

18. Soloff, L.A. Arrhythmias following infusions of fatty acids. Am. Heart J. 80:671-674, 1970.

THE MECHANISM OF THE "LUNG LESION" IN SHOCK[1]

Jack L. Ratliff, LCDR, MC, USNR[2], John R. Fletcher, LCDR, MC, USN[3], Erwin F. Hirsch, CDR, MC, USN[4], and Charles J. Kopriva, LCDR, MC, USNR[5]

United States Navy Surgical Research Unit, Naval Support Activity, Station Hospital, Da Nang, Republic of Vietnam

The pulmonary insufficiency often associated with various forms of shock has attracted considerable attention only recently. Its incidence in critically injured patients from our highways and the battlefields of Southeast Asia has spurred considerable speculation and research. So great is the interest in this area that in 1968 the National Research Council conducted a conference on pulmonary complications of nonthoracic trauma. Several similar conferences have been held since then. Although this conference focuses more broadly on the subject of shock, the lung lesion in shock deserves careful consideration.

What, then, is the nature of the "lung lesion" in shock and what mechanisms are responsible for its genesis? Pulmonary injury follows a great variety of stress forms. This discussion will be

---

[1]Funded in part by the Office of Naval Research, Subtask M4305.05. 3007, and Office of Naval Research Grant NR105.621.

[2]Department of Surgery, University of Mississippi Medical Center, Jackson, Mississippi.

[3]Department of Surgery, Naval Hospital, Bethesda, Maryland

[4]Department of Surgery, Harvard Medical School, Boston, Massachusetts

[5]Division of Experimental Surgery, Naval Medical Research Institute, Bethesda, Maryland.

limited to hypovolemia and sepsis. Whether the pulmonary response to stress is specific for the insult remains to be established.

The anatomical lesion seen in the lung after septic or hemorrhagic shock has been characterized differently by three groups of investigators. Embolic phenomena and pulmonary arterial spasm have been the focus of the first (precapillary) school of thought, utilizing subprimate models (1,10,12,13,15,18,19). Ultrastructural pulmonary capillary changes in various shock states (capillary), involving both subhuman primates and humans, have been described by electron microscopists (2,3,7,9,12,17,19). Pulmonary venous capillary spasm has been indicted by some investigators in subprimate models (postcapillary) (8,10,11,14,16).

Varying results from laboratories across the country suggest emboli, metabolic by-products, or hypoperfusion as the stimulus for these changes. At this time the concept of the lung lesion in septic or hemorrhagic shock is a matter of much speculation.

While the authors were associated with the Navy Surgical Research Unit in Southeast Asia, they participated in studies of both hemorrhagic and septic shock. Relevant to this discussion were three patient groups which we studied in detail: (a) five wounded soldiers in hemorrhagic shock, (b) five in septic shock, and (c) six wounded but nonshocked controls.

METHODS

The hemorrhagic shock study group consisted of five young servicemen (Americans) who (a) had two or more extremity amputations from booby trap injury, (b) were without thoracic, abdominal, head, or burn injury, and (c) presented in shock with blood pressures below 80 mm Hg systolic. No patient was presented with a tourniquet in place, and we estimate that the average period of shock lasted between 30 minutes and 1 hour. No fluids had been administered in the field, and no data were available concerning vital signs before arrival at our station hospital. Debridement and resuscitation were carried out immediately under general anesthesia, after which catheters were inserted in the pulmonary artery, superior vena cava, and a radial artery. Blood samples were drawn twice daily for the first 2 days, then once daily for 3 days. Initial sampling was performed immediately after catheter insertion, usually less than 2 hours after termination of the surgical procedure. The studies and measurements taken (relevant to this discussion) included pressures from all three catheters, including pulmonary arterial wedge pressures; blood gas estimates from the radial, pulmonary arterial, and pulmonary arterial wedge positions; cardiac outputs measured by the dye dilution technique;

TABLE 1

COMPARISON OF CARDIOVASCULAR PARAMETERS BETWEEN HEMORRHAGIC SHOCK AND CONTROL PATIENTS

Parameters	Group: Hemorrhagic Shock	Group: Controls	*P* value
Arterial pO_2 (mm Hg)	486	504	>0.10
O_2 consumption (cc/min)	218	175	<0.05
Cardiac output (liters/min)	7.2	7.5	>0.60
Transpulmonary shunt (%)	14.2	14.2	—
Central venous pressure (cm saline)	4.2	6.37	<0.005
Pulmonary measurements			
Mean arterial pressure (mm Hg)	11.5	11.2	>0.70
Arterial wedge pressure (mm Hg)	4.4	5.7	>0.10
Vascular resistance (dyne-cm^{-5})	87.8	60.5	<0.005
Peripheral vascular resistance (dyne-cm^{-5})	1179	962	<0.005

blood culture; and coagulation studies. All sample periods were begun after the patient had been on 100% oxygen for at least 20 minutes; otherwise the patient's FIO_2 (fraction of inspired oxygen) consisted of whatever gas mixture was required to maintain an arterial pO_2 above 60 mm Hg.

The septic shock group consisted of five soldiers with multiple extremity or abdominal injuries but no burns, head injuries, or thoracic wounds. Each patient accepted in this group had clinical sepsis and positive blood cultures. All underwent the same studies, twice daily, as described above for the hemorrhagic shock group.

The control study group comprised six soldiers who presented with minor extremity injuries requiring general anesthesia for debridement and hospitalization for at least 5 days. Before operation, each was fully informed about the nature and risks of our study and thereafter voluntarily underwent the same sampling procedures as the other two groups.

RESULTS

No complications were encountered in the control or the hemorrhagic shock groups. However, two of the patients in septic shock died during the study period. Coagulation studies revealed no differences between the three groups.

Hemorrhagic Shock

Relatively few differences were noted between the test results of the control group and those of the hemorrhagic group (Table 1). Oxygen consumption was high in the hemorrhagic group. The cardiac output was stable and equal to that in the control group even though there was ablation of one half to one third of the body mass. Transpulmonary shunting was not only the same in the groups, but did not change between sample periods within the same sample group. Central venous pressure and peripheral vascular resistance are thought to reflect conservative rehydration and replacement in these postshock patients. The elevation of pulmonary vascular resistance is contrary to what has been observed in more severe shock in subhuman primate models (4,6). These primates underwent a drop in pulmonary vascular resistance after induction of shock; it returned toward normal soon after reinfusion. In our patients, the elevation in values was greatest initially (Table 2). Our data support the concept of change in the precapillary pulmonary vascular bed after massive soft-tissue injury and hemorrhagic shock. On the basis of wedge pressure measurements in this study group, our observations do not agree with canine catheterization data which have been interpreted to suggest pulmonary venous capillary spasm as etiologic.

To improve our management of various kinds of shock, we must identify, understand, and learn to control the lethal cycle or cycles activated in each. We do not mean to understate the real and formidable clinical problem of post-traumatic pulmonary in-

TABLE 2

COMPARISON OF PULMONARY VASCULAR RESISTANCE
BETWEEN THE HEMORRHAGIC SHOCK AND CONTROL PATIENTS

Sample period	Mean PVR ($dyne\text{-}cm^{-5}$)		
	Hemorrhagic Shock	Controls	*P* value
1	132	61	<0.01
2	64	66	>0.50
3	72	55	>0.50
4	90	62	>0.10
5	89	51	>0.10
6	70	71	>0.50
7	96	53	<0.05

PVR = pulmonary vascular resistance.

sufficiency, which certainly does exist. Based on our experience in these studies, our knowledge of the literature, and more recent data from studies on baboons (4,6), we do not believe that the "lung lesion" in hypovolemic shock has been clearly identified as a major link in such a cycle. When combined with fat embolism, sepsis, over-hydration, etc., the resulting pulmonary insufficiency certainly may contribute to the death of patients in hemorrhagic shock.

Septic Shock

Clinical sepsis, unlike experimental sepsis, is a state of continual showers of bacteria, bacterial by-products, and/or degraded host tissues. The intensity and timing of these insults vary so that we really study a nonnormal patient's response to repeated and uncontrolled insults.

Table 3 compares the data from the control and septic groups. Arterial desaturation correlated with pulmonary shunting. Oxygen consumption was high. Pulmonary arterial pressure and resistance

TABLE 3

COMPARISON OF CARDIOVASCULAR PARAMETERS BETWEEN SEPTIC SHOCK AND CONTROL PATIENTS

Parameter	Group: Septic shock	Group: Controls	*P* value
Arterial pO_2 (mm Hg)	331	504	<0.001
O_2 consumption (cc/min)	266	175	<0.001
Cardiac output (liters/min)	10.2	7.5	<0.001
Transpulmonary shunt (%)	21.9	14.2	<0.001
Central venous pressure (cm saline)	4.7	6.37	<0.05
Pulmonary measurements			
Mean arterial pressure (mm Hg)	14.5	11.2	<0.001
Arterial wedge pressure (mm Hg)	6.2	5.7	>0.60
Vascular resistance (dyne-cm^{-5})	73.8	60.5	<0.05
Peripheral vascular resistance (dyne-cm^{-5})	779	962	<0.001

were high, but so was the cardiac output. High cardiac output with low central venous pressure and peripheral vascular resistance suggests peripheral vasodilatation or precapillary shunting in these patients. Poor correlation was found between the onset or peaks of febrile episodes and the above-listed parameters. For this reason, we wonder whether any correlation actually exists between the patient in septic shock and the conventional injection model—subprimate (11) or subhuman primate (5)—in the laboratory.

Reference will be made to the mechanism of lung injury in

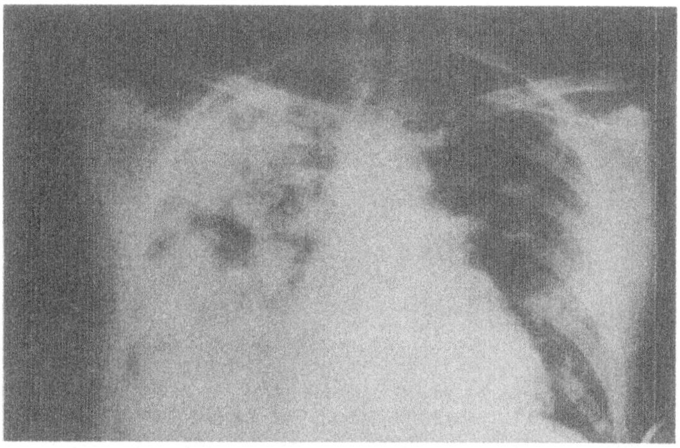

FIG. 1. Chest film 1 day before death in a patient with septic shock.

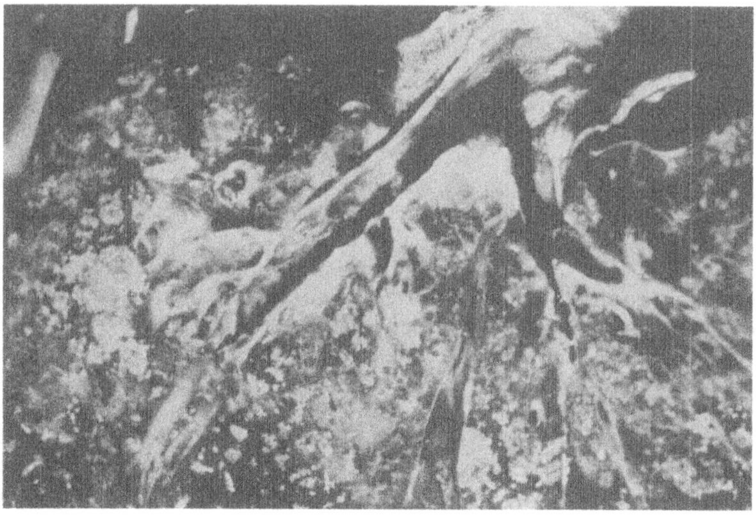

FIG. 2. Cut section of lung at autopsy from the same patient (see Fig. 1), showing hematogenous pneumonia.

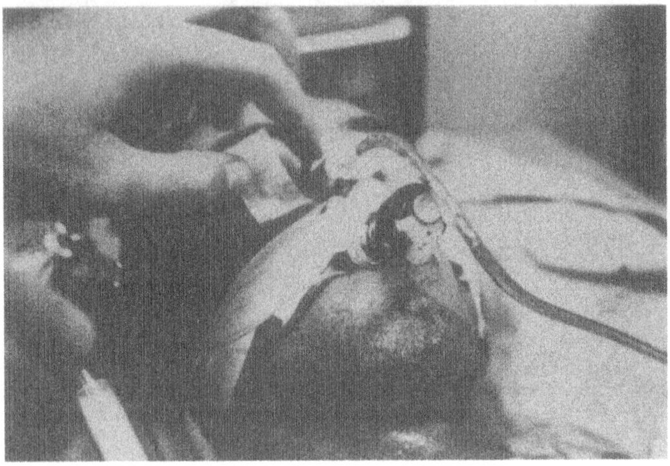

FIG. 3. Overt pulmonary edema as an agonal event in the same patient (see Figs. 1 and 2).

sepsis later. Grossly and by light microscopy, these patients had hematogenous pneumonia (Figs. 1 and 2), and agonally developed protein-rich pulmonary edema (Fig. 3) despite normal pulmonary arterial wedge pressures.

Mechanisms of the Lung Lesion in Septic Shock

Samples of blood were drawn and analyzed from the pulmonary artery wedge position during each sample period to help establish the accuracy of wedging. The data were fairly consistent, reflecting excellent gas exchange and respiratory alkalosis in the control and hemorrhagic shock groups. Occasionally, in patients with septic shock, different results were encountered. As seen in Table 4, occasional samples from the wedge position of septic patients with wide alveolar-arterial gradients yielded very high pO_2 values. X-ray films and autopsy studies of the patients in septic shock with peripheral arterial desaturation revealed hematogenous pneumonia. One explanation for the high pO_2 values would be that the wedge samples were drawn through areas of normal lung which were surrounded by intermixed areas of consolidation and shunting. An alternate explanation for the findings is that if the clear areas seen by x-ray and autopsy examinations contained diffuse endothelial damage with interstitial edema, rapid flow through these capillary beds would not allow adequate equilibration time and

TABLE 4

BLOOD GAS STUDIES ON SEPTIC SHOCK PATIENTS

PRD	# PT.	ARTERIAL			VENOUS			WEDGE		
		pO_2	pCO_2	pH	pO_2	pCO_2	pH	pO_2	pCO_2	pH
1	2	536	29	7.445	59	27	7.410	388	14	7.595 bc
3	2	388	28	7.480	45	33	7.375	388	19	7.580 bc
4	2	372	30	7.390	47	33	7.310	449	16	7.560 c
	4	186	31	7.520	40	27	7.530	480	10	7.860 ce
	5	423	37	7.540	45	40	7.440	388	37	7.405 d
5	1	103	31	7.475	51	35	7.470	460	23	7.680 ace
	2	505	35	7.400	51	39	7.400	572	24	ac
	3	444	34	7.495	56	36	7.485	428	23	7.585 ac
	4	147	33	7.410	38	33	7.450	432	15	7.640 ce
6	2	423	31	7.410	51	35	7.375	286	11	7.650 bc
7	2	439	24	7.500	50	32	7.440	444	15	7.680 c
8	3	418	27	7.480	62	26	7.445	397	15	7.620 bc
	4	105	29	7.490	41	39	7.410	334	10	7.850 bc
9	3	371	24	7.530	47	30	7.470	371	23	7.490 d
	4	202	31	7.555	43	32	7.550	295	13	7.780
10	4	58	39	7.540	34	40	7.495	291	12	7.880 bc

Note: PRD = sample period; #PT. = patient number.
(At sample period 5, Patient #1 had a normal cardiac output.)

[a]The pCO_2 of these samples suggests relatively rapid withdrawal through normal lung.

[b]Contamination with pulmonary arterial blood suggested.

[c]Characteristic of slow withdrawal through normal lung.

[d]Suggestive of sampling through an area of shunting.

[e]Fair oxygen tension in septic patients (sample from wedge position) with high alveolar-arterial oxygen difference.

therefore would yield hypoxic samples. Complete equilibration could occur through interstitial edema with slow retrograde flow, and samples with high pO_2 values would be obtained. This chance observation suggests that, if random pulmonary venous samples were drawn in an appropriate septic animal model which had peripheral arterial oxygen desaturation, we might determine whether diffuse endothelial (toxic, chemical) damage or focal (embolic or arteriolar spastic) damage had occurred, and we might thereby gain information as to the mechanism of the "lung lesion" in the septic patient.

We went to Vietnam having been warned of the "shock lung" phenomenon. Indeed, over 20 patients died of postoperative pulmonary insufficiency in our hospital in one 8-month period. Over half of the cases occurred over 1 week after injury, and over half of the 20 patients died of rapidly progressing pneumonia and sepsis. The remainder died of aspiration, fat embolism, blast injury, or massive crystalloid overload.

SUMMARY

After nearly a year of surgical practice in an active combat zone, we could not identify a single case of posthemorrhagic shock pulmonary insufficiency. We did document a small but statistically significant rise in the pulmonary arterial pressure of a group of patients presenting in hemorrhagic shock.

Pulmonary insufficiency associated with sepsis in the same theater took the form of progressive hematogenous pneumonia, which does not lend itself well to comparison with septic shock models as currently employed. Suggestions to help elucidate the mechanism of pulmonary damage with septic shock have been made.

NOTE

The opinions or assertions contained herein are the private ones of the authors and are not to be construed as official or reflecting the views of the Navy Department or the Naval service at large.

REFERENCES

1. Allardyce, B., H.F. Hamit, T. Matsumoto, and R.V. Mosely. Pulmonary vascular changes in hypovelemic shock: Radiography of the pulmonary microcirculation and the possible role of platelet embolism in increasing vascular resistance. J. Trauma 9:403-411, 1969.

2. Barkett, V.M., J.J. Coalson, and L.J. Greenfield. Early effects of hemorrhagic shock on surface tension and ultrastructure of canine lungs. Johns Hopkins Med. J. 124:86-94, 1969.

3. Barkett, V.M., J.J. Coalson, and L.J. Greenfield. Effects of

pulmonary denervation on canine lung structure and surfactant after hemorrhagic shock. J. Trauma 11:248-254, 1971.

4. Buckberg, G.D., and A.R. Dowell. The effects of hemorrhagic shock and pulmonary ischemia on lung compliance and structure in baboons. Surg. Gynecol. Obstet. 131:1065-1072, 1970.

5. Buckberg, G.J., J. Chon, and C. Darling. *Escherichia coli* bacteremic shock in conscious baboons. Ann. Surg. 173: 122-130, 1971.

6. Buckberg, G.D., C.A. Lipman, J.A. Hahn, M.J. Smith, and J.A. Hennessen. Pulmonary changes following hemorrhagic shock and resuscitation in baboons. J. Thorac. Cardiovasc. Surg. 59: 450-460, 1970.

7. Coalson, J.J., L.B. Hinshaw, and C.A. Guenter. The pulmonary ultrastructure in septic shock. Exptl. Mol. Pathol. 12: 84-103, 1970.

8. Cook, W.A., and W.R. Webb. Pulmonary changes in hemorrhagic shock. Surgery 64:85-94, 1968.

9. Henry, J.N., J.H. McArdle, H.J. Scott, and F.N. Gurd. A study of the acute and chronic respiratory pathophysiology of hemorrhagic shock. J. Thorac. Cardiovasc. Surg. 54:666-681, 1967.

10. Horwitz, D.L., C.M. Herman, and R. Moquin. Coagulation changes of septic shock in the baboon. Fed. Proc. 29:381, 1970.

11. Kuida, H., L.B. Hinshaw, R.P. Gilbert, and M.B. Visscher. Effect of gram-negative endotoxin on pulmonary circulation. Am. J. Physiol. 192:335-344, 1957.

12. Lim, R.C., Jr., F.W. Blaisdell, S.H. Choy, J.R. Goodman, and A.D. Hall. Pulmonary microvascular changes following regional shock: A clinical and experimental study. Bull. Soc. Intern. Chir. 27:22-28, 1968.

13. Lowery, B.D., C.T. Cloutier, and L.C. Carey. Blood gas determinations in the severely wounded in hemorrhagic shock. Arch. Surg. 99:330-338, 1969.

14. Sealy, W.C., S. Ogino, A.M. Lesage, and W.G. Young. Functional and structural changes in the lung in hemorrhagic shock. Surg. Gynecol. Obstet. 122:754-760, 1966.

15. Steiner, A.K., M. Allgower, P. Matter, J. Meine, W. Hunter,

and S.M. Perren. Circulatory changes after local tissue destruction by electric heat. J. Surg. Res. 11:23-32, 1971.

16. Sugg, W.L., W.D. Craver, W.R. Webb, and R.R. Ecker. Pressure changes in the dog lung secondary to hemorrhagic shock: Protective effect of pulmonary reimplantation. Ann. Surg. 169:592-598, 1969.

17. Teplitz, C. The ultrastructural basis for pulmonary pathophysiology following trauma: Pathogenesis of pulmonary edema. J. Trauma 8:700-703, 1968.

18. Veith, F.J., J.W.C. Hagstrom, A. Panossian, L. Nehlsen, and J.W. Wilson. Pulmonary microcirculatory response to shock, transfusion, and pump-oxygenator procedures: A unified mechanism underlying pulmonary damage. Surgery 64:95-109, 1968.

19. Wilson, J.W., N.B. Ratliff, and D.B. Hackel. The lung in hemorrhagic shock. Am. J. Pathol. 58:337-351, 1970.

IRREVERSIBILITY IN THE POST-TRANSFUSION PHASE OF HEMORRHAGIC SHOCK

Benjamin F. Rush, Jr., M.D.

Department of Surgery, College of Medicine and Dentistry of New Jersey, New Jersey Medical School, Newark, New Jersey

The concept of irreversibility in shock was popularized by Wiggers (94) about two decades ago. He demonstrated that, if dogs are bled enough to create profound hypotension, early replacement of normal blood volume results in survival, while late replacement is followed by a gradual drop in blood pressure and death—despite post-treatment restoration of blood pressure to normal and a normal blood volume. Wiggers called this latter phase "normovolemic shock" and indicated that it was resistant to all modes of therapy then current. Some feel that this concept is of little use in describing clinical shock, stating (a) that human shock is rarely permitted to reach the levels used in canine experiments, (b) that no such clear-cut moment exists in clinical shock when irreversibility supervenes, and (c) that, in any case, the dog is an unacceptable model for human shock (64). However, the concept of irreversibility persists as a challenge to many investigators and appears to have outgrown the old connotations of the experimental model, reflecting instead the current state of the art. Thus, clinical shock which fails to respond to all the agents we command is irreversible. Most clinicians will agree that therapy fails (with eventual death of the patient) much later in clinical shock today than it did two decades ago, when the concept was introduced.

CLINICAL MEASURES WHICH SEEM TO POSTPONE IRREVERSIBILITY

The success or failure of the clinical agents which have been tried in an attempt to defer irreversibility in shock (both laboratory and clinical) offers some etiologic clues to this state (Table 1). Vasopressors have enjoyed a long and unjustified grip

TABLE 1

CLINICAL AGENTS USED TO EXTEND REVERSIBILITY
IN POST-TRANSFUSION HEMORRHAGIC SHOCK

Treatment	Effectiveness	References
Vasopressors	-	6,23
Vasodilators	±	24,69,88
Blood	+	70
Correction of acidosis	+	51
Buffered saline	+	12,13,63,65,77
O_2 and mechanical respiration	+	51
Inotropic cardiac stimulants	+	87
Corticosteroids	±	2,37,45,67,74,95

Note: - = ineffective; + = effective; ± = in dispute. The clinical effectiveness of both vasodilators and corticosteroids is in dispute, but the former are rarely used, while the latter are frequently administered.

on clinical treatment of hypovolemic shock. As long ago as World War I, it was realized that vasopressors given over a sufficient period actually produce shock. Numerous laboratory experiments have indicated that animals in irreversible shock die sooner rather than later when treated with vasopressors (6,23). While it is apparent that the *sine qua non* of hemorrhagic shock therapy is to replace the lost blood, transfusion in an amount which exceeds that lost sometimes appears to improve survival in clinical shock (70).

Another agent which has received major attention in the past 10 years is saline. Data from experiments on the dog (65,77,96), cat (12), and rat (13,63) indicate that administration of buffered saline solutions will resuscitate animals in the "normovolemic" phase of hemorrhagic shock which otherwise would presumably have died. In the clinic, apparent improvement of patients treated with saline solutions may stem from replacement of occult transudates in traumatized areas. In the laboratory, however, the response is not so easily explained. The popular interpretation revolves around the whole complex of changes which occur in tissue ischemia with increasing capillary permeability and the question of intracellular translocation of fluids (33,34,76). Other measures of apparent clinical benefit are: correction of acidosis (16), administration of cardiac inotropic stimulants such as isoproterenol (87), respiratory support with mechanical ventilators and oxygen (51), and the use of corticosteroids. Some claim that corticosteroids act as vasoactive agents (37,95), while others suggest that they support metabolism of the cell membrane (2,45,67). Vasodilators generated a brief period of interest when it was suggested that inappropriate vasoconstriction in the vessels led to increased blood sequestration in shock (69). No consistent, convincing clinical response has been noted in patients in shock (24).

Wiggers' monograph in 1950 (94) identified the principal events in irreversible shock as failure of the peripheral vascular tree, consequent peripheral pooling of blood, and concurrent myocardial failure. Other factors considered were increased capillary and terminal vessel permeability, breakdown of intracellular metabolic processes, and release of factors into the circulation from hypoxic tissues which depress function in other tissues and cells. After two decades, we are still trying to evaluate these various mechanisms.

INCREASED CAPILLARY PERMEABILITY

Increased capillary permeability, with a shift of protein and fluid from capillaries to the interstitial space (49,61), is often assumed to contribute to the progression of shock (Table 2). Such increasing permeability has no effect in tissue and cannot be detected until hydrostatic pressure within the damaged capillary is elevated toward normotensive levels (61). The average closing pressure is about 30 mm Hg, and little flow occurs in the capillary bed in animals maintained in shock at this level (54). At this perfusion pressure, large areas of the capillary bed are perfused little or not at all. Tissue oxygen levels drop precipitously, approaching zero in the extremities (42). Large amounts of lactic acid, an effective agent in producing capillary permeability, accumulate in local tissues during this period of stagnant anoxia (81). Histamine, serotonin, and various lysozymes are also released during shock and have the potential of injuring endothelium and increasing capillary permeability (9,61,83,99). With reestablishment of normal blood volume in the dog after hemorrhagic hypotension, thoracic duct lymph flow rises markedly (38). Labeled albumin injected intra-arterially appears much more rapidly in lymph (38). Both observations are interpreted as indirect evidence

TABLE 2

EVIDENCE FOR INCREASED CAPILLARY PERMEABILITY
IN POST-TRANSFUSION HEMORRHAGIC SHOCK

Observation	Interpretation	References
Increased tissue mediators	+	9,61,83,99
Increased thoracic duct flow	+	38
Increased hematocrit	+	21,89
Red cell aggregation	±	31,97
Electron microscopy:		
Endothelial changes	±	2
Interstitial edema	±	2,22

Note: + = observation strongly supported; ± = evidence exists both for and against observation.

of increased capillary permeability. Red cell aggregation in small vessels may be due to obstruction of distal sphincters or can suggest a loss of plasma volume and a clumping of cells as they are stranded in distal peripheral vessels. Loss of serum protein by capillary leakage would cause a decrease in serum protein if the protein were lost in excess of water, or if water returned to the large vessels more rapidly than protein. Likewise, the albumin-globulin ratio would be altered if there were a differential loss of albumin compared to globulin. None of these changes is seen, however. This suggests that, if capillary leakage is a major problem, the proportion of water and protein remains the same as in the serum; moreover, both the water and protein being returned to the large vessels via the thoracic duct contain the same constituents as the plasma. Loss of plasma to the interstitial space would be expected to increase the hematocrit value. Indeed, this is seen in splenectomized dogs immediately after restoration of the lost blood at the end of the hypotensive period in shock models (89). A rise in the hematocrit of the microcirculation compared to the control circulation has also been noted in humans during shock (21).

TABLE 3

EVIDENCE FOR PERIPHERAL POOLING OF BLOOD
IN POST-TRANSFUSION HEMORRHAGIC SHOCK

Observation	Interpretation	References
Microphotography of small vessels	+	31,97
Two-phase dilution curve	±	29,64,97
Gross changes in organ size and color	±	31,64,97

Note: + = observation strongly supported; ± = evidence exists both for and against observation. While the phenomenon seems generally accepted, there is still much dispute regarding regional anatomical and species differences.

Electron microscopy has demonstrated gaps in the endothelium which could permit the passage of plasma, and changes in the interstitial spaces of some organs have been described which suggest interstitial edema (2). Certainly, the interstitial edema resulting from local tissue trauma depletes the total blood volume. Presumably a generalized leakage of fluid from the capillary bed would accomplish the same change. Liberal fluid replacement in patients in the post-shock period, either with plasma or generous amounts of buffered saline solutions, would serve to repair this deficiency—perhaps accounting for some of the effectiveness of these solutions. In animal experiments, the drop in blood pressure generated by histamine can be largely suppressed if the animals have been pretreated with large amounts of saline solution before the injection of histamine (B.F. Rush, unpublished data).

POOLING OF BLOOD

Pooling of blood with red cell aggregation and increase in venular size (31,97) has been regularly seen in peripheral tissues of a number of species during late shock, after return of blood (Table 3). This is a common phenomenon in dogs, with an accompanying plethora which is grossly visible in the liver and the duodenum (64,83). The dog has, however, an inferior vena caval sphincter which is absent in primates; many feel that this particular response is peculiar to the dog and to other animals with similar inferior vena caval anatomy (64). Still, photomicrography of the mesentery of species without the inferior vena caval sphincters also demonstrates late small vessel dilation (97). Shoemaker has pointed to a two-phase dilution curve of chromium-tagged red cells, suggesting a slow and rapid phase of mixing in the postshock normotensive period (86). Moore and others have not been able to confirm this (64). Some degree of pooling and sequestration of blood seems to be accepted by most investigators as a feature of hemorrhagic shock, but its degree and importance remain unresolved. Again, the use of liberal transfusions and additional infusions of saline solution may act as a defense against these changes.

INTRAVASCULAR CLOTTING

Intravascular clotting (35) or aggregates of fibrin and platelets (15) are frequently found in dogs during the irreversible phase of hemorrhagic shock if heparin is not used in the shock model. Hardaway (35,36) has conducted extensive experiments on this phenomenon and speculates about its role in human shock. Certainly hemorrhagic shock changes blood viscosity (39) and increases endothelial stickiness (61). Aggregation of red cells has been described in the microcirculation both clinically and experimentally during shock. Intravascular clotting in the microcirculation would help to explain some of the problems with irreversible ischemia and increased peripheral resistance. On the other hand, canine blood seems to have a special propensity to clot when exposed to glass and when manipulated in the fashion usually used in experimental models (78). Such clots are rarely observed histologically in man after death in hemorrhagic shock (4); perhaps this represents the most telling argument against the concept.

SHIFTS OF INTERSTITIAL FLUIDS

Laboratory investigations by Shires (85) first drew attention to an apparent decrease in the interstitial fluid volume during shock states (Table 4). Since his first reports, a host of papers have confirmed and refuted the initial data (20,29,77,86). The reports have been confusing enough to finally reflect on the dilution method itself. One can question whether the equilibration required by various dilution methods is not too slow and clumsy a technique to evaluate the dynamic changes which occur in the experimental animal receiving intravenous fluids after a period of hypotension (59). More direct data from electron micrography suggest the occurrence of intracellular swelling, especially in the mitochondria (22). This may be interpreted as an influx of fluid from the interstitial space, or it may reflect a simple translocation of fluid within the cell. ATP is known to be required to fuel the sodium pump, and high-energy phosphate compounds disappear

TABLE 4

EVIDENCE FOR SHIFT OF INTERSTITIAL FLUID INTO CELLS IN POST-TRANSFUSION HEMORRHAGIC SHOCK

Observation	Interpretation	References
Decreased interstitial fluid pressure	+	32
Increased interstitial K^+ and Mg^{++}	+	7,33
Increased intracellular sodium (RBCs)	+	19
Decreased ECF (dilution studies)	±	20,29,59,77,85,86
Decreased tissue ATP	±	55,91,92
Intracellular edema *in vivo* and *in vitro*	±	2,22,40
Mitochondrial swelling	±	22
Decreased transmembrane potential	±	14

Note: + = observation strongly supported; ± = evidence exists both for and against observation. While most agree that this fluid shift occurs, many have felt it to be an agonal event occurring long after hope of reversing the shock state was lost. More recent evidence seems to favor an earlier shift of fluids.

almost entirely from cells after 1 or 2 hours of ischemia (55,91, 92). Presumably, if the pump fails, an isotonic shift of sodium into the cells can occur, with an outward shift of potassium (14). Serum potassium concentration rises late in the post-transfusion shock period, but it rises much earlier and to a much higher level in samples of interstitial water, either withdrawn from "Guyton capsules" or from capillary wicks in muscular tissue (79). Cellular swelling in the presence of hypoxia is a commonly known phenomenon and has been observed repeatedly (26). This failure of methods for examining localized tissues to yield results which parallel many of the reported results of dilution techniques is of continuing interest. Some suggest that while the intracellular phase of distribution of appropriate isotopes in the normotensive shock phase remains the same, a rapid and slow equilibration of a steady state occurs with decrease of the rapid phase after shock (86). Some evidence exists that collagen may adsorb sodium from interstitial fluid in ischemia, another phenomenon which will effectively change interstitial osmolarity and promote intracellular translocation of water. This latter mechanism has been proposed by Moyer and Butcher (65), who suggest that the effectiveness of buffered sodium solutions in the shock state relates primarily to sodium content rather than to volume. This is supported by Fulton, who demonstrated that strips of implanted collagen adsorb substantial amounts of sodium and water during hypovolemic and normovolemic shock (28).

During the post-transfusion phase in shock models, increased negativity of interstitial fluid pressure has been observed by several investigators using a number of techniques (32). This finding suggests a loss of fluid from interstitial space. Increased intracellular sodium has been demonstrated by direct examination of red blood cells in late shock (19). Since the sodium space as measured by dilution studies appears not to change, some workers have assumed that both water and sodium must move into the cell. It has been suggested that the use of saline infusions in the therapy of shock is effective because of the alleviation of an interstitial fluid deficit which would be less adequately accomplished by the use of whole blood (34,84). Some have also proposed that the presumed effectiveness of cortisone stems from its ability to support the metabolism of cellular membranes and that the pharmacologic doses utilized will prolong the period of active partitioning of cellular fluids in the presence of hypoxia.

MYOCARDIAL FAILURE

The role of the myocardium in hemorrhagic shock has been under investigation for many years. Crowell and Guyton (17) have stimulated some of the more recent discussions; they believe that myocardial failure is the major factor in irreversibility. This conclusion is based on the following concepts: First, irreversibility occurs and can be identified in animal experiments by the reversal of flow in a blood reservoir held at a level which maintains hypotensive shock. When the animal stops bleeding into the reservoir and, instead, the blood begins to return to the animal, the irreversible state has been assumed to be reached. Second, this moment of irreversibility seems to correlate with the development of an oxygen debt calculated at approximately 120-140 ml/kg (18, 44). Third, a major target organ for this oxygen deficiency is assumed to be the heart; left-sided heart failure is initiated at the point of flow reversal, as indicated by a sudden rise in left auricular pressure which persists and increases to infinity over a period of time despite return of blood to the animal and of blood pressure to normotensive levels. In his early observations, Wiggers (94) also indicated that myocardial failure played a role in some of his dogs in irreversible shock; however, he felt that this could account for only a third of the deaths and that other factors were responsible in the remainder. Many have observed that, after "irreversibility" has been reached, the heart can still produce a normal output when transfusion brings the blood volume back to normal. However, in the failing heart (and often in the heart after hemorrhagic shock), a higher left atrial pressure is required to achieve any given level of cardiac output. In the period of irreversibility, left atrial pressure continues to increase in order to maintain cardiac output. With persistent transfusion, left auricular pressure may increase markedly as death supervenes.

The heart muscle cell is endowed with abundant mitochondria, reflecting the immense need of this organ for metabolic energy. Unlike most organs (including skeletal muscle), the heart extracts lactic acid as one of its prime substrates for oxidative metabolism (25). In the course of severe hypotension, however, anaerobic glycolysis reverses this process so that even the heart begins to produce lactic acid rather than consume it, indicating a dependence on anaerobic glycolysis for its energy. That some mitochondria do not recover during or after transfusion is suggested by the persistently depressed levels of ATP in hemorrhagic shock (91). Left ventricular work, coronary flow, and left ventricular oxygen consumption remain below control values during the normovolemic phase (25). Blood levels of pyruvate and lactate remain significantly elevated during this same period. Case and others (15) have shown that left atrial pressure falls to normal if the left descending coronary artery is perfused at normal arterial pressures in the presence of low systemic arterial pressure.

Possibly, factors extrinsic to the myocardium may also suppress function during the normovolemic phase of shock as indicated by the myocardial depressant factor which has been identified in serum during shock (50). This appears to arise from the pancreas and may be related to the lysosomal enzymes.

In clinical shock, our attempts to support the failing heart are based primarily on the use of inotropic stimulants (87). Beta-adrenergic stimulants, such as isoproterenol, have found the greatest favor. Blocking the alpha-stimulating component of epinephrine with phenoxybenzamine while taking advantage of the beta-stimulating component has also been advocated. Recent evidence suggests that the hypoxic myocardium responds better to beta-adrenergic stimulation if additional glucose is present (1,10). Digitalis has been suggested as an additional agent, but its benefits have not been clearly established.

METABOLIC DETERIORATION

A dramatic breakdown of the metabolic machinery occurs in the post-transfusion phase of metabolic shock (27,43,47,55) (Table 5). Examination of the serum reveals a progressive accumulation of many metabolites, indicating both increasing catabolism and a failure of anabolism in the tissues. Free fatty acids are increased, and almost all circulating amino acids increase in concentration (46). Lactic acid rises, and acidosis becomes progressively more severe (80). Potassium and magnesium, primarily intracellular fluid constituents, gradually rise. Serum glucose levels first rise precipitously and then gradually fall toward the final phase of the shock period. Hydrolytic enzymes appear in increasing concentration, including cathepsins, alkaline phosphatase, and beta-glucuronidase (3,9,72,79). In addition to these lysosomal enzymes, cytoplasmic enzymes (such as creatine phosphokinase) leak into the circulating blood (79). Most of these changes have been known to exist for many years. The more recent analyses of lymph and soft tissues indicate that serum concentrations represent only the tip of the iceberg, and that many intracellular substances appear in much higher concentrations in interstitial fluid during the late phase of shock (9,34). The increased presence of this "flotsam and jetsam" of intracellular enzymes in the interstitial fluids and systemic circulation leads to speculation concerning toxicity which may be produced (82). Glenn *et al.* (30) indicate that the infusion of purified lysosomal enzymes at a level found in late shock will reproduce many of the features of the shock syndrome.

Some superb analyses of serum biochemistry in shock have been done by Stoner and Threlfall (92), Engle (27), and others (60). Recently, emphasis on this part of the shock picture has been rekindled, with the opportunity to examine tissue cellular and subcellular biochemistry. Most subcellular analyses have tended to confirm the conclusions drawn from previous findings in the serum, but the changes revealed by these more direct measurements are usually greater than those found in serum (9,33,48).

Anaerobic glycolysis obviously occurs in ischemic tissues. The Krebs cycle contributes very little to energy production; incorporation of amino acids and fat into the metabolic cycle of the cell is almost abolished. Despite the return to normal blood volume, most of the derangements of the metabolic process persist in the irreversible state, indicating persisting ischemia of peri-

TABLE 5

EVIDENCE OF CELLULAR DETERIORATION IN POST-TRANSFUSION HEMORRHAGIC SHOCK

Observation	Interpretation	References
Appearance of cytoplasmic enzymes in plasma and interstitial fluids	+	79
Appearance of lysosomal enzymes in plasma and interstitial fluids	+	3,9,30,72,79
Disappearance of cellular ATP	+	8,11,43,55
Uncoupling of mitochondrial oxidation	+	8,56,57,58
Electron microscopic observation of vacuolization of mitochondria and disruption of lysozymes	+	2,22,40

Note: + = observation strongly supported. As is the case for interstitial fluid shift into the cells, recent observations identify biochemical and structural changes in the cell much earlier than previously thought.

pheral tissues or the failure of cells to utilize oxygen conventionally, even when it is available (8,11,47,55-58).

A loose coupling of mitochondrial respiration has been detected within an hour after the onset of severe hemorrhagic hypotension. Some theorize that an uncoupled respiration may form part of the irreversible shock syndrome (8,56-58). Electron microscopy combined with histochemistry indicates a number of major changes in the cell structure, including membrane-bound cytoplasmic vacuoles, loss of nucleochromatin, and leakage of endogenous magnesium and pyrimidine nucleotides (2,22,40). Diffusion of enzymes from the lysosomal particles occurs (9). Thus far, therapy designed to alter or ameliorate the biochemical changes in late shock has defied the ingenuity of the clinician and the investigator. Aside from corticosteroids as a possible membrane stabilizer and buffers to combat acidosis, no other agents have shown promise. Some efforts have been exerted to identify metabolic intermediates, which, if given in large amounts, might reverse some of these processes and the accompanying biochemical deterioration. Infusions of succinate, alpha-ketoglutarate and glucose-6-phosphate have been tried without success. Administration of glucose during shock seems to be of some benefit in dogs (62). Some have claimed that ATP infusions during experimental shock are beneficial (53, 93), but it is difficult to explain how molecules of this size would enter cells.

SUMMARY

The changes observed in the so-called irreversible phase of hemorrhagic shock have been reviewed briefly. These include increasing capillary permeability, pooling and stagnation of blood, shifts of interstitial fluid, myocardial failure, and biochemical deterioration. How current modes of therapy relate to the reversal of some of these changes is also considered. Obviously, the interrelationships among these changes are of great importance. Most of them will intensify the others, with creation of a feedback mechanism in which ischemia provokes metabolic derangements, which then provoke capillary and membrane permeability, which leads to further loss of function of myocardium and other organs, which creates further ischemia. The excursions of this inherently unstable state escalate until death occurs.

In the field of shock, we are overwhelmed with a massive amount of data, thus far rather poorly correlated. We are still ignorant of the hierarchy of the various changes. Which really occurs first? Where do we need to direct our therapy to prevent the next step? The identification of target organs most likely to fail first is also a major, unresolved consideration. Which organs should be supported initially in order to stop the cycle of deterioration? What new gains may accrue from something as conceptually simple as a pump oxygenator to support the failing heart in shock, or as subtle as an infusion of the appropriate metabolic intermediary at just the right point in the shock syndrome?

In any case, the point of irreversibility in clinical shock has been moved further and further into the area of profound and late shock during the past decade. We expect that it will continue to be moved in this direction (64).

REFERENCES

1. Amsterdam, E.A., D. Foley, R. Zelis, T. Lais, and D.T. Mason. Effects of inotropic and metabolic interventions on myocardial mechanics during severe hypoxia. Clin. Res. 19:302, 1971.

2. Ashford, T., C. Palmerio, and J. Fine. Structural analogue in vascular muscle to the functional disorder in refractory traumatic shock and reversal by corticosteroid: Electron microscopic evaluation. Ann. Surg. 164:575, 1966.

3. Attar, S., J. McLaughlin, P. Hanashiro, and R.A. Cowley. The kallikreins in human shock and trauma. Surg. Forum 22:11, 1971.

4. Attar, S., P. Hanashiro, A. Mansberger, J. McLaughlin, H. Firminger, and R.A. Cowley. Intravascular coagulation: Reality or myth? Surgery 68:27, 1970.

5. Bacalzo, L.V., Jr., A.L. Cary, L.D. Miller, and W.M. Parkins. Methods and critical uptake volume for hemorrhagic shock in rats. Surgery 70:555, 1971.

6. Bainbridge, F.A., and J.W. Trevor. Memorandum upon surgical shock and some allied conditions. Brit. Med. J. 1:381, 1917.

7. Baue, A., M.A. Worth, and M.M. Sayeed. Alterations in activated magnesium and sodium plus potassium adenosine triphosphatase and the Krebs cycle in hemorrhagic shock. Surg. Forum 21:8, 1970.

8. Baue, A., and M.S. Mohammed. Alterations in the functional capacity of mitochondria in hemorrhagic shock. Surgery 68: 40, 1970.

9. Bell, M., A.H. Herman, R. Egdahl, E.E. Smith, and A.M. Rutenburg. Role of lysosomal disruption in the development of refractory shock. Surg. Forum 21:10, 1970.

10. Bing, O.H.L., W.W. Brooks, and J.V. Messer. Mechanical benefits and hazards of isoproterenol during myocardial hypoxia. Clin. Res. 17:305, 1971.

11. Bounous, G., N.G. Sutherland, A.H. McArdle, and F.N. Gurd. The prophylactic use of an "elemental" diet in experimental hemorrhagic shock and intestinal ischemia. Ann. Surg. 166: 312, 1967.

12. Brand, E.D., T.K. Suh, and M.C. Avery. Reversal of postoligemic shock in the cat by hypervenobaric massive fluid therapy. Am. J. Physiol. 211:1232, 1966.

13. Butcher, H.R., Jr., and A. Braitberg. Hemorrhagic shock in rats: A method of therapeutic bioassay. Arch. Surg. 98: 685, 1969.

14. Campion, D.S., L.J. Lynch, F.C. Rector, Jr., N. Carter, and G.T. Shires. Effect of hemorrhagic shock on transmembrane potential. Surgery 66:1051, 1969.

15. Case, R.B., J.J. Sarnoff, P.E. Waithe, and L.C. Sarnoff. Intra-arterial and intravenous blood infusion in hemorrhagic shock. JAMA 152:208, 1953.

16. Cloutier, C.T., B.D. Lowery, and L.C. Carey. Acid-base disturbances in hemorrhagic shock. Arch. Surg. 98:551, 1969.

17. Crowell, J.W., and A.C. Guyton. Evidence favoring a cardiac mechanism in irreversible hemorrhagic shock. Am. J. Physiol. 201:893, 1961.

18. Crowell, J.W., and E.E. Smith. Oxygen deficit and irreversible hemorrhagic shock. Am. J. Physiol. 206:313, 1964.

19. Cunningham, J.N., G.T. Shires, and Y. Wagner. Changes in intracellular sodium and potassium content of red blood cells in trauma and shock. Am. J. Surg. 122:650, 1971.

20. Cunningham, J.N., G.T. Shires, and Y. Wagner. Cellular transport defects in hemorrhagic shock. Surgery 70:215, 1971.

21. Doty, D.B., and M.H. Weil. Comparison of microcirculatory and central hematocrit as measures of circulatory shock. Surg. Gynecol. Obstet. 124:1263, 1967.

22. De Palma, R., Y. Harano, A.V. Robinson, and W.D. Holden. Structure and function of hepatic mitochondria in hemorrhage and endotoxemia. Surg. Forum 21:3, 1970.

23. Drucker, W.R., and H.K. Wright. The use of vasopressors in hemorrhagic shock. In: *Shock and Hypertension,* edited by L.C. Mills and J.H. Moyer. New York: Grune & Stratton, 1965, p. 401.

24. Eckenhoff, J.E., and L.H. Cooperman. Clinical application of phenoxybenzamine in shock and vasoconstrictive states. Surg. Gynecol. Obstet. 121:483, 1965.

25. Edwards, W.S., A. Siegal, and R.J. Bing. Studies on myocardial metabolism. III. Coronary blood flow, myocardial oxygen consumption, and carbohydrate metabolism in experimental hemorrhagic shock. J. Clin. Invest. 33:1646, 1954.

26. Enerson, D.M. Cellular swelling. I. Hypothermia, graded hypoxia and the osmotic effects of low-molecular-weight

dextran on isolated tissues. Ann. Surg. 163:169, 1966.

27. Engel, F.L. The significance of the metabolic changes during shock. Ann. N.Y. Acad. Sci. 55:381, 1952.

28. Fulton, R.L. Adsorption of sodium and water by collagen during hemorrhagic shock. Ann. Surg. 172:861, 1970.

29. Gillett, D.J., and F.J. Halmagyi. Red cell circulation in irreversible shock in sheep and dogs. J. Surg. Res. 10: 443, 1970.

30. Glenn, T.M., J.R. Morris, A.M. Lefer, A.M. Lopez-Rasi, W.W. Ferguson, T.S. Serate, and S.L. Wangensteen. Influence of lysosomal enzymes on circulatory function. Surg. Forum 22:14, 1971.

31. Green, H.D. Physiology of peripheral circulation in shock. Fed. Proc. 20:61, 1961.

32. Guyton, A.C. A concept of negative interstitial pressure based on pressures in implanted perforated capsules. Circ. Res. 12:399, 1963.

33. Hagberg, S., H. Haljamae, and H. Rockert. Shock reactions in skeletal muscle. III. The electrolyte content of tissue fluid and blood plasma before and after induced hemorrhagic shock. Ann. Surg. 168:243, 1968.

34. Haljamae, H. "Hidden" cellular electrolyte responses to hemorrhagic shock and their significance. Rev. Surg., Sept.-Oct., 1970, p. 315.

35. Hardaway, R.M., and F.H. Weiss. Intracapillary clotting as the etiology of shock. Arch. Surg. 83:851, 1961.

36. Hardaway, R.M., W.H. Brune, E.F. Geever, J.W. Burns, and H.P. Mock. Studies on the role of intravascular coagulation in irreversible hemorrhagic shock. Ann. Surg. 155:241, 1962.

37. Harrison, T.S., R.C. Chawla, and R.S. Wojtalik. Steroidal influences on catecholamines. N. Engl. J. Med. 279:136, 1968.

38. Hidai, K.R., R.W. Hopkins, and F.A. Simeone. Studies of thoracic duct lymph in hemorrhagic shock. In: *Lymph and the Lymphatic System*. Springfield, Ill.: Charles C Thomas, 1969, p. 260.

39. Hissen, W., R.L. Swank, L. Lino, and G.V.F. Seaman. Physio-

chemical changes in circulating canine blood on exsanguination or administration of histamine. Surg. Gynecol. Obstet. 122:1003, 1966.

40. Holden, W.D., R.G. DePalma, W.R. Drucker, and A. McKalen. Ultrastructural changes in hemorrhagic shock: Electron microscopic study of liver, kidney, and striated muscle cells in rats. Ann. Surg. 162:517, 1965.

41. Hollenberg, N.K., J.R. Waters, M.R. Toews, R.O. Davies, and M. Nickerson. Nature of cardiovascular decompensation during hemorrhagic hypotension. Am. J. Physiol. 219:1476, 1970.

42. Hunt, T.K., B.H. Zederfeldt, T.K. Goldstick, and W.B. Conolly. Tissue oxygen tension during controlled hemorrhage. Surg. Forum 18:3, 1967.

43. Jones, C.E., and Crowell, J.W. Energy base loss in shock. Fed. Proc. 26:331, 1967.

44. Jones, C.E., J.W. Crowell, and E.E. Smith. A cause-effect relationship between oxygen deficit and irreversible hemorrhagic shock. Surg. Gynecol. Obstet. 127:1, 1968.

45. Kibbey, I.I., F.E. D'Amour, and D.L. Smith. Effect of ACTH on rate of oxygen consumption in experimental traumatic shock. Am. J. Physiol. 174:241, 1953.

46. La Brosse, L.H. Plasma amino acids in normal humans and patients with shock. Surg. Gynecol. Obstet. 125:516, 1967.

47. Lazarus, H.M., A.H. Herman, A.M. Rutenburg, and R.H. Egdahl. Hepatic nuclear ribonucleic acid synthesis in hemorrhagic shock. Surg. Forum 21:14, 1970.

48. Lemieux, M.D., R.N. Smith, and N.P. Couch. Electrometric surface pH of skeletal muscle in hypovolemia. Am. J. Surg. 117:627, 1969.

49. Lewis, D.H., and L. Appelgren. Capillary transport function in skeletal muscle in hemorrhagic shock. Surg. Forum 20: 7, 1969.

50. Lovett, W.L., S.L. Wangensteen, T.M. Glenn, and A.M. Lefer. Presence of a myocardial depressant factor in patients in circulatory shock. Surgery 70:223, 1971.

51. Manger, W.M., G.G. Nahas, D. Hassam, D.V. Habif, and E.M. Papper. Effect of pH control and increased O_2 delivery in

the course of hemorrhagic shock. Ann. Surg. 156:503, 1962.

52. Marks, L.J., D.W. King, and H.F. McCarthy. Physiological role of cortisol in the plasma volume response to hemorrhage. Surgery 61:422, 1967.

53. Massion, W.H. Value of high-energy compounds in the treatment of shock. Am. J. Surg. 110:342, 1965.

54. Matsumoto, T., R.M. Hardaway, and J.E. McClain. Microcirculation in hemorrhagic shock with relationship to blood pressure. Arch. Surg. 95:911, 1967.

55. McArdle, A.H., D. Mavrias, G. Bounous, and F.N. Gurd. Energy production in the dog intestine following hemorrhagic shock. Surg. Forum 19:8, 1968.

56. Mela, L., L.V. Bacalzo, R.R. White, IV, and L.D. Miller. Shock-induced alterations of mitochondrial-energy-linked functions. Surg. Forum 21:8, 1970.

57. Mela, L., L.V. Bacalzo, Jr., and L.D. Miller. Defective oxidative metabolism of rat liver mitochondria in hemorrhagic and endotoxin shock. Am. J. Physiol. 220:571, 1971.

58. Mela, L., K. Olofsson, L.D. Miller, L.V. Bacalzo, and R.R. White, IV. Effect of lysosomes and hypoxia on mitochondria in shock. Surg. Forum 22:19, 1971.

59. Middleton, E.S., R. Mathews, and G.T. Shires. Radiosulphate as a measure of the extracellular fluid in acute hemorrhagic shock. Ann. Surg. 170:174, 1969.

60. Migone, L. Mètabolic aspects of shock. In: *Shock: Pathogenesis and Therapy: An Internation Symposium*, Stockholm, June, 1961.

61. Miles, A.A. Local and systemic factors in shock. Fed. Proc. 20:141, 1961.

62. Moffat, J.G., J.A. King, and W.R. Drucker. Tolerance to prolonged hypovolemic shock: Effects of infusion of an energy substrate. Surg. Forum 20:8, 1968.

63. Monafo, W.W., T.L. Wachtel, and F. Deitz. Bioassay of hemorrhagic shock in rats. Arch. Surg. 98:275, 1969.

64. Moore, F.D. Relevance of experimental shock studies to clinical shock problems. Fed. Proc. (Suppl. 9) 20:227, 1960.

65. Moyer, C.A., and H.R. Butcher. *Burns, Shock and Plasma Volume Regulation.* St. Louis: C.V. Mosby Co., 1967.

66. Moyo, C.T., J.B. Dossetor, and L.D. MacLean. Hemodialysis in the treatment of shock. J. Surg. Res. 4:3801, 1964.

67. Nagy, S., K. Tarnoky, and G. Petri. Effect of a water-soluble corticosteroid analogue in experimental hemorrhagic shock. J. Surg. Res. 4:62, 1964.

68. Naylor, B.A., M.H. Welch, A.W. Shafer, and C.A. Guenter. Oxyhemoglobin dissociation in hemorrhagic and endotoxic shock. Clin. Res. 18:631, 1970.

69. Nickerson, M., and S.A. Carter. Protection against acute trauma and traumatic shock by vasodilators. Can. J. Biochem. Physiol. 37:1161, 1959.

70. Prentice, T.C., J.M. Olney, Jr., C.P. Artz, and J.M. Howard. Studies of blood volume and transfusion therapy in the Korean battle casualty. Battle Casualties in Korea; Studies of the Surgical Research Team 2:114, 1956.

71. Randall, H.T. The shifts of fluid and electrolytes in shock. Ann. N.Y. Acad. Sci. 55:412, 1952.

72. Reich, T., B.M. Dierolf, and B.M. Reynolds. Plasma cathepsin-like acid proteinase activity during hemorrhagic shock. J. Surg. Res. 5:116, 1965.

73. Reich, M.P., and B. Eiseman. Tissue oxygenation following resuscitation with crystalloid solution following experimental acute blood loss. Surgery 69:928, 1971.

74. Replogle, R.L., H. Kundler, M. Schottenfeld, and S. Spear. Hemodynamic effects of dexamethasone in experimental hemorrhagic shock: Negative results. Ann. Surg. 174:126, 1971.

75. Robb, H.J. The role of microembolism in the production of irreversible shock. Ann. Surg. 158:685, 1963.

76. Rothe, C.F. Heart failure and fluid loss in hemorrhagic shock. Fed. Proc. 29:1854, 1970.

77. Rush, B.F., Jr. Treatment of experimental shock: Comparison of the effects of norepinephrine, Dibenzyline, dextran, whole blood and balanced saline solutions. Surgery 61: 938, 1967.

78. Rush, B.F., Jr., and R.J. Wilder. Renal necrosis and mortality in hemorrhagic shock: Effects of heparin and plastic or glass systems. Surgery 58:720, 1965.

79. Sacks, E.I., J. Fewel, J. Hsieh, and B.F. Rush, Jr. Electrolyte and enzyme gradients in plasma, lymph and "interstitial" fluid during shock. Surg. Forum 21:44, 1970.

80. Schloerb, P.R., C.E. Peters, G.K. Cage, J.C. Kearns, and J.K. Lam. Evaluation of the sulfate space as a measure of extracellular fluid. Surg. Forum 18:39, 1968.

81. Schumer, W. Lactate studies of the dog in oligemic shock. J. Surg. Res. 8:491, 1968.

82. Schumer, W., S.K. Kapica, and T.L. Teng. Validity of the lysosomal theory in oligemic shock. Arch. Surg. 99:325, 1969.

83. Selkurt, E.E. Status of investigative aspects of hemorrhagic shock. Fed. Proc. 29:1832, 1970.

84. Selkurt, E.E., and R.F. Rothe. Critical analysis of experimental hemorrhagic shock models. Fed. Proc. 20:30, 1961.

85. Shires, T., F.T. Brown, P.C. Conizano, and N. Somerville. Distributional changes in extracellular fluid during acute hemorrhagic shock. Surg. Forum 11:15, 1960.

86. Shizgal, H.M., G.A. Lopez, and J.R. Gutelius. Extracellular fluid volume changes following hemorrhagic shock. Surg. Forum 18:35, 1968.

87. Shoemaker, W.C., and F. Iida. Studies on the equilibrium of labelled red cells and T-1824 in hemorrhagic shock. Surg. Gynecol. Obstet. 114:539, 1962.

88. Shoemaker, W.C., and R.S. Brown. The dilemma of vasopressors and vasodilators in the therapy of shock. Surg. Gynecol. Obstet. 132:51, 1971.

89. Simeone, F.A. Experimental hemorrhagic shock and irreversibility. In: *Shock and Hypotension,* edited by L.C. Mills and J.H. Moyer. New York: Grune & Stratton, 1965.

90. Stallworth, J.M., H. Ramirez, B.A. Barrington, Jr., and R.R. Bradham. Hypovolemic shock microcirculatory changes during and after specific therapy. Am. Surg. 169:694, 1969.

91. Staples, D., C. Topuzlu, and E. Blair. A comparison of ATP

levels in hemorrhagic and in endotoxin shock. Clin. Res. 16:555, 1968.

92. Stoner, H.B., and C.J. Threlfall. *The Biochemical Response to Injury*. Oxford: Blackwell, 1960.

93. Talaat, S.M., W.H. Massion, and J.A. Schilling. Effects of adenosine triphosphate administration in irreversible hemorrhagic shock. Surgery 55:813, 1964.

94. Wiggers, C.J. *Physiology of Shock*. New York: The Commonwealth Fund, 1950.

95. Wilson, R.F., and R.R. Fisher. The hemodynamic effects of massive steroids in clinical shock. Surg. Gynecol. Obstet. 127:769, 1968.

96. Wolfman, E.F., Jr., S.A. Neill, D.K. Heaps, and G.D. Quidema. Donor blood and isotonic salt solution: Effect on survival after hemorrhagic shock and operation. Arch. Surg. 86: 869, 1963.

97. Zweifach, B.W. Microcirculatory derangements as a basis for the lethal manifestations of experimental shock. Brit. J. Anaesthesiol. 30:466, 1958.

98. Zweifach, B.W., A.L. Nagler, and W. Troll. Some effects of proteolytic inhibitors on tissue injury and systemic anaphylaxis. J. Exptl. Med. 113:437, 1961.

99. Zweifach, B.W. Functional deterioration of terminal vascular beds in irreversible hemorrhagic shock. Ann. N.Y. Acad. Sci. 55:370, 1952.

HISTAMINE RELEASE IN ENDOTOXIN SHOCK: EFFECT OF DEXAMETHASONE ADMINISTRATION

William Schumer, M.D.

Department of Surgery, College of Medicine, University of Illinois at the VA West Side Hospital, Chicago, Illinois

Informal Presentation[1]

We have been doing some work in our laboratories with immunological factors and histamine. It has been proposed that bacterial endotoxins possess little or no intrinsic toxic activity, but that they exert their myriad pathophysiological effects by an antigenic action (12). Weil and Spink reported a marked resemblance between the effects of anaphylactic and endotoxic shock (14). When Lichtenstein and associates incubated endotoxin from *Veillonella alcalescens* or *Serratia marcescens* with guinea pig complement, they were able to produce an anaphylatoxin which had a contractile effect on guinea pig ileum (8). This action was significantly inhibited by antihistamines, indicating a histamine release. In this connection, Hinshaw and co-workers found that plasma histamine increased after induction of endotoxic shock (5). The role of histamine in anaphylactic shock has been well documented (7), but its role in endotoxic shock has received scant attention. The research efforts of our laboratory have been directed toward the elucidation of the mechanism and treatment of septic shock. Therefore, we decided to study the conditions required for *Escherichia coli* endotoxin-induced histamine release and then the effect of the potent anti-endotoxic agent, dexamethasone, on this releasing activity (4).

In the present investigation, we used the rat peritoneal cavity as a test system. White male rats, weighing 165-225 g,

---

[1]This manuscript appears here as presented at the symposium, with minor editorial revisions.

TABLE 1

HISTAMINE CONTENT IN PLASMA OF ENDOTOXIN-CHALLENGED RATS

Treatment	No. rats	Histamine (ng/ml)[a]	Increment or decrement[b]	P value[c]
Saline (0.5 ml)	5	158	—	—
Endotoxin (12 mg/kg)	5	216	+58(+27%)	<0.01
Endotoxin + dexamethasone (25 μg/kg)	5	110	-48(+44%)	<0.05

[a]Plasma histamine content was measured 1 hour after treatment. Mean values are given.

[b]Compared to control levels (ng/ml) before treatment.

[c]Student's "t" test.

were adrenalectomized and 48 hours later were injected intraperitoneally with 25 ml of modified Tyrode's solution by means of a cannula. In control animals, the lateral tail vein was injected with 0.5 ml of saline. Experimental animals similarly received *E. coli* endotoxin solution (12 mg/kg, Difco) either alone or containing dexamethasone sodium phosphate (25 μg/kg, Merck Sharpe and Dohme). A zero time sample of peritoneal exudate was withdrawn through the cannula. At 1 hour after challenge, plasma was analyzed for histamine by Shore's spectrofluorometric method (11). Concomitantly, the peritoneal cavity was opened and a 4-ml sample removed. Both peritoneal samples were analyzed for histamine according to Norn's method (10).

Table 1 shows that 1 hour after endotoxin challenge, plasma histamine concentration rose, supporting the findings of Hinshaw and co-workers (5). Dexamethasone given simultaneously with endotoxin completely suppressed plasma histamine release and significantly decreased the plasma histamine content below control levels. During the same period, histamine in the peritoneal exudate increased twofold over control levels; dexamethasone reduced the peritoneal exudate histamine by 40% (Table 2). It has been reported that glucocorticoids inhibit the hypersensitivity phenomenon at

TABLE 2

HISTAMINE CONTENT OF RAT PERITONEAL EXUDATE AFTER ENDOTOXIN CHALLENGE

Treatment	No. rats	Histamine (ng/ml)[a] Initial values	After 1 hr	Increment	*P* value[b]
Saline (0.5 ml)	8	34.0	42.2	+8.2	—
Endotoxin (12 mg/kg)	8	34.5	59.1	+24.6	<0.01
Endotoxin + dexamethasone (25 μg/kg)	9	34.1	52.0	+17.9	<0.05

[a]Mean values (nanograms/ml of exudate).

[b]Student's "t" test comparing rats treated with endotoxin and dexamethasone to saline-treated rats.

the level of antibody production (1,9). Yet, once immunity is established, they suppress the cytopathogenic response partially or not at all (2,3). Recently, however, Jennings showed that glucocorticoids can interfere with the lytic response of sensitized cells by forming an unstable association with immune reactants. He proposed that steroids block the combination of complement with the antigen-antibody complex (6).

An *in vitro* study using peritoneal exudate cells from intact rats was performed to establish the requirements for histamine release by endotoxin, and to evaluate the effect of dexamethasone on this activity. Preliminary results revealed that endotoxin alone was ineffective in releasing histamine. However, upon addition of reconstituted lyophilized guinea pig serum and magnesium chloride, a consistent increment in free histamine was observed. Guinea pig serum alone did not cause histamine release. After incubation of endotoxin with guinea pig serum, formation of the histamine-releasing factor could be inhibited by either decreasing the temperature to 4°C, by adding ethylenediaminetetraacetic acid, or by heating at 100°C for 5 minutes. This histamine-releasing factor could be separated from endotoxin and serum by filtering with a CF50A membrane ultrafilter (Amicon Corp.,

Lexington, Mass.). The filtrate, containing molecules below 50,000 molecular weight, revealed the histamine-releasing activity. This supports the contention that endotoxin induces the histamine release through the formation of anaphylatoxin (8).

The effect of dexamethasone on the histamine-releasing activity was determined by the incubation of guinea pig serum with saline, endotoxin, and dexamethasone. Evidently, the histamine-releasing activity generated by incubation of serum with endotoxin is only minimally depressed when dexamethasone is added after incubation. However, if it is added before incubation, histamine release is significantly diminished.

Further support for the dexamethasone effect was provided by determining the amount of intracellular histamine. This was calculated according to the following scheme: the cells were sedimented and histamine concentration in the supernatant was measured. Subtracting this value from total histamine yielded quantitation of intracellular histamine. Figure 1 reveals that the generation of anaphylatoxin results in a three- to fourfold decrease in intracellular histamine levels. Experiments in which anaphylatoxin generation was inhibited by dexamethasone showed a decrease in intracellular histamine content to one-half the control value. These data would support a proposal that dexamethasone prevents the generation of anaphylatoxin from complement, thus reducing histamine release. A second but not exclusive alternative has been proposed by Surján and Csaba (13), *i.e.*, that dexamethasone may lyse immature acid-mucopolysaccharides which bind histamine, resulting in a lower percentage of free histamine. The lytic effect hypothesis was supported by our experiments in which dexamethasone alone was incubated with serum and the resulting mixture was used to challenge the peritoneal exudate. The results revealed free histamine levels below saline control levels (Fig. 2). This effect was also noted in the *in vivo* plasma histamine determinations (Table 1).

In our determination of intracellular and free histamine, we found that their sum never equalled the total histamine, the residual being denoted as "bound" histamine. The nature of this extracellular "bound" histamine is unknown, but it supports the possibility that a combination of histamine with heparin or other acid-mucopolysaccharide occurs, since the proportion of this fraction increases significantly over saline controls when either anaphylatoxin or dexamethasone is present (Fig. 3).

From these observations, we propose that dexamethasone interferes with histamine release by preventing the generation of anaphylatoxin when administered in close temporal proximity to endotoxin, and that these findings may help explain the anti-endotoxic

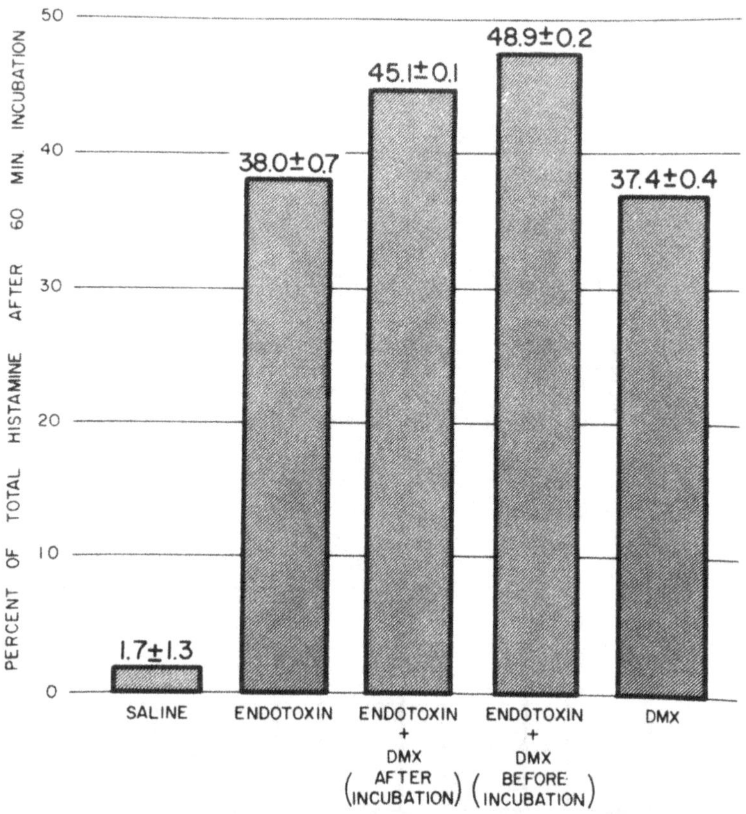

FIG. 1. *In vitro* intracellular histamine in peritoneal mast cell exudate. Control tubes containing 6.3 ml of reconstituted guinea pig serum (Hyland, Costa Mesa, Calif.) were incubated for 60 minutes at 37°C with 0.5 ml of saline. Experimental tubes contained serum with 0.5 ml (2.6 mg) endotoxin solution, 0.5 ml endotoxin solution with 4 μg dexamethasone added after incubation but before challenge, 0.5 ml endotoxin solution with dexamethasone added before incubation and challenge, and 0.5 ml of dexamethasone solution. Twenty nanomoles of magnesium chloride was added to each tube before incubation. After incubation, 20 ml of freshly pooled peritoneal exudate from intact rats was added, and tubes were incubated for 60 minutes at 37°C. Values shown represent the percentage of calculated intracellular histamine in the exudate.

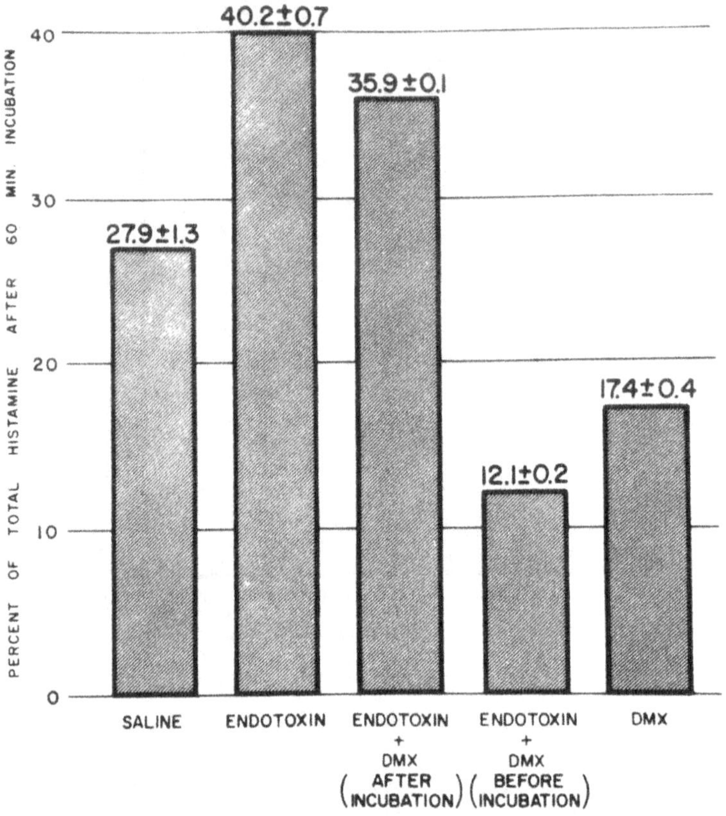

FIG. 2. *In vitro* free histamine in peritoneal mast cell exudate. Free histamine concentration in the exudate after challenge is expressed as a percentage of total histamine after a correction for guinea pig serum histamine. (For experimental details, see legend for Fig. 1.)

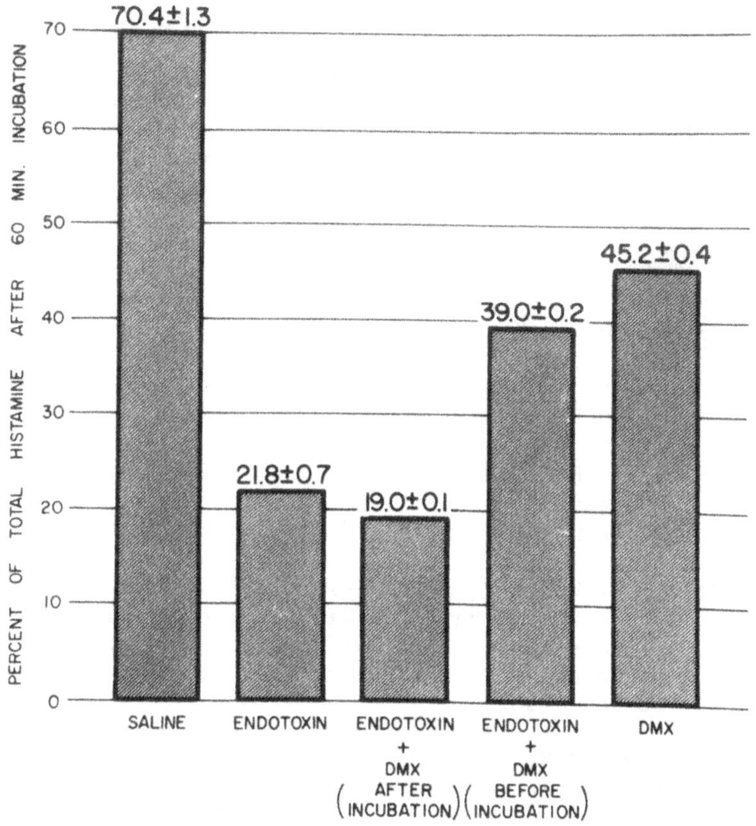

FIG. 3. *In vitro* "bound" histamine in peritoneal mast cell exudate. Values shown represent the percentage of calculated histamine appearing as "bound". (For experimental details, see legend for Fig. 1.)

properties ascribed to this drug. If the role of histamine in endotoxic shock could be clarified, our observations would support the contention that steroids must be administered in the early stages of septic shock.

When this work was presented, Dr. Hinshaw stated that he gave antihistamines to animals in septic shock and was unable to improve their survival rate. Just recently, we did a study in which rats were given compound 48/80, causing degranulation of the mast cells. We used a technique developed by West which reduced the histamine content to 10% of the original amount. We then gave these adrenalectomized, histamine-depleted animals 25 μg/kg endotoxin. Ordinarily, this dose causes 100% mortality, but only 30% of our animals died.

It is our impression from these studies that endotoxin exerts its effect primarily through an immunological factor, probably complement or an antigen-antibody reaction.

REFERENCES

1. Bjorneboe, M., E.M. Fischel, and H.C. Stoerk. The effect of cortisone and adrenocorticotrophic hormone on the concentration of circulating antibody. J. Exptl. Med. 93:39, 1951.

2. Blumer, H., M. Richter, F. Cua-Limg, and B. Rose. Precipitating and nonprecipitating antibodies in the primary and secondary immune responses: Rate of decline, anaphylaxis-sensitizing capacity, and the effect of cortisone. J. Immunol. 88:669, 1962.

3. Fischel, E.E., J.H. Vaughan, and C. Photopoulos. Inhibition of rapid production of antibody by cortisone: Study of secondary response. Proc. Soc. Exptl. Biol. Med. 81:344, 1952.

4. Fukuda, T., and N. Hata. Mechanisms of endotoxin shock in rats and the anti-endotoxic effect of glucocorticoids and endotoxin-conditioning. Japan J. Physiol. 19:509, 1969.

5. Hinshaw, L.B., J.A. Vick, C.H. Carlson, and Y. Fan. Role of histamine in endotoxin shock. Proc. Soc. Exptl. Biol. Med. 104:379, 1960.

6. Jennings, J.F. The effect of hydrocortisone on immune lysis of cells induced by cytotoxic antibody and complement *in vitro*. J. Immunol. 96:409, 1966.

7. Lecomte, J. In: *CIBA Foundation Symposium on Histamine*, edited by G.E.W. Wolsteinholme and C.M. O'Connor. Boston: Little, Brown & Co., 1956, p. 173.

8. Lichtenstein, L.M., H. Gewurz, N.F. Adkinson, Jr., H.S. Shin, and S.E. Mergenhagen. Interactions of the complement system with endotoxic lipopolysaccharide: The generation of an anaphylatoxin. Immunology 16:327, 1969.

9. Malkiel, S., and B.J. Hargis. The effect of ACTH and cortisone on the quantitative precipitin reaction. J. Immunol. 69:217, 1952.

10. Norn, S. Effect of histamine liberators on rat peritoneal mast cells and influence of antirheumatic agents. Acta pharmacol. toxicol. 25:281, 1966.

11. Shore, P.A., A. Burkhalter, and V.H. Cohn, Jr. A method for the fluorometric assay of histamine in tissues. J. Pharmacol. Exptl. Therap. 127:182, 1959.

12. Stetson, C.A., Jr. Studies on the mechanism of the Shwartzman phenomenon: Similarities between reactions to endotoxins and certain reactions of bacterial allergy. J. Exptl. Med. 101: 421, 1955.

13. Surján, L., Jr., and G. Csaba. Effect of prednisolone on anaphylactic reaction of peritoneal mast cells of the rat. Z. Mikro. Anat. Forsch. 80:321, 1969.

14. Weil, M.H., and W.W. Spink. A comparison of shock due to endotoxin with anaphylactic shock. J. Lab. Clin. Med. 50: 501, 1957.

DOPAMINE IN THE TREATMENT OF SHOCK

Linda L. Shanbour, Ph.D.

Program in Physiology, The University of Texas Medical School at Houston, Houston, Texas

Various agents have been advocated in the treatment of shock, and certain advantages and disadvantages attend the use of each. The problem is complicated because the underlying mechanism of shock is not understood. In order to quantitate the effects of septic shock in the laboratory, *Escherichia coli* endotoxin has been administered to the dog and monkey. Since most studies have been conducted on the dog I will limit this discussion to the canine species, recognizing fully that shock in primates may be different.

The development of systemic hypotension, after the injection of lethal doses of endotoxin, may be accounted for by decreases in total peripheral resistance (9,15,17) and cardiac output (15,17, 35). Many studies have been conducted on the heart during endotoxic and hemorrhagic shock (1,6,7,9,12,21,25). The majority suggest that cardiac tissue suffers no direct toxic damage, and most effects can be attributed to low blood flow and diminished tissue perfusion. Recent studies by Hinshaw and colleagues support this conclusion (13). Many substances, such as histamine, are released during shock and have deleterious effects on pre- and postcapillary segments (3,5,14). In general, there is net dilation of precapillary and net constriction of postcapillary segments. This leads to progressive decrease in total peripheral resistance and in venous return, with subsequent decrease in cardiac output. The primary drop in arterial pressure is caused by a decrease in venous return (21,35). Hinshaw *et al.* (16) have shown that the decrease in venous return is caused mainly by hepatosplanchnic pooling which results from hepatic venous constriction. Because of the decrease in circulating blood volume, blood flow to the kidneys decreases, with subsequent retention of waste products. Another major region which is affected is the splanchnic bed. With decreased splanchnic blood flow, the gut wall becomes necrotic, with subsequent release of toxic substances from the gut which further prolong the shock condition. Any agent or combination of agents which would alleviate these conditions would have potential therapeutic value in the clinic.

Dopamine (3,4-dihydroxyphenethylamine) has many interesting properties. Its effects on the peripheral vasculature are highly variable and species-dependent. In the dog, dopamine, when administered in doses which do not affect mean blood pressure, elicits peripheral vasoconstriction and selective vasodilation in the renal, superior mesenteric, and celiac vascular beds (8). Dopamine exerts direct actions on the heart (2,18,23). It increases cardiac output by both inotropic and chronotropic effects. Its effects are dose-related. Administration of 2-4 μg/kg body weight has little or no cardiac effect and produces slight pressor-depressor responses. A dose of 8-16 μg/kg increases the contractile force of heart muscle and the heart rate, with more pronounced effects on blood pressure. At higher doses, 32-64 μg/kg, marked increments are observable in heart contractile force, heart rate, and systemic arterial pressure (23). Use of alpha- and beta-adrenergic receptor blocking agents in experimentally induced shock suggest that the pressor effect of dopamine is due to both beta-inotropic action on the heart and alpha-adrenergic receptor stimulation in the peripheral vasculature (4). Its vasodilatory properties appear to result from beta-adrenergic receptor stimulation, with the exception of renal and splanchnic beds. Dopamine produces vasodilation of these two beds which is not blocked by beta-adrenergic receptor blocking agents (36). Dopamine infusion in water-loaded dogs increases Na^+, K^+, and osmolal excretion, as well as *p*-aminohippurate and inulin clearances (24).

An increasing number of clinical studies indicate that dopamine exerts beneficial effects in patients in various shock states (10,11,19,20,22,34). In a representative study, MacCannel *et al.* administered dopamine to 11 hypotensive patients, six of whom had signs of postinfection, cardiogenic, or neurologic shock (20). Most of these patients had received prior medication and showed no significant improvement. However, when dopamine was infused, peripheral circulation and urinary output was improved in five cases, and an additional five showed improvement in one of these. Dopamine infusion increases sodium excretion in patients with severe congestive heart failure (11). In contrast to other sympathomimetic amines, dopamine increases glomerular filtration rate and renal plasma flow (32). Dopamine has never been reported to produce bradycardia in man.

Studies in our laboratory have been concerned with exploring the actions of dopamine in the endotoxin-shocked dog. In a series of studies designed to evaluate the cardiovascular effects, a venous return preparation was used in which peripheral effects could be separated from cardiac effects (27-30). In this preparation, the cardiac inflow was held constant. Intra-atrial infusions of dopamine (17-34 μg/kg/minute) increased venous return and mean systemic arterial pressure. Dopamine prevented pooling during the infusion time. With these infusion rates, tachycardia and decreased portal vein pressure were evidenced.

Since the major site of pooling in the dog is the liver, additional studies were conducted to evaluate the effects of dopamine on the isolated, perfused canine liver (31). Dopamine infusion produced marked reductions in liver weight before endotoxin administration and continued reductions at slower rates afterwards. No significant changes occurred in portal venous or hepatic venous resistances. Dopamine increased hepatic artery constriction. The mechanism of liver shrinkage is postulated to be primarily due to active contraction of the sinusoidal linings of the liver.

Since dopamine exerted marked beneficial effects on the heart and liver, extensive studies were conducted to evaluate the effects of dopamine on renal hemodynamics and function (32). However, contrary to the other studies, pre- and post-treatment of shocked animals with dopamine failed to significantly improve any of the measured parameters. It was necessary to block the constrictor action of dopamine with the alpha blocking agent, phenoxybenzamine, and to administer dextran for volume replacement. The combination of dopamine with phenoxybenzamine and dextran significantly increased renal blood flow, decreased renal resistance, increased glomerular filtration rate, and increased urine flow. These studies point to the importance of a combination of agents rather than a single agent for beneficial results in the treatment of shock.

Similar actions are suggested when the effects of dopamine infusion on the splanchnic bed are evaluated (33). When dopamine is infused into the superior mesenteric artery of a dog in hemorrhagic shock, mesenteric blood flow further decreases. In the normal dog, phenoxybenzamine reverses the dopamine responses of the mesenteric bed to those of pure vasodilation (no transient constriction was observed). The beta-receptor blocking agent, propranolol or haloperidal, which has been suggested as a specific blocking agent for the dopamine receptor (26), failed to attenuate the mesenteric responses to dopamine.

These studies suggest that dopamine alone is insufficient in the treatment of shock patients and that a combination of agents,

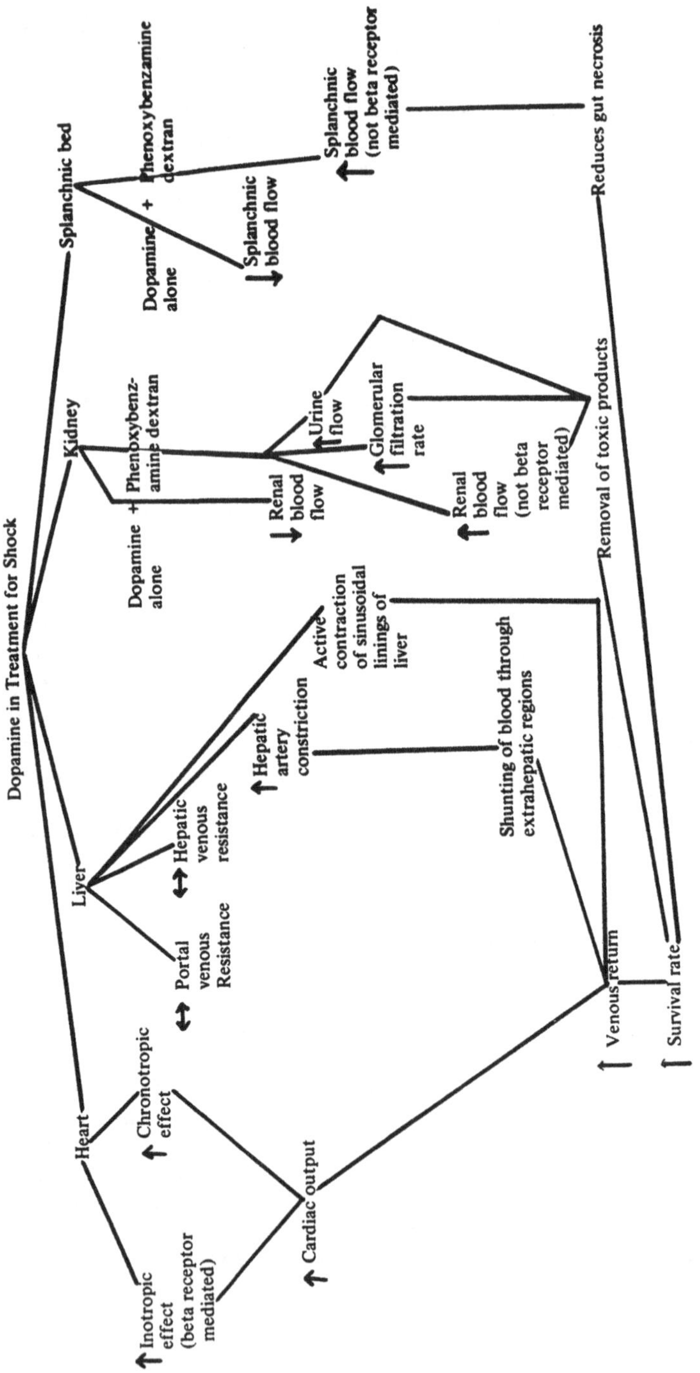

FIG. 1. Suggested mode of action of dopamine during treatment for shock.

such as dopamine, phenoxybenzamine, and dextran, is more desirable. In addition, a buffering agent should be included to reduce the degree of acidosis which is typically observed.

Survival studies in which dopamine alone was infused in 12 intact, nonperfused dogs suggest a survival benefit from dopamine since a greater percentage of treated animals survived (50%, compared to 17%) (30). This percentage is predicted to increase when dopamine is administered with a combination of agents, such as those suggested.

Figure 1 illustrates a suggested mode of action of dopamine during treatment for shock. Inotropic and chronotropic effects on the heart would increase cardiac output which, in turn, would contribute to an increase in venous return. An increase in hepatic artery constriction would result in the shunting of blood through extrahepatic regions. This, together with active contraction of the sinusoidal linings of the liver, would aid in increasing the venous return. Dopamine, used in combination with phenoxybenzamine and dextran, would increase renal blood flow, glomerular filtration rate, and urine flow. Toxic products thus would be more adequately removed. The combination of dopamine, phenoxybenzamine, and dextran would increase splanchnic blood flow and reduce potential gut necrosis. Increase in venous return, removal of toxic products, and reduced gut necrosis would increase survival rate.

SUMMARY

Although dopamine shows promise as a valuable therapeutic agent in the treatment of various forms of shock, it is still under experimental investigation. If, indeed, dopamine has clinical value, it will probably be most effective when administered in combination with other agents.

REFERENCES

1. Alican, F., M.L. Dalton, Jr., and J.D. Hardy. Experimental endotoxin shock. Am. J. Sur. 103:702-708, 1962.

2. Black, W.L., and E.L. Rolett. Dopamine-induced alterations in left ventricular performance. Circ. Res. 19:71-79, 1966.

3. Brake, C.M., L.B. Hinshaw, and T.E. Emerson. Alteration of vascular responses to endotoxin by adrenergic blockage. Am. J. Physiol. 207:149-151, 1964.

4. Carvalho, M., J.K. Vyden, H. Berstein, H. Gold, and E. Corday. Hemodynamic effects of 3-hydroxytyramine (dopamine) in experimentally induced shock. Am. J. Cardiol. 23:217-223, 1969.

5. Chien, S., and L. Krakoff. Hemodynamics of dogs in histamine shock, with special reference to splanchnic blood volume and flow. Circ. Res. 12:29-39, 1963.

6. Crowell, J.W.,and A.C. Guyton. Evidence favoring a cardiac mechanism in irreversible hemorrhagic shock. Am. J. Physiol. 201:893-896, 1961.

7. Ebert, R.V., and R.S. Abernathy. Septic shock. Fed. Proc. 20:179-184, 1961.

8. Eble, J.N. A proposed mechanism for the depressor effect of dopamine in the anesthetized dog. J. Pharmacol. Exptl. Ther. 145:64-70, 1964.

9. Frohlich, E.D., J.B. Scott, and E.S. Dooley. Hemodynamic alterations due to *Salmonella typhosa* endotoxin with special reference to the coronary vascular bed. J. Clin. Invest. 41:147-152, 1962.

10. Gifford, R.M., K.L. MacCannell, J.L. McNay, and J.A. Haas. Changes in regional blood flows induced by dopamine and by isoproterenol during experimental hemorrhagic shock. Can. J. Physiol. Pharmacol. 46:847-851, 1968.

11. Goldberg, L., R. McDonald, Jr., and A. Zimmerman. Sodium diuresis produced by dopamine in patients with congestive heart failure. New Engl. J. Med. 269:1060-1064, 1963.

12. Guyton, A.C., and J.W. Crowell. Dynamics of the heart in shock. Fed. Proc. 20:51-60, 1961.

13. Hinshaw, L.B., L.T. Archer, J.A. Miller, L.J. Greenfield, and C.A. Guenter. Absence of direct action of endotoxin on myocardial tissue. Physiologist 13: 222, 1970.

14. Hinshaw, L.B., T.E. Emerson, Jr., P.F. Iampietro, and C.M. Brake. A comparative study of the hemodynamic actions of histamine and endotoxin. Am. J. Physiol. 203:600-606, 1962.

15. Hinshaw, L.B., R.P. Gilbert, H. Kuida, and M.B. Visscher. Peripheral resistance changes and blood pooling after endotoxin in eviscerated dogs. Am. J. Physiol. 195:631-634, 1958.

16. Hinshaw, L.B., D.A. Reins, and R.J. Hill. Response of iso-

lated liver to endotoxin. Can. J. Physiol. Pharmacol. 44:529-541, 1966.

17. Hinshaw, L.B., J.A. Vick, L.E. Wittmers, D.M. Worthen, D.L. Nelson, and O.P. Swenson. Changes in peripheral resistance in endotoxin shock. Proc. Soc. Exptl. Biol. Med. 108: 24-27, 1961.

18. Holmes, J.C.,and N.O. Fowler. Direct cardiac effects of dopamine. Circ. Res. 10:68-72, 1962.

19. Horwitz, D., S.M. Fox, and L.I. Goldberg. Effects of dopamine in man. Circ. Res. 10:237-243, 1962.

20. MacCannell, K.L., J.L. McKay, M.B. Meyer, and L.I. Goldberg. Dopamine in the treatment of hypotension and shock. New Engl. J. Med. 275:1389-1398, 1966.

21. MacLean, L.D.,and M.H. Weil. Hypotension (shock) in dogs produced by *E. coli* endotoxin. Circ. Res. 4:546-556, 1956.

22. McDonald, R., Jr., L. Goldberg, J. McNay, and E. Tuttle, Jr. Effects of dopamine in man: Augmentation of sodium excretion, glomerular filtration rate, and renal plasma flow. J. Clin. Invest. 43:1116-1124, 1964.

23. McDonald, R.H.,and L.I. Goldberg. Analysis of the cardiovascular effects of dopamine in the dog. J. Pharmacol. Exptl. Ther. 140:60-66, 1963.

24. Meyer, M.B., J.L. McNay, and L.I. Goldberg. Effects of dopamine on renal function and hemodynamics in the dog. J. Pharm. Exptl. Ther. 156:186-192, 1967.

25. Palmerio, C., S.C. Ming, E.D. Frank, and J. Fine. Cardiac tissue response to endotoxin. Proc. Soc. Exptl. Biol. Med. 109:773-776, 1962.

26. Rossum, J.M., van. The significance of dopamine-receptor blockade for the mechanisms of action of neuroleptic agents. Arch. Intern. Pharmacodyn. Ther. 160: 492-494, 1966.

27. Shanbour, L.L., and L.B. Hinshaw. Effects of dopamine infusion in endotoxin shock in the dog. Fed. Proc. 28:271, 1969.

28. Shanbour, L.L., and L.B. Hinshaw. Mechanism of action of dopamine in endotoxin shock. Basel: *Fourth International Congress on Pharmacology*, 1969, p. 315.

29. Shanbour, L.L., and L.B. Hinshaw. Cardiovascular effects of dopamine in endotoxin shock. Physiologist 12;354, 1969.

30. Shanbour, L.L., and L.B. Hinshaw. Cardiac and peripheral effects of dopamine infusion in endotoxin shock in the dog. J. Pharmacol. Exptl. Ther. 170:108-116, 1969.

31. Shanbour, L.L., and L.B. Hinshaw. Effects of dopamine on the liver before and following administration of endotoxin. Can. J. Physiol. Pharmacol. 47:923-928, 1969.

32. Shanbour, L.L., R.D. Lindeman, L.T. Archer, S.H. Tung, and L.B. Hinshaw. Improvement of renal hemodynamics in endotoxin shock with dopamine, phenoxybenzamine and dextran. J. Pharmacol. Exptl. Ther. 176:383-388, 1971.

33. Shanbour, L.L., and D. Parker. Comparative and competitive effects of dopamine and other catecholamines on the splanchnic bed. (In preparation).

34. Talley, R.C., L.I. Goldberg, C.E. Johnson, and J.L. McNay. A hemodynamic comparison of dopamine and isoproterenol in patients in shock. Circulation 39:361-378, 1969.

35. Weil, M.H., L.D. MacLean, M.B. Visscher, and W.W. Spink. Studies on the circulatory changes in the dog produced by endotoxin from gram-negative microorganisms. J. Clin. Invest. 35:1191-1198, 1956.

36. Yeh, B.K., J.L. McNay, and L.I. Goldberg. Attenuation of dopamine renal and mesenteric vasodilation by haloperidol: Evidence for a specific dopamine receptor. J. Pharmacol. Exptl. Ther. 168:303-309, 1969.

LIVER METABOLISM AND ENERGY PRODUCTION IN *Staphylococcus aureus* SEPTIC SHOCK IN MICE[1]

Ian M. Smith, M.D., and Kanai L. Mukherjee, Ph.D.

Infectious Disease Division, Department of Internal Medicine, University of Iowa Hospitals, Iowa City, Iowa

In 5-28% of septic shock patients in different series, infections with gram-positive organisms were responsible for the sepsis. Most were caused by *Staphylococcus aureus* (5,15). Extensive studies have been made of the many toxins produced by staphylococcal cells. Experimental studies have also been made of infections in animals, but the subtle biochemical interactions between host metabolism and a challenging infection with *S. aureus* have received scant attention (6). We have felt that nothing less than whole bacteria, with their many chemical products, and the whole living animal should be the objects of study initially. Our experiments have demonstrated the importance of hepatic metabolism, particularly in relation to glycolysis and mitochondrial function (36).

MATERIALS AND METHODS

Albino white Swiss mice of the Rockland Swiss Webster strain were delivered regularly to the laboratory from Arthur Sutter, Springfield, Missouri. Four or more days were allowed to elapse for equilibration before the mice were used for the experiments. The mice weighed 26±3 g; they were housed 10 to a cage, fed Purina Mouse Chow, and given water *ad libitum*. Food was withheld for the 16 hours preceding the experiment unless otherwise noted.

Infection was produced with the hemolytic, coagulase-positive Smith strain of *S. aureus*. This strain, originally phage-type

---

[1]This research was supported by grants from the USPHS (AI 04046) and the Iowa Thoracic Society.

44A/42E (also called SA 235), was isolated from a patient with osteomyelitis in 1930, and has been maintained in our laboratory by regular *in vitro* transfer.

The staphylococci were prepared for injection as follows. A 4-hour culture of the staphylococci was made in brain-heart infusion broth (Difco) at 37° C. Petri dishes with infusion broth agar were flooded with 0.3 ml of 4-hour growth and incubated at 37° C overnight. The confluent growth was washed off in 3 ml of distilled water and 0.1 ml of this material (10^9 cells) was used as the intraperitoneal challenge.

Bacteria were enumerated on solid media by plating dilutions with a standard volume platinum loop. Homogenates of organs were made in 5 ml of distilled water in Pyrex tubes with Teflon grinders which were attached to an electric motor.

Blood was collected from the mice by beheading them with scissors. All chemical estimations were made within 30-60 minutes. Pools of blood were made from two to five mice. In some selected estimations, blood was obtained by cardiac puncture.

Values obtained "at death" were the result of challenging 10 mice. When two died, the remaining eight were killed to harvest blood or organs. Otherwise, the eight mice would have died within a span of 45 minutes.

Treatment Model

Chemicals used for treatment were all given subcutaneously 1 hour after challenge. All reagents were chemically pure or of USP standards. Initially, control experiments were performed by equal-volume treatments with saline or sucrose. However, because they never differed from those performed on animals not so controlled, they were abandoned. The quantity injected subcutaneously was a 1:16 dilution of an LD_{50} of the substance being tested.

The data were analyzed by comparing the time from challenge until death for 10 control animals with the time to death for 10 treated animals. A statistical analysis was also made by the chi-square method. The level of significance used was $P \leq 0.05$.

Systolic blood pressures were measured by a modification of the radioisotope tail-cuff technique described by Hicks and associates (10). Mitochondrial suspensions were prepared by the method of Schneider and Hogeboom (26), except that the initial nuclear fraction was separated at 1,000 x *g* and the subsequent supernatant containing the mitochondria was centrifuged at 10,000 x *g*. The mitochondrial fraction obtained at 10,000 x *g* was resuspended and washed twice in 0.25 M sucrose solution. Electron microscopy confirmed the purity of mitochondria prepared by this method.

The respiratory rate of the mitochondria from the various organs was determined by standard Warburg manometric techniques. All results of respiratory rates were the average from duplicate samples, with measurements starting after a 10-minute equilibration period. Later studies were made using an oxygen polarograph.

Mitochondrial function was quantitated by nitrogen determinations using the standard micro-Kjeldahl technique. All mitochondrial activity was expressed as $QO_2(N)$, representing the microliters of oxygen consumed per hour per milligram of mitochondrial nitrogen. Later mitochondrial studies were made by oxygen polarography (Gilson Medical Electronics). Lipids and lipid fractions were measured by the methods described by Henry (9). Total fatty acids were determined as methyl esters by gas-liquid chromatography (Hewlitt Packard #5750) after separation by thin-layer chromatography.

RESULTS

The model used in these studies has been developed over a period of years; we find it useful and dependable. Because it differs in many respects from other infection models, a detailed description is included.

Our investigations have shown a constant number of staphylococci in the bodies of moribund and dead mice regardless of the inoculation route or the dose of staphylococci within the range of 10^7 to 10^{11} bacteria (31,34). Inocula of 10^6 or fewer bacteria kill irregularly or are nonfatal. When they do kill, however, the number of bacteria at death is the same as when the regularly fatal dose is administered. This critical lethal dose of staphylococci has also been noted by Sellers and LeMaistre (27). It is not possible to choose an LD_{50} of staphylococci which will predictably kill 50% of the animals at a predetermined time. A dose of 10^9 bacteria intraperitoneally, however, will always prove lethal to 90-100% of the animals at 270±20 minutes. Therefore, this work was confined to the use of large dose (0.1 ml = 10^9 organisms) to produce intraperitoneal infection. Multiplication of the inoculated staphylococci, from 10^9 to 10^{10} or higher, occurs during the challenge period. The need to challenge with a high dose of inoculum to produce a predictable number of deaths in a predetermined interval has also been noted by Saslaw in his experiments with Macaca monkeys (25). Guenter and Hinshaw have used a similarly high number of microorganisms in other experiments with monkeys (8). Death is not caused by extracellular products alone, as shown by the nonlethality of broth culture filtrates in large doses and by the failure of bacteria enclosed in an intraperitoneal Millipore filter chamber to cause death. Animals with such chambers can live 336 hours or longer, but chamber leaks are common. The chamber contains 10^8 to 10^9 bacteria when removed at autopsy—a quantity of bacteria which would kill at 4-6 hours if injected directly into the peritoneum (34). The need for whole bacteria rather than exotoxins is also shown by the production of death by the protoplasmic fraction of *S. aureus* separated by the Servall-Ribi refrigerated cell fractionator (35) or by the use of trypsin nafcillin digestion and Sephadex column separation (11). In general, we have avoided the use of single toxins, as this method has already been shown to be inadequate in studies of death from anthrax, where three toxins act symbiotically and each toxin individually cannot kill (30). Staphylococci produce many toxins, and the arbitrary choice of any one could and has led to unsuccessful studies of the cause of death. The whole bacteria and the protoplasmic extract are both heat-labile, and therefore they differ from endotoxin.

The shortest period between challenge and death has been 60 minutes after intravenous injection of 10^{11} bacteria (34). We believe this indicates that death is not a direct toxic event from the chemicals in the challenge material, but that it involves some interaction with host systems.

The mice develop shock during the 4.5-hour study period. Animals dying of *S. aureus* challenge become profoundly hypothermic, with a rectal temperature of 37.2° C (99° F). In an hour or so, this falls to 32.8° C (91° F), and to 25° C (77° F) at death. Urine production virtually ceases. Normal mice produce 1.4 ml urine per hour and mice in staphylococcal shock produce 0.42 ml urine per hour. The systolic blood pressure (measured by release of intraperitoneally injected radioactive material into the tail when a cuff is deflated) falls from a normal value of 112 mm Hg to 76 mm Hg (24). The blood volume obtainable by free bleeding after decapitation is reduced from a normal of 0.38 ml to 0.27 ml. During the same period, the hematocrit rises from 43% to 67%. Blood viscosity is increased, clot retraction ceases, and platelets fall from 154,000 to 53,000/cu mm.

After the bacteriologic variables were standardized, the model infection was studied by a variety of biochemical methods (Table 1). The blood, carcass, and then the various organs were examined successively. The liver, in particular, demonstrated a number of profound changes.

At death from *S. aureus* challenge, the blood was found to have significantly increased levels of inorganic phosphorus, alkaline phosphatase, and transaminase (4). These changes were

TABLE 1

BIOCHEMICAL VALUES IN MICE AT DEATH FROM INTRAPERITONEAL INFECTION WITH *S. aureus* (10^9)

	BLOOD		CARCASS		LIVER	
	Normal	At Death	Normal	At Death	Normal	At Death
Sugar (mg%)	52.7±12.2	35.8±14.5	58.6±13.2	18.8± 9.9[a]	124± 49	15± 0[a]
Inorganic phosphorus (mg%)	9.7± 0.7	12.8± 1.7[a]	9.0± 6.9	21.2± 0.8[a]	25.6± 7.1	44.8±21.9[a]
Alkaline phosphatase (Sigma units/100 ml)	3.9± 0.2	54.0±24.4[a]	53.7±11.6	40.3±19.0	26.3± 8.0	42.5±15.0
Sodium (mEq/liter)	149.8± 3.1	145.1± 3.0	29.1±15.8	23.5± 7.2	—	—
Cholesterol (mg%)	139.0±33.8	106.0±28.3	31.1±11.2	10.8±10.5[a]	33.2±20.0	32.1±22.0
Total protein (gm%)	5.6± 0.5	5.1± 0.8	1.73± 0.5	1.07± 0.6	34.0±13.2	27.9± 8.1
Glutamic oxaloacetic transaminase (Sigma-Frankel units/100 ml)	166.0±48.7	227 ±64.3[a]	1937±1503	2583±1166[a]	11,200±5500	7800±6200
Glycogen	—	—	2667± 353	1669± 663[a]	5620± 336	1279± 425[a]

[a]Significant, $P \leq 0.05$.

not caused by heat-killed bacteria or by *S. epidermidis*. A study of the biochemistry of the carcass (12) showed a striking fall in glucose, cholesterol, and total protein. These changes and other changes were also produced by heat-killed bacteria. The fall in carcass glucose could be reversed by penicillin treatment. Loss of glucose was not directly due to bacterial growth; this was apparent from the fact that, when the animal was killed shortly after challenge in the usual way and the carcass was stored at 37° C, there was no loss of glucose. Separate analysis of the liver, kidney, lung, spleen, heart, adrenal glands, brain, and muscle showed that the glucose change occurred in the liver and that the significant rise in inorganic phosphorus at death was present only in the liver and adrenal glands. Separate studies of glycogen metabolism showed significant losses from the liver, brain, and muscle and a significant gain of glycogen in the kidney, lung, spleen, and heart at death from staphylococcal infection (13).

Other studies were then made of various phosphate fractions in different organs of normal and infected mice between challenge and death from *S. aureus* (16). The most marked changes occurred in the liver. Inorganic phosphate increased progressively with a concomitant fall of soluble organic phosphates, which largely represented high-energy phosphates and sugar phosphates. Phosphoproteins and phospholipids, on the other hand, remained unaltered. Consequently the ratio of inorganic phosphate or organic phosphate increased significantly.

When oxygen metabolism was studied in normal and infected mice, the infected animals increased their oxygen consumption near death. An additional increase in late oxygen consumption was noted when the animals breathed 100% oxygen, suggesting that oxygen needs exceeded the capabilities of the transport system (23). Oxygen therapy in concentrations of 20-100% was not helpful; the same concentrations at 2 or 3 atmospheres were also without benefit. A reduced concentration of oxygen (10%) with nitrogen at atmospheric pressure significantly prolonged the life of infected mice. Further benefit was derived by treatment with 10% or 20% oxygen at 0.6 atmospheres of pressure. The effect was not due to the change in the concentration or pressure of nitrogen (1).

The increase in the concentration of inorganic phosphate in the liver and a decrease in the concentration of both organic phosphates (partly consisting of the high-energy nucleotides) and glucose suggested that derangements in oxidative phosphorylation might exist. Studies of mitochondrial metabolism (23) showed that uncoupling of oxidative phosphorylation occurred mainly in the liver. Further uncoupling was not possible by the addition of dinitrophenol in concentrations which usually uncoupled normal mitochondria. This uncoupling was accompanied by a progressive change of lacy "high-energy" mitochondria to chunky "low-energy" mitochondria on electron microscopy. Such changes have been described by Green and his colleagues (17).

An examination of lipid metabolism (18) at intervals from the onset of infection to 120 minutes in a 260-minute infection showed a significant decrease in total serum cholesterol, phospholipids, and triglycerides, with a concomitant increase of cholesterol and phospholipid fractions in the liver. Fats accumulate in the liver early in infection. The ratio of ester cholesterol to free cholesterol, however, decreases in both serum and liver secondarily to a rise in free cholesterol in the infected mice. Free fatty acids accumulate in the infected blood with a loss of glyceride fatty acids and free fatty acids from the liver. Free fatty acids are probably not utilized because of the hypoglycemic state of the diseased mice. Mild ketosis is also noted. The saturated fatty acids (palmitic and stearic) increase more than the unsaturated fatty acids (oleic, linoleic, and arachidonic). It became apparent that the imbalance of the long-chain fatty acids in the body of the host might lead to mitochondrial damage and uncoupling.

Recently preliminary experiments (19) have been done with normal mouse liver mitochondria in reaction media with 100 μg/ml of different fatty acids. Saturated fatty acid (palmitic) will uncouple mitochondria more effectively than unsaturated fatty acid (oleic). We were able to produce uncoupling in normal mitochondria and almost none in the mitochondria from infected livers, which were assumed to be already uncoupled. In studies *in vitro*, when we duplicated the increased ratio of palmitic to oleic acid seen in the serum from naturally infected mice, the serum from infected mice would also uncouple normal mouse mitochondria but not mitochondria from the livers of infected mice.

In staphylococcal infections, the lethal constituent resides in *S. aureus* protoplasm and not in the cell wall (35). Mice can be killed by certain separated protoplasmic fractions of *S. aureus* cells separated in a column of Sephadex G-100 (11). We are presently studying the effects of these fractions on the mouse serum palmitic-oleic acid ratios and other lipid parameters.

Credibility is lent to these observations by the potential reversibility of the staphylococcal infection by chemical treatments. Subcutaneous treatment with carefully titrated doses of a variety of chemicals will significantly delay death in mice challenged intraperitoneally with *S. aureus* (37). Successful treatments are accomplished with the following: glucose and other hexoses (14), phosphate as Sorenson's buffer, olive oil (glyceryl trioleate), 1/6 M sodium lactate, sodium bicarbonate, high-dose cortisol, chlordiazepoxide (Librium), diphenylhydantoin (Dilantin), fresh liver extract, testosterone (38), glycine, arginine, glutamic acid, and nicotinamide (39). Fifty-nine varied chemical treatments were ineffective in prolonging life of infected mice. Fasting for 16 hours (32), dinitrophenol, thyroxine (33), and insulin shortened the life span of mice infected with *S. aureus*.

DISCUSSION

Despite extensive work and characterization of various staphylococcal exotoxins, the mechanism of death from *S. aureus* infection is unknown. It has recently become possible, however, to state the problem in more exact biochemical terms.

The concept of a critical lethal dose has been defined for death from *Salmonella* in mice (3). Others agree with our concept (27,7) of a similar occurrence in staphylococcal death, although one disagreement appears in the literature (without compelling evidence to support that divergence of opinion)(2). Evidence from the indwelling intraperitoneal diffusion chamber is against death from the diffusible products of the staphylococci as the only lethal cause. At present, we are willing to keep an open mind about which toxin is lethal, and we prefer to avoid pinpointing any of the many known toxins.

In dogs, it has been possible to monitor hepatic circulation (40) and to show a two-compartment flow in response to the injection of *S. aureus* exotoxin. Although this might explain some of the hepatic chemical changes, we have thus far been unable to adapt the methodology to mice.

Defective oxygen transport was suggested to us when mice were taken from room air to 100% oxygen at the time of the convulsion, which usually led to death. This change in ambient pO_2 prolonged their lives 30±10 minutes, suggesting an acute tissue hypoxia. Removal of the mice from 100% oxygen at 290 minutes inevitably caused rapid death. Mice in 100% oxygen consumed more oxygen than those in 20% oxygen. All these facts support the repayment of an oxygen debt and suggest that oxygen needs exceeded the capabilities of the transport system functioning with room air. Shoemaker and his colleagues (29) have shown that oxygen consumption values in septic shock patients, while not generally abnormal in terms of accepted normal values, are, nonetheless, inadequate in terms of the real needs of these patients. Siegel *et al.* (28) have also suggested an unrequited disparity between oxygen demand and supply.

Uncoupling of oxidative phosphorylation was first described by Niselovskaya and Paderma in 1964 (20) *in vivo* and confirmed by us in 1967. Similar observations have been made *in vitro* by Rahal *et al.* in 1967 (21) and 1970 (22).

A comparison of septic shock caused by gram-negative (*E. coli*) and gram-positive (staphylococcal) organisms in rhesus monkeys showed that the cardiac output was higher and the peripheral resistance was lower, however, 30-60 minutes after challenge in a 16% lethal infection. Measurements taken after a longer interval showed that responses became similar in both groups (8). Therefore, it is important to study both types of septic shock to define more clearly biochemical similarities and differences.

By continually going from carcass to tissue and then to tissue components, and from whole staphylococci to defined lethal components, we hope we can avoid premature conclusions which are artifactual.

Presently, antiobiotic therapy can reduce the death rate from *S. aureus* septicemia in man from 80-90% in untreated patients to 25-35%. To further improve survival, host resistance will have to be maintained by other nonantibiotic ancillary means which are directed toward either the maintenance of biochemical normality or the blockage of the lethal interaction of staphylococcal toxins and energy-accumulating mechanisms, particularly in the liver. This support of host mechanisms will be necessary for 2-4 days to allow adequate time for the proper interaction to occur between accumulated staphylococci in the infected host and the therapeutic antibiotics. Carefully monitored patients in septic shock have been maintained by attention (28,29) to their cardiopulmonary status and to an adjustment of alkalosis or later acidosis. It would now appear possible to monitor carbohydrate and lipid metabolism in these patients, to monitor the other changes noted in murine experiments, and then to apply the lessons learned to the clinical situation. Liver biopsies should allow us to study the nature of the mitochondria found and the percentage of coupled and uncoupled mitochondria at different stages of staphylococcal shock.

Recent studies on lipid metabolism and uncoupling of oxidative phosphorylation in liver mitochondria lead us to a number of definitive studies which may unravel the complex interaction of the chemically active *S. aureus* cells and the infected host.

SUMMARY

After intraperitoneal challenge with 10^9 cells of *S. aureus*, the mice in these experiments died in septic shock within 270±20 minutes. The mice died when a critical number of bacteria ($10^{9.5}$ to $10^{10.5}$) had accumulated at any site in the carcass. Millipore filter chamber studies indicated that whole cells were necessary. Biochemical analysis of the blood and organs of this LD_{90} model showed a loss of glucose and an increase of inorganic phosphorus which was not noticeable in the liver. There was evidence of increased oxygen usage with defective oxygen transport. Treatment with low-concentration oxygen (10%), low pressure oxygen (0.6 atmospheres), or both prolonged life in these infected mice. A study of mitochondrial metabolism showed uncoupling of oxidative phosphorylation also most noticeable in the liver. This oxygen waste without energy accumulation is a continuous process associated with a change in the character of the mitochondria. In the blood, fatty acids accumulated and the ratio of saturated (palmitic and stearic) to unsaturated fatty acids (oleic, linoleic, arachidonic) increased. Uncoupling of oxidative phosphorylation could be induced in normal mouse liver mitochondria by suspending them in reaction media with artificially selected ratios of fatty acids or in naturally occurring infected mouse serum. Mitochondria from the livers of infected mice could not be further uncoupled by these maneuvers. The heat-labile lethal effect of the staphylococci for mice resides in the bacterial cell protoplasm and not in the cell wall.

REFERENCES

1. Barnwell, P., S. Sopher, R.R. Flickinger, C.H. Rhoden, and I.M. Smith. Treatment of *Staphylococcus aureus* infections in mice with oxygen at various pressures and concentrations. Am. Rev. Resp. Dis. 94:755-760, 1966.

2. Bartell, P.F., T.E. Orr, A. Gelfan, and P. Iono. Experimental infections of mice with *Staphylococcus aureus*: Evidence against alpha toxin and the terminal size of the bacterial population as determinants of lethality. J. Infect. Dis. 118:481-490, 1968.

3. Berry, L.J., and D.S. Smythe. Some metabolic aspects of host-parasite interactions in the mouse typhoid model. Ann. N.Y. Acad. Sci. 88:1278-1286, 1960.

4. Counts, G.W., I.M. Smith, J.I. Routh, E. Ch. Hazard, and J.F. McTavish. Biochemical changes in lethal staphylococcal infections in mice. Nature 191:783-786, 1961.

5. Ebert, R.V., and R.S. Abernathy. Septic shock. Fed. Proc. Suppl. No. 9:179-184, 1961.

6. Elek, S.D. *Staphylococcus pyogenes and Its Relation to Disease*. London: Livingston, 1959.

7. Gorrill, R.H., and E.M. McNeill. Staphylococcal infection in

the mouse. I. The effect of route of inoculation. Br. J. Exp. Pathol. 44:404-415, 1963.

8. Guenter, C.A., and L.B. Hinshaw. Comparison of septic shock due to gram-negative and gram-positive organisms. Proc. Soc. Exp. Biol. Med. 134:780-783, 1970.

9. Henry, R.J. *Clinical Chemistry: Principles and Techniques.* New York: Harper & Row, 1964.

10. Hicks, J.D., P. Giltman, and J. Fye. A new method of measuring blood pressure in mice. Lancet 2:930-932, 1965.

11. Kong, Y.L., and I.M. Smith. Further purification of *Staphylococcus aureus* protoplasmic lethal factor. To be published.

12. Lindell, S.S., I.M. Smith, J.I. Routh, and M. Delle. Biochemical analyses of the carcass in lethal staphylococcal infections of mice. Nature 197:155-157, 1963.

13. Lindell, S.S., I.M. Smith, J.W. Nelson, M. Delle, and J.I. Routh. Locus of biochemical changes in mice dying of staphylococcal infection. Nature 201:185-187, 1964.

14. Lindell, S.S., S. Sopher, and I.M. Smith. Carbohydrate treatment of severe *Staphylococcus aureus* infections in mice. Rev. Lationoam. Microbiol. 8:14-23, 1967.

15. MacLean, L.D., W.G. Mulligan, A.P.H. Maclean, and J.H. Duff. Patterns of septic shock in man: A detailed study of 56 patients. Ann. Surg. 166:543-558, 1967.

16. Mukherjee, K.L., S.S. Lindell, I.M. Smith, and J.I. Routh. The phosphate fractions of *Staphylococcus aureus* infected mice. J. Infect. Dis. 115:278-284, 1965.

17. Mukherjee, K.L., I.M. Smith, and R. Barker. Oxidative phosphorylation with *Staphylococcus aureus* infection. Experientia, in press.

18. Mukherjee, K.L., A.K. Bhattacharyya, R.M. Smith, T. Mueller, and I.M. Smith. Changes in the lipid metabolism of mice challenged with a lethal infection of *Staphylococcus aureus.* To be published.

19. Mukherjee, K.L., and I.M. Smith. Long-chain fatty acids and uncoupling of oxidative phosphorylation by *Staphylococcus aureus* infection. To be published.

20. Niselovskaya, L.I., and E.M. Paderma. Oxidative phosphorylation in the liver of guinea pigs poisoned with staphylococcal toxin. Fed. Proc. 23:536, 1964.

21. Rahal, J.J., M.E. Plant, and L. Weinstein. Effect of purified staphylococcal alpha toxin on active sodium transport and aerobic respiration in the isolated toad bladder. J. Clin. Invest. 47:1603, 1968.

22. Rahal, J.J., G.T. Keusch, and L. Weinstein. Uncoupling of oxidative phosphorylation by purified staphylococcal alpha toxin. J. Lab. Clin. Med. 75:442-448, 1970.

23. Rhoden, C.H., L. Lowry, S. Rabinovich, and I.M. Smith. Mitochondrial oxygen metabolism in lethal staphylococcal infection. Am. Rev. Resp. Dis. 100:699-705, 1969.

24. Rhoden, C.H., D.B. Leeper, I.M. Smith, T.C. Evans, and B.R. Duling. Blood pressure changes in mice after lethal staphylococcal infection and endotoxin challenge. To be published.

25. Saslaw, S., and H.N. Carlisle. Staphylococcal infection in normal and splenectomized monkeys. Proc. Soc. Exp. Biol. Med. 123:565-571, 1966.

26. Schneider, W.C., and G.H. Hogeboom. Intracellular distribution of enzymes. V. Further studies on the distribution of cytochrome in rat liver homogenates. J. Biol. Chem. 183:123, 1950.

27. Sellers, T.F., and C.A. LeMaistre. Experimental staphylococcal infection in mice: Observations on the effects of inoculum size, strain variation, penicillin, and cortisone. J. Lab. Clin. Med. 55:199-215, 1960.

28. Siegel, J.H., M. Greenspan, and L.R.M. Del Guercio. Abnormal vascular tone, defective oxygen transport and myocardial failure in human septic shock. Ann. Surg. 165:504-517, 1967.

29. Shoemaker, W.C., K.J. Printen, R.S. Brown, J.J. Amato, J.S. Corey, S. Youssef, J.M. Reinhard, and A.E. Kark. Use of segmental physiologic measurements for evaluation and therapy of uncomplicated septic shock. Gurg. Gynecol. Obstet. 131: 245-254, 1970.

30. Smith, H. Biochemical challenge of microbial pathogenicity. Bact. Rev. 32:164, 1968.

31. Smith, I.M., and R.J. Dubos. The behavior of virulent and

avirulent staphylococci in the tissues of normal mice. J. Exp. Med. 103:87-108, 1956.

32. Smith, I.M., and R.J. Dubos. The effect of nutritional disturbances on the susceptibility of mice to staphylococcal infections. J. Exp. Med. 103:109-118, 1956.

33. Smith, I.M., and R.J. Dubos. The effect of dinitrophenol and thyroxin on the susceptibility of mice to staphylococcal infection. J. Exp. Med. 103:119-126, 1956.

34. Smith, I.M., A.P. Wilson, E. Ch. Hazard, W.K. Hummer, and M.E. Dewey. Death from staphylococci in mice. J. Infect. Dis. 107:369-378, 1960.

35. Smith, I.M., S.S. Lindell, and J.I. Routh. Death in mice induced by *Staphylococcus aureus* protoplasm. Nature 205: 1318-1319, 1965.

36. Smith, I.M. Metabolic response of the host to staphylococcal infection. Ann. N.Y. Acad. Sci. 128:335-350, 1965.

37. Smith, I.M., S.S. Lindell, E. Ch. Hazard, and S. Rabinovich. Chemical treatments of staphylococcal infections in mice. Nature 211:720-722, 1966.

38. Smith, I.M., S.S. Lindell, and E. Ch. Hazard. Inhibitory action of the testosterone and liver extract on staphylococcal infections in mice. Nature 211:722-723, 1966.

39. Smith, I.M., A. Lopez-S., J. Gell, and P. Tarr. Amino acid metabolism in murine lethal staphylococcal infection. In: *Proceedings of the Sixth International Congress of Chemotherapy,* Tokyo, 1970.

40. Vetto, R.M., F.O. Belzer, R.C. Rogers, K.A. Robertson. A dye dilution study of the hepatic circulation during staphylococcus toxin shock. Surg. Gynecol. Obstet. 121:1263-1268, 1965.

MYOCARDIAL METABOLISM DURING ACUTE HEMORRHAGIC OR ENDOTOXIC SHOCK[1]

John J. Spitzer, M.D., Judy A. Spitzer, Ph.D., J. T. Weng, M.D., and John C. Scott, Ph.D.

Department of Physiology and Biophysics, Hahnemann Medical College, Philadelphia, Pennsylvania

In both hemorrhagic and endotoxic shock, a diminished venous return is probably responsible for the decreased cardiac output. Although the heart eventually fails in both types of shock, it is unclear whether cardiac failure is responsible for the irreversibility of the condition. Also, it is unknown whether alterations of myocardial metabolism precede cardiac failure and, if so, whether they are due to or simply a reflection of myocardial hypoxia.

The present experiments were designed to (a) determine whether early changes in myocardial metabolism may be demonstrated after the hemorrhagic or endotoxic insult, (b) ascertain whether any metabolic signs of myocardial hypoxia appear in the early phase of shock, and (c) contrast the metabolic changes that appear after hemorrhagic hypotension with those following endotoxin administration.

MATERIALS AND METHODS

Two groups of experiments were performed, each using nine dogs. The methodologic details are described elsewhere (5,7); hence only the major features of the experimental protocol will be described here.

Food was withheld from all dogs for about 16 hours before

[1]Supported by the U.S. Navy Themis Project and by Grants HE03130 and HE04916 from the National Heart Institute.

the studies were begun. Before each experimental procedure, the dog was anesthetized with sodium pentobarbital. Simultaneous arterial and coronary sinus blood samples were taken during the control period and after the experimental insult.

Coronary blood flow was determined by the ^{131}I iodoantipyrine method. ^{14}C-1-C palmitate was infused continuously throughout the experiments so that changes in free fatty acid (FFA) metabolism could be evaluated. In addition to FFA flux, myocardial uptake and oxidation and lactate uptake were measured.

In the first group of dogs, the coronary sinus was catheterized under manual control after thoracotomy. No heparin was administered to these animals. After control blood samples were drawn, each dog was bled until hemorrhagic loss reached an average of 4.4% of the body weight. The experimental blood samples were obtained about 45 minutes after the blood pressure stabilized. In the second group of animals, the coronary sinus catheter was placed under fluoroscopic control and kept patent by a continuous drip of dilute heparin. After control samples were drawn, *E. coli* endotoxin was injected intravenously. The experimental samples were obtained about 1 hour later.

The data were expressed as percent changes during the experimental period, compared to the control values. The mean percent changes of the two groups of dogs are contrasted in the figures. The numerical values of the data upon which the calculations were based may be found in previous publications (5,7).

RESULTS

Figure 1 compares the changes in a number of hemodynamic parameters after hemorrhage or endotoxin administration. One can see that the changes in both groups of animals were similar. Mean arterial blood pressure and cardiac output decreased by 40-50%, while the heart rate remained unchanged. Coronary blood flow and vascular resistance decreased by about 30%, while total peripheral resistance changed very little.

Left ventricular CO_2 production diminished markedly in both groups of dogs (Fig. 2). Changes of hematocrit occurred in the opposite direction, indicating hemodilution after hemorrhage and hemoconcentration after endotoxin administration.

A comparison of changes in FFA metabolism between the two groups is shown in Figure 3. While the arterial FFA concentration showed nonsignificant changes in both groups, the changes in FFA flux and in myocardial FFA extraction ratio were quite different

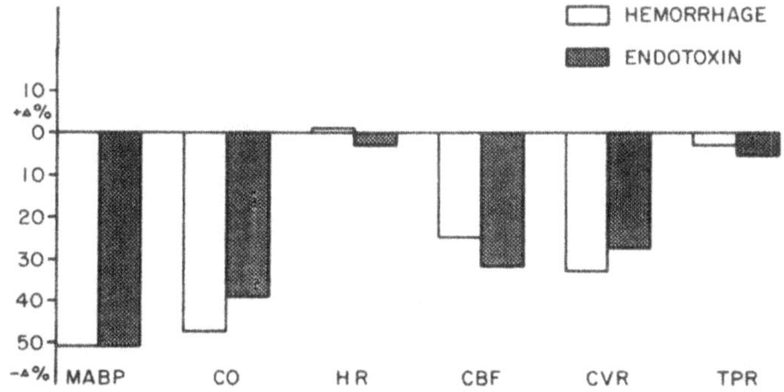

FIG. 1. Comparison of changes in hemodynamic parameters after hemorrhage or endotoxin administration. MABP = mean arterial blood pressure; CO = cardiac output; HR = heart rate; CBF = coronary blood flow; CVR = coronary vascular resistance; TPR = total peripheral resistance.

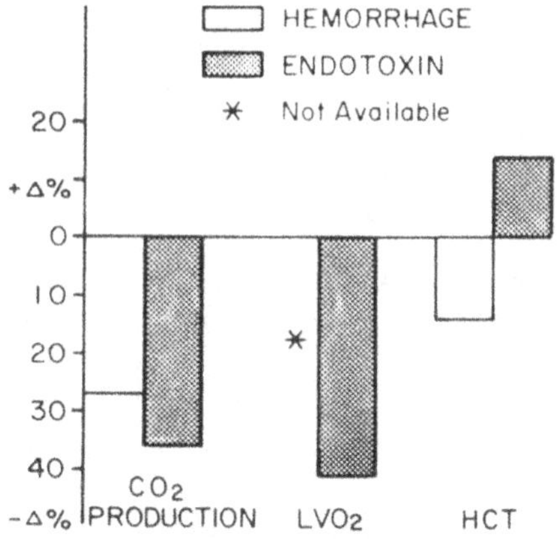

FIG. 2. Changes in left ventricular CO_2 production, O_2 consumption, and arterial hematocrit after hemorrhage or endotoxin administration.

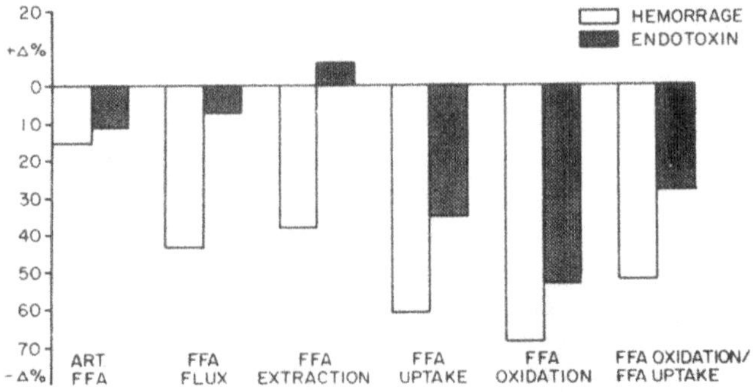

FIG. 3. Comparison of changes in arterial FFA, total body FFA flux, and myocardial FFA metabolism after hemorrhage or endotoxin administration.

in the two groups of experiments. Both of these parameters decreased markedly after hemorrhage but showed no significant changes after endotoxin administration. Although the direction of change in both myocardial FFA uptake and oxidation was the same in both groups, the percent changes of these parameters were larger after hemorrhage than after endotoxin injection. The difference is especially marked when the fraction of myocardial oxidation/uptake is considered.

Although arterial lactate increased markedly after both insults (Fig. 4), hemorrhagic hypotension was accompanied by a much more pronounced change (+366%) than endotoxin administration (+137%). Changes in myocardial lactate uptake were similar in both groups. The myocardium extracted the same fraction of the arterial lactate both before and after the experimental intervention in both groups of animals. However, changes in arterial glucose concentration differed. The mean concentration rose after hemorrhage but had a tendency to fall after injection of endotoxin.

The contribution of FFA to metabolic CO_2 production by the heart decreased and that of lactate increased after the experimental insult in both groups of dogs (Fig. 5). The changes were more marked after hemorrhage than after the administration of endotoxin.

DISCUSSION

These studies indicate that, early in hemorrhagic hypotension and relatively soon after endotoxin administration, changes in myocardial metabolism take place. The changes in both experimental

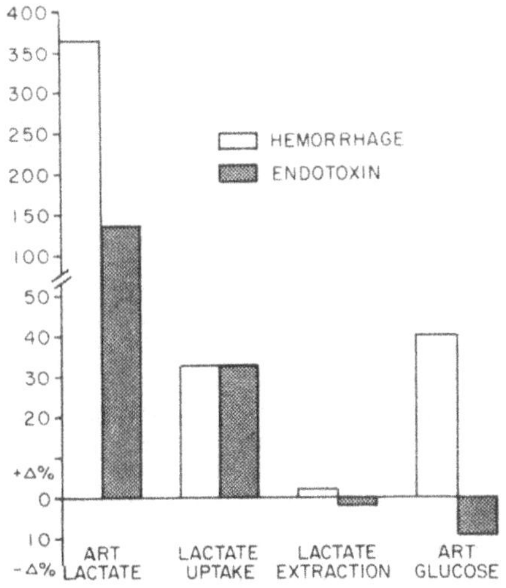

FIG. 4. Changes in arterial lactate and glucose and myocardial lactate uptake after hemorrhage or endotoxin administration.

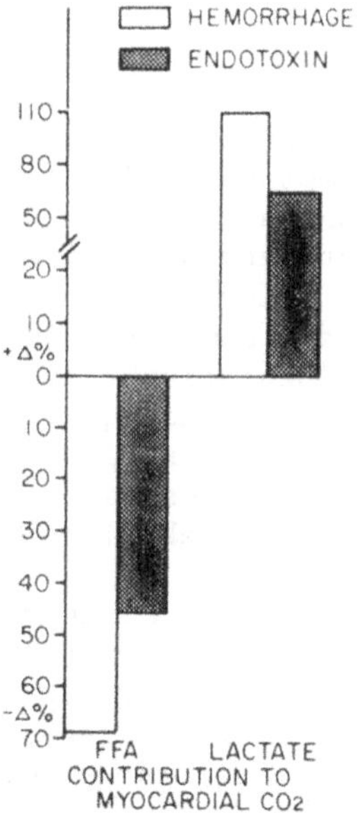

FIG. 5. Changes in FFA and lactate contribution to myocardial CO_2 production after hemorrhage or endotoxin administration.

models are similar, consisting of a decreased reliance on plasma FFA as oxidative substrates and an increased contribution of lactate to myocardial metabolism. Although the early changes in myocardial metabolism may not be quantitatively identical during hemorrhagic hypotension and after endotoxin administration, the direction of the alterations is remarkably similar. The only major exception is represented by the myocardial extraction of FFA, which decreases significantly after hemorrhage but remains unchanged after endotoxin administration.

On the other hand, changes in metabolite parameters that reflect total body metabolism were dissimilar. Total body FFA flux decreased significantly after hemorrhage—which is consistent with previous findings in anesthetized dogs (8)—but remained unchanged after injection of endotoxin. Whether the discrepancy is due to differences of adipose tissue perfusion (and thus FFA release) or to the removal of FFA by actively metabolizing tissues remains to be ascertained. The different directional changes in arterial glucose level are consistent with previous findings (1) indicating a prevalent hypoglycemia after endotoxin administration in dogs.

Since lactate utilization was quite high in both groups of animals after the experimental insult, and because one of the first signs of metabolic hypoxia in the heart is considered to be a diminished lactate utilization or an actual lactate output by the myocardium (4), evidence of metabolic hypoxia was concluded to be absent in these studies (5). The myocardial changes described in this paper may be due to one or a combination of the following: decreased metabolic demands imposed on the heart, secondary effects of peripheral hypoxia, and increased availability of blood lactate for metabolic utilization. It is, perhaps, not too suprising that the principal cardiac metabolic adjustments to the two forms of shock are similar, since the main cardiac stress in both cases (although brought about by different mechanisms) is also similar, *i.e.*, an inadequate venous return. Thus, despite some differences in hemodynamic responses, an insufficient perfusion of the peripheral tissues is primarily responsible for the changes in myocardial metabolism.

Since excessive concentration of intracellular FFA may have a deleterious effect on myocardial function, especially when the availability of O_2 is limited (2,3,6), it is appropriate to consider the utility of the metabolic changeover in the myocardium in the early phases of hemorrhagic or endotoxic shock.

SUMMARY

Alterations in myocardial substrate utilization were found in anesthetized dogs after acute hemorrhagic hypotension was induced or endotoxin was administered. Myocardial uptake and oxidation of free fatty acids were greatly diminished, and the contribution of free fatty acids to myocardial energy metabolism decreased markedly. At the same time, lactate became important as an energy source. There was no metabolic sign of myocardial hypoxia. The directional changes of myocardial metabolism were similar under the two experimental conditions.

REFERENCES

1. Berk, J.L., J.F. Hagen, W.H. Beyer, and M.J. Gerber. Hypoglycemia of shock. Ann. Surg. 171:400-408, 1970.

2. Henderson, A.H., A.S. Most, W.W. Parmley, R. Gorlin, and E.H. Sonnenbleck. Depression of myocardial contractility in rats by free fatty acids during hypoxia. Circ. Res. 26:439-449, 1970.

3. Kurien, V.A., P.A. Yates, and M.F. Oliver. Free fatty acids, heparin, and arrhythmias during experimental myocardial infarction. Lancet 2:185-187, 1969.

4. Scheuer, J., and N. Brachfeld. Coronary insufficiency: Relation between hemodynamic, electrical, and biochemical parameters. Circ. Res. 18:178-189, 1966.

5. Scott, J.C., J.T. Weng, and J.J. Spitzer. Myocardial metabolism during endotoxic shock. In: *Neurohumoral and Metabolic Aspects of Injury*, edited by A.G.B. Kovách, B. Stoner, and J.J. Spitzer. New York: Plenum Press, in press.

6. Severeid, L., W.E. Connor, and J.P. Long. The depressant effect of fatty acids on the isolated rabbit heart. Proc. Soc. Exptl. Biol. Med. 131:1239-1242, 1969.

7. Spitzer, J.J., and J.A. Spitzer. Myocardial metabolism in dogs during hemorrhagic shock. Am. J. Physiol., in press.

8. Spitzer, J.J., and J.A. Spitzer. Plasma lipid changes during hemorrhagic shock. J. Trauma, in press.

METABOLIC CHANGES IN HEMORRHAGIC SHOCK

Arisztid G. B. Kovách, M.D.

Experimental Research Department, Medical University of Budapest, Budapest, Hungary

Before discussing our results on the metabolic changes in reversible and irreversible hemorrhagic shock, I wish to make a comment on the presentation of Dr. Horwitz. Our work (5) has shown that the blood flow in canine subcutaneous adipose tissue during hemorrhage drops to approximately 10% of the resting level and often ceases completely. Using the same experimental procedure, the decrease in blood flow in adipose tissue is more pronounced than in other organs, including skeletal muscle, myocardium, kidney, liver, hypothalamus and intestine. Furthermore, the outflow rate of free fatty acids from the subcutaneous adipose tissue is not elevated despite a presumably high sympathicoadrenal activity, which may have promoted lipolysis. Arterial free fatty acids do not rise during hemorrhage. This finding may indicate that the reactions in subcutaneous adipose tissue also reflect the responses in adipose tissue from other anatomic regions. In addition, the arterial glycerol concentration rises significantly during bleeding.

In view of the fact that adipose tissue provides the largest energy source for an organism, the difficulty in augmenting the release of free fatty acids may adversely affect the organism during hemorrhagic shock by failing to meet its energy requirements. Under such conditions, it may be important to maintain the delivery of free fatty acids at normal or increased levels. One way to accomplish this may be to administer alpha-adrenergic blocking agents or beta-adrenergic stimulating drugs (7). The possible therapeutic value of such treatment deserves further study.

Our experiments on the metabolic changes in hemorrhagic shock were performed partly last year in Dr. Chance's laboratory at the University of Pennsylvania and, prior to that, at the Medical University of Budapest. In earlier studies on rats in traumatic shock (2), we found that severe adynamia and impaired reflexes can be observed in shock while the energy-rich phosphate content of the brain still remains normal. However, normal concentrations of ATP and creatine phosphate do not necessarily imply that the rate of oxidative phosphorylation is normal. It was demonstrated that the rate of synthesis of energy-rich phosphates in the brain was decreased despite normal concentrations (4). The electrical activity of the brain in both hemorrhagic and tourniquet shock decreased considerably. Activity was impaired at a blood pressure of 55 mm Hg. After a period of 30 minutes at 35 mm Hg, activity ceased, and only isoelectric readings were recorded. After retransfusion, the electrical activity did not return, although the blood pressure was normal. Phenoxybenzamine pretreatment diminished the impairment of the electrocorticographic activity and increased the survival rate of dogs in hemorrhagic shock (3).

Reversal of the hypoxic electrocorticographic changes depends largely on the available oxygen, blood flow, and duration of hypoxia. Before and during hemorrhage, we found no difference in regional blood flow changes between the untreated group and the phenoxybenzamine-pretreated group, although this drug prevented the adverse electrocorticographic changes. We then investigated the possibility of differences in regional oxygen utilization in the brain. The pO_2 in the hypothalamus and frontal cortex was measured polarographically with microelectrodes. We found a continous and progressive decrease in pO_2 during bleeding to below 20% of the initial value (6). After reinfusion, the pO_2 in both the hypothalamus and the frontal cortex remained at this low level despite a significant elevation in local blood flow. These results suggested that oxygen utilization increased after hemorrhage. In the phenoxybenzamine-treated group, the pO_2 showed fewer changes during the hypotensive period and returned to normal after reinfusion. This suggests that the protective effect of the drug may be related to a local metabolic action. We have found that phenoxybenzamine reduced the metabolic activity of isolated rat liver mitochondria, so that states III and IV respiration as well as uncoupled dinitrophenol-activated respiration were reduced (8). The protective action of phenoxybenzamine in hemorrhagic shock may be due to its metabolic anti-uncoupling activity along with its alpha-adrenergic pharmacological actions. Isolated mitochondria from rat liver and kidney suggested defects at the subcellular level.

At the University of Pennsylvania, Dr. Chance developed a double fluorometer for the simultaneous measurement of flavin and pyridine nucleotide fluorescence in suspensions of isolated mitochondria and oxidation-reduction changes in perfused rat liver. Optical methods have the distinct advantage of monitoring cellular and subcellular parameters without disrupting the tissue. Their application is limited in the presence of hemoglobin, however, because of its strong absorption band in the range of visible light. A close correlation between a blue fluorescence excited at 366 nm and the content of reduced pyridine nucleotides of various tissues has been established (1). It was previously shown that changes in fluorescence intensity, excited on the liver surface by 366 nm light, represent oxidation-reduction changes in both mitochondrial and the extramitochondrial NAD systems. Studies of the absorbance and fluorescence changes indicate that a yellow fluorescence, excited at 436 nm, results from certain oxidized flavoproteins which are predominantly due to mitochondrial flavoproteins.

In our experiments, gluconeogenesis, oxygen uptake, and flavin and pyridine nucleotide oxidation-reduction changes were followed in perfused rat livers in control and hemorrhagic shock experiments. The gluconeogenesis of the liver is significantly inhibited in early shock states, followed by uncoupled respiration. Later, during the development of irreversible shock, oxygen delivery and consumption in hepatic tissue becomes progressively more reduced. In this state, the tissue is incapable of restoring its ATP content. Phenoxybenzamine pretreatment protected the experimental animals against shock which elicited both uncoupled respiration and inhibition of gluconeogenesis.

As previously shown, dinitrophenol (1 mg/kg) elevates oxygen consumption significantly in the intact animal and elevates its sensitivity to shock. The effect of dinitrophenol on metabolic rate and on shock sensitivity is significantly reduced in phenoxybenzamine-treated rats and dogs.

We conclude that tissue metabolism is seriously affected in hemorrhagic shock. Uncoupled respiration and later depressed tissue oxygen consumption develops. Phenoxybenzamine protection against irreversible hemorrhagic shock can be explained primarily by its metabolic (anti-uncoupling) effect. In late irreversible shock, in addition to low blood flow perfusion and inadequate oxygen delivery, inefficient oxygen utilization aggravates the local hypoxia. Our experiments demonstrated that through adequate control of metabolic processes, mortality was significantly reduced in ordinarily irreversible hemorrhagic shock.

REFERENCES

1. Chance, B., *et al.* Personal communication.

2. Kovách, A.G.B., A. Fonyó, and E. Kovách. Cerebral phosphate metabolism in traumatic shock. Acta. Physiol. Acad. Sci. hung. 16:157-164, 1959.

3. Kovách, A.G.B., and A. Fonyó. Metabolic responses to injury in cerebral tissue. In: *The Biochemical Response to Injury*, edited by H.B. Stoner and C.I. Threlfall. Oxford: Black-Well Scientific Publications, 1960, pp. 129-160.

4. Kovách, A.G.B., and A. Fonyó. Incorporation of P into the rat's brain during traumatic shock. Acta Physiol. Acad. Sci. hung. 27:27-31, 1965.

5. Kovách, A.G.B., S. Rosell, P. Sándor, E. Koltay, E. Kovách, and N. Tomka. Blood blow, oxygen consumption, and free fatty acid release in subcutaneous adipose tissue during hemorrhagic shock in control and phenoxybenzamine-treated dogs. Circ. Res. 26:733-741, 1970.

6. Kovach, A.G.B. The function of the central nervous system after hemorrhage. J. Clin. Pathol. (Suppl. 4) 23:202-212, 1970.

7. Kovách, A.G.B., S. Rosell, P. Sándor, E. Koltay, M. Hámori, and E. Kovách. Influence of adrenergic beta-receptor activity on blood flow and free fatty acid release in canine subcutaneous adipose tissue during hemorrhagic shock. Arch. exper. Path. u. Pharmakol. 268:140-147, 1971.

8. Kovách, A.G.B., E. Koltay, A. Fonyó, and E. Kovách. Effect of phenoxybenzamine on the respiration of isolated rat liver mitochondria. Biochem. Med. 5:384-390, 1971.

DISCUSSION: SESSION II

DR. L.R.M. DEL GUERCIO, *Panel Moderator (Livingston, N.J.):* Obviously, we can't tie this all together for you. It would be a miracle if, with presentations such as these, we were able to come up with a unified theory of shock. What I would like to do first is read to you the questions that Dr. Valeri had posed and then, just to fill in for him, present some of the concepts of DPG and oxygen delivery to the tissues, because I think it's an important concept and fits into the area of metabolism.

Dr. Valeri asks, first, what are the mechanisms influencing oxygen transport and oxygen tissue delivery in endotoxic and hemorrhagic shock? And, second, what is the role of altered oxyhemoglobin dissociation in shock, including the role of 2,3-DPG?

As you know, it's long been known that blood stored in ACD solutions over an extended period does not follow the standard Bohr effect as far as the oxyhemoglobin dissociation curve is concerned. There is an abnormal shift of the curve to the left, meaning that it requires a lower oxygen tension in order to release the same proportion or percentage of oxygen, regardless of the pH or temperature of the blood at that particular time. The Benesches, working at Columbia University, showed, several years ago, that this effect could be related to the level of 2,3-DPG within the red cell. This organic phosphate is present in all tissues but it's particularly rich within the red cell in association with hemoglobin. Mole for mole, the concentration of 2,3-DPG almost equals that of hemoglobin itself. Somehow, the 2,3-DPG enables the release of oxygen from the hemoglobin at lower oxygen tensions than would be ordinarily possible. The exciting aspects of this, in relation to shock, were demonstrated by Miller at the Society of University Surgeons a couple of years ago, when he showed that, in certain cases of septic shock, patients had abnormal shifts of the oxyhemoglobin dissociation curve to the left outside of the effect of pH and temperature. In these situations, part of the AV difference narrowing that we see in septic shock may be related to low concentrations of DPG. Therefore, if one could manipulate the dissociation curve by transfusing with cells rich in DPG, or by pharmacological means, one might benefit the patient by widening the arteriovenous oxygen difference through the mechanism of encouraging oxygen release to the tissues at a high tissue pO_2. This would make oxygen more available to the cells and improve the oxygen gradient at the cellular level. The question regarding therapy was answered, to some extent, in subsequent papers of Miller's group. They showed that newborn infants with problems of oxygen transport, which proved to be related to 2,3-DPG, benefited from exchange transfusions of fresh blood. However, there has been no absolute demonstration that, in hemorrhagic shock, massive transfusion of old ACD blood reduces oxygen consumption. No one has been able to prove that a low red cell 2,3-DPG level is detrimental to oxygen delivery at the tissues.

From a teleological standpoint, it's an attractive proposal to explain some of the findings in Vietnamese war casualties, where soldiers receiving massive transfusions of ACD blood after hemorrhagic shock had narrow arteriovenous oxygen differences. They were building up oxygen debts, as demonstrated by increased lactate, even though cardiac output was high, oxygen capacity was normal, and oxygenation of the arterial blood was normal. The mixed venous blood was still coming back highly saturated. Proving this mechanism on a clinical or even an experimental basis is very difficult. It gets down to some of the problems that Dr. Kovách has presented to you regarding that very narrow gradient of oxygen tension from the cell membrane to the mitochondrion itself. How much of a gradient has to exist before you begin to run into problems of oxygen delivery to the mitochondrion? It's complicated by the fact that Dr. Rita McConn and I showed that, in septic shock, the shift of the dissociation curve (*i.e.*, the non-Bohr shift) is not necessarily related to low levels of DPG alone, but is probably related, as well, to shifts in sodium and potassium into the red cells themselves. Bartels has shown that the intracellular concentration (the sum of the concentration of sodium and potassium) is an important factor in the release of oxygen, and the red cell doesn't care what the pH of the plasma is. The factor which determines the position of the dissociation curve in relation to pH is the pH within the red cell rather than the plasma pH. We cannot assume, in the shock state, that the relationship between plasma pH and intracellular pH is similar, particularly in view of some of the membrane defects that have been alluded to by Dr. Rush.

What we are dealing with is another concept in the chain of delivery of oxygen, from its uptake in the lungs, to its transport in the blood, and, finally, to its release by hemoglobin into the tissues. All of the presentations here have, of course, raised many more questions about the place of oxygen consumption in shock, itself. And what we're facing is our inability to conceive of the efficiency of oxygen utilization and transport. Even total oxygen consumption is not a good enough measurement, when we realize now that uncoupling of oxidative phosphorylation has probably been detected in clinical states. Many of the clinical investigators here have described situations in which the terminal event appeared to be a massive increase in oxygen consumption at a time when the patient was obviously falling apart at the seams. What was really happening was that the governor of cellular bioenergetics had gone haywire, oxygen was being consumed, but adenosine triphosphate was not being replenished for the performance of cellular work. I think, in our discussion now, we ought to consider all of this in context. We've started out with discussion of oxygen transport in the lung, the metabolism of the lung, the uptake of oxygen, shunting, and anatomic pathways to explain the clinical phenomena in shock. The problem of which comes first, injury to the cell membrane with increased capillary permeability or direct injury to the mitochondrion, itself, has been mentioned. The important thing about our discussion is that we're beginning to see methods which arrive at some answers in a more direct way. Ultimately, we're going to be forced to measure the kinetics of the availability of oxygen at the cellular level and demonstrate the direct effects of various types of shock.

Now, I'd like to throw the discussion open to the audience. The questions you've been accumulating can be directed at the specific members of the panel.

DR. K.G. SWAN *(Washington, D.C.)*: I'd like to direct a question to Dr. Schumer. He has postulated that histamine is perhaps one of the mediators of shock and maybe one of the final common pathways. I see that Gene Jacobson is here now, and he can correct me if I'm wrong, but I believe that in 1963 or 1964, in the Journal of Clinical Investigation, he reported a study in dogs in which he depleted them of a variety of possible vasoactive mediators, including histamine with compound 48/80. He found, contrary to your findings, that there was no protection from endotoxin shock. Does this suggest that we have a different methodology, do we have a species difference, or how would you explain the differences in the two studies?

DR. W. SCHUMER *(Chicago, Ill.)*: All I can say is that we performed the experiments in the rat, and those were the findings. We have to assume that there probably is a species difference. There are a number of other similar findings. James Vick recently found that hemodynamic changes occur after infusion of endotoxin in the dog. He measured histamine associated with these changes and found a correlative liberation of histamine. The controversy provoked by these studies warrants further investigations. The discrepancies between the findings of Drs. Vick and Jacobson may represent a difference in methodology. In my case, it may be a difference of species.

DR. C.M. HERMAN *(Bethesda, Md.)*: I think this whole concept of endotoxin membrane activity is a terribly important one. It's particularly interesting in regard to the red cell. In this respect, Dr. Del Guercio, I wonder if we could explore a little bit more and perhaps get you to speculate about the mechanism by which endotoxin damage to the red cell membrane might, in turn, lead to a shift of this dissociation curve to the left in the absence of lysosomal membranes within the red cell and in an unnucleated cell in which the oxygen uptake and release is the major feature. Are you postulating that it's damage to the membrane pump which leads to an intracellular alkalosis, thereby producing a left shift? Or do you have some other thought in mind?

DR. DEL GUERCIO: I think that could well be happening, and it's an attractive concept. It's more important to demonstrate, first, that this could be a significant mechanism for the narrow arteriovenous oxygen difference in septic shock and also in cases of massive transfusion. I personally feel this is going to be an important area. Preliminary evidence of ours indicates that this may be one of the most important actions of massive doses of steroids. *In vitro* (and in a few cases, *in vivo*), we've been able to demonstrate a temporal relationship between the shift of the dissociation curve of red cells in patients with septic shock in a more favorable direction, with improvement in oxygen consumption under these circumstances. But to prove that this is the case is quite difficult. It's going to be much easier to work out the kinetics of membrane function in red cells. There are many people working in this area who have been approaching the problem of red cell metabolism from numerous other standpoints. If uncoupling of oxidative phosphorylation is occurring, maybe piling up of oxygen is detrimental, as suggested by Dr. Ian Smith this afternoon. Dr. Smith, do you have any comments on the role of the availability of oxygen in states of uncoupling?

DR. I.M. SMITH *(Iowa City, Iowa):* No, I'm sorry, I don't but there was a comment in our leading medical journal, Time Magazine, about a year ago in relation to some work on traumatic shock in Russia, where they were using reduced concentrations and pressures of oxygen. I have not been able to find any other reference to this in the literature.

DR. DEL GUERCIO: Dr. Shanbour, what do you think about the role of the red cell membrane in states of endotoxic shock?

DR. L.L. SHANBOUR *(Houston, Texas):* Just looking at all these factors and particularly the point you made on the importance of the sodium/potassium shift, I think this shift can be explained by a direct membrane effect, and probably many of the changes can be accounted for by membrane phenomena. I would like to ask about something that hasn't been brought up yet—that is, whether individuals who are experts in this area can possibly comment on the probability of the endotoxin directly altering membrane structure. Possibly Dr. Alaupovic can comment on this.

DR. P. ALAUPOVIC *(Oklahoma City, Okla.)*: I cannot really answer these questions, but I would like to continue this discussion by asking a pertinent question; namely, can endotoxin actually attach itself to the red cell membrane? It seems to me that we've seen data on this, this morning, indicating that no binding of endotoxin to red blood cells occurred. This binding takes place, really, on the platelet membrane rather than on the red cell itself. Again, let me say that the important thing is what is being used: Is it fragments of endotoxin in these experiments or is it the entire intact molecule? I think this makes a terrific difference. One has to define, really, the source and the chemical characteristics of these endotoxin preparations.

DR. D.L. HORWITZ *(Chicago, Ill.)*: We did some studies, a while ago, which relate to this subject of how endotoxin interacts with the red cell membrane (In: *Sixth European Conference on Microcirculation*, Basel: Karger, 1971). These were studies of changes in red cell surface charge as measured by electrophoretic mobility. In these studies, we found a definite decrease in red cell surface charge in animals subjected to *E. coli* bacteremia. Similar experiments done on animals in hemorrhagic shock showed no difference. So, I think there is some interaction there. Now, it was interesting that we could only observe this decrease in red cell surface charge if the red cell electrophoretic mobility was measured when the red cells were suspended in their own plasma. If we did this in saline-washed red cells, it did not happen. Consequently, either something in the plasma or something related to the plasma was also necessary to get this effect.

DR. DEL GUERCIO: I've been wracking my brain to see if there is some way that, at the metabolic level, we can tie together traumatic and hemorrhagic shock in relation to endotoxic shock, from the standpoint of hypoxic injury to the cell membrane and endotoxin injury. Does anyone on the panel have any ideas about this, or have I missed something?

DR. B.F. RUSH, JR. *(Newark, N.J.)*: I would like to at least supplement what you have said for this reason: I think you have underlined that there is a difference between traumatic and hemorrhagic shock. While I'm sure this is quite clear to all of us, it somehow seems to get buried in conferences like this. One begins to talk about changes induced by endotoxin as though they may be the same as changes induced by the hypoxia of ultimate trauma and hemorrhage. Now, the common pathways in the end may be the same. But, certainly, the way the system or the way the injury starts must be different. It appears to most of us that the hypoxic injury plus the accumulating metabolites of pleural perfusion are the agents we are most concerned with in traumatic shock and hemorrhagic shock. In endotoxin shock, on the other hand, there is some evidence that the injury may occur very early and that the membrane and cell changes may precede the evolution of the rest of the syndrome.

DR. E.D. JACOBSON *(Houston, Texas):* A couple of comments. First, on work with dogs, we demonstrated that depletion of tissue stores of histamine with either chronic administration of reserpine or with a combination of compound 48/80 and cortisol failed to alter essential hemodynamic responses to endotoxin in dogs. Similarly, we were unable to alter these basic responses of the circulation in animals pretreated with massive doses of the antihistaminic, diphenhydramine—doses which blocked the circulatory responses to histamine itself. Furthermore, we showed, in dogs, that there was no rise in circulating levels of histamine after injection of endotoxin. This has been corroborated in other laboratories. And, lastly, the infusion of large doses of histamine does not duplicate in dogs the essential circulatory responses to endotoxin. So, for these reasons, we felt that histamine probably was not the trigger mechanism involved in the circulatory response to endotoxin in the shocked animal. I might note that certainly there could be species differences. Now, for example, on the physiological level, histamine may be important in regulating gastric secretion in rats. On the other hand, the data in dogs are very convincing that histamine plays no role in the regulation of the production of gastric juice. And just one point for Dr. Alaupovic: that is, in liver tissue we have some evidence that endotoxin does bind to the membrane fraction.

DR. DEL GUERCIO: Bill, do you have any rebuttal?

DR. SCHUMER: Yes; however, we may again be dealing with species differences. Survival in the rat after histamine release by treatment with compound 48/80 is very infrequent. A dose of 8 to 10 mg of 48/80 will kill the rat by what we would term histamine shock. We measured the histamine levels and found that they increased as much as 100%. I have not used the dog as an experimental model for this study, but we do find that the rat is very sensitive to increased histamine levels, and that it dies in a similar way as in endotoxin shock. Dr. Weil did some work in this area and found similarities between anaphylactic, histamine, and endotoxin shock. The final proof of the relationship of histamine and shock will be found only by further investigation.

DR. DEL GUERCIO: Dr. Kovách, were you able to detect any molecular signals from histamine with the surface fluorometry techniques? Can you fill us in on any of this?

DR. A.G.B. KOVÁCH *(Budapest, Hungary):* I would think it would be possible to measure the effect of histamine on these mechanisms.

DR. ROSENBLUTH *(Oklahoma City, Okla.):* What is the perfusate used in these preparations of yours?

DR. KOVÁCH: The perfusion medium was Krebs-Henseleit bicarbonate buffers containing 4% bovine serum albumin (fraction V, Sigma). The buffer was dialyzed against two changes of Krebs-Henseleit bicarbonate buffers and filtered through Millipore filters (0.45-micron porosity) before use. After saturation with an O_2-CO_2 mixture (95:5), the pH was adjusted to 7.4. Substrate for gluconeogenesis was 10 mM lactate.

DR. M.H. WEIL *(Los Angeles, Calif.)*: With respect to some of the similarities between anaphylactic shock and the acute response to endotoxin, a series of reactions take place which have close similarities—not only the suddenness of the response (the hematological response) but, as Dr. Schumer said, the immediate appearance of histamine. I must admit that, back in the early 50's in Dr. Visscher's laboratory, we used bioassays with all the hazards of bioanalytical techniques at that particular time. We demonstrated the close relationship to the decrease in platelet concentration, leukopenia, and the lesions which were reminiscent of those described as early as 1902, I believe, for which Professor Doctor Reecher got the Nobel prize. So, I think a relationship exists there. The proper argument might be whether histamine has a biological action of its own. There are gross parallels between the anaphylactic reaction and the reaction to endotoxin. Both are accompanied, under experimental conditions, by the liberation of histamine which is demonstrable in blood.

I have one other comment, Dr. Del Guercio, that's really addressed to Dr. Gump. I want to be sure that I do understand his position correctly. I gather that it is on the basis of your studies in the intact human patient, Dr. Gump, and by measuring actually oxygen consumptions under your canopy, that you have been somewhat disappointed in looking for close relationships between oxygen consumption or changes in oxygen consumption in the intact human patient during shock and the presumed reduction in oxygen consumption that you would anticipate. Am I correct in interpreting your comments?

DR. F.E. GUMP *(New York, N.Y.)*: Yes. The exceptions that I didn't mention are patients who are hypothermic or unconscious. The underlying problem, of course, is that all these measurements, put in terms of per meter square, have to be related to a predicted normal value. It's important to keep that in mind because the predicted normal value varies between fairly wide limits. Because we are dealing with a wide range of normal values, it is often difficult to say whether oxygen consumption is actually below or above normal.

DR. WEIL: There is no question but that it becomes extremely difficult, over the clinical course of a patient, to really demonstrate reductions in oxygen consumption. And yet, I would be concerned if we left this afternoon having one of our basic trusts violated (if I might put it that way)—namely, that a rather fundamental defect on which we ordinarily agree is reduction in effective perfusion, and that perhaps the best way to determine this reduction is to measure oxygen consumption. When Dr. Crowell and Dr. Guyton first established the relationship between oxygen consumption (or oxygen debt, as they defined it in the dog) and mortality some years ago, they described a rather refined relationship between the calculated oxygen deficit and survival of the animal. More recently, Howard Whigham, in our own laboratory, used rather refined conditions in which the temperatures of animals were kept constant and there were relatively short life histories. The relationship between oxygen consumption and hemorrhage was demonstrated very nicely. In the course of these studies, lactate production was also implicated. The findings were reminiscent of the work of Huckaby.

Certainly, the energy kinetics at the cellular and subcellular levels are of the greatest moment. However, the energy requirements of any organism (particularly the human organism), under uncontrolled conditions of activity, fever, exposure, and treatment, may not give us a sufficiently uncontaminated signal. Under experimental conditions, the one thing that we can hold on to is that the perfusion deficit which is the fundamental effect of shock, is accompanied by a parallel reduction in oxygen availability in comparison to the oxygen need. This is reflected in some of the gross metabolic changes that we observe, including the acidosis. Am I right, Dr. Gump, if I hold onto that rather primitive concept?

DR. W.C. SHOEMAKER *(New York, N.Y.):* I would agree with the general consensus and the concept that Dr. Weil recently alluded to about the importance of oxygen consumption. However, Cuthbertson demonstrated this in 1931—a fact, I think, that has also been lost sight of, possibly even in Dr. Gump's recent review of that subject. What I would like to raise exception to is the conclusion that oxygen consumption is not diminished early in shock, in contrast to what Cuthbertson observed in very sophisticated units, where the patient only gets there two weeks after the fact. If you are going to look at the pattern of events, it is quite fair, under the circumstances that have been studied, to say that there is no decrease in oxygen consumption in the middle and late stages. I think you have to leave it quite open, though, that in the early period, there may be (as, indeed, it has been demonstrated) a diminution in oxygen consumption associated with a diminished oxygen availability.

DR. DEL GUERCIO: It's not actual oxygen consumption, but it's the efficiency of oxygen utilization that is important. One must know not only requirements but energy costs to the organism at any particular time of delivering 1 cc of oxygen for utilization by the cell. Even though oxygen consumption may be elevated, this may occur at very low efficiency for any of the numerous reasons which have been mentioned this afternoon. The inefficiency of the pulmonary gas exchange mechanism, the inefficiency of the circulation from the standpoint of the heart or peripheral vasculature, or the inefficiencies related to shifts in the dissociation curve, somewhere along the line, require that a penalty be paid by the organism for these decreases in efficiency. I think that only when we have a means of measuring this in man will we be able to say to Dr. Shoemaker, "Okay, at Stage 1 or Stage A, this patient is in trouble because he is utilizing oxygen inefficiently, either at a cellular level or at a more easily handled level, which is that of the blood itself." Does anyone else have any comments on this basic conflict?

DR. RUSH: I'll add one point which has come up several times today. That is, if you do indeed have uncoupling, the relationship of oxygen consumption to energy production is, of course, destroyed; whatever one measures, in terms of oxygen consumption, loses its parallel.

DR. GUMP: I've been very interested to hear that there may be uncoupling seen in actual clinical studies. It comes as a surprise. However, it doesn't destroy the relationship between oxidation and heat production, and if it does take place, then the body heat content would have to rise.

DR. DEL GUERCIO: You are implying that core body temperature generally drops under those circumstances.

DR. GUMP: It doesn't seem to go up.

DR. J.L. RATLIFF *(Jackson, Miss.):* Total body calorimetry would have to really be used to look at how much heat's being produced, though. Nobody has done that in the whole patient with sepsis.

DR. GUMP: You could either look at it as an increase in body heat content. Or, if you want to say the body heat content stays the same, the only other explanation would be a large increase in body heat loss.

DR. RATLIFF: The radiator surely works better under some circumstances than it does under others, however; that wouldn't be an irrational assumption. Without total body calorimetry, you really don't know how much heat you are producing. The core temperature doesn't really give you that picture.

DR. GUMP: I don't think that's true. In other words, there

is no question about the fact that if you oxidize the fuel in a bomb calorimeter or in the body, the amount of heat produced is the same.

DR. RATLIFF: That's true, but if your skin vessels are dilated and you're radiating your heat rapidly, your core temperature won't get to the same level that it will if your peripheral vessels go into spasm and you hold onto all of that heat. We've all seen neurosurgical patients whose skin gets cold and yet, their core temperature is 105° F. The only way to get it down is to promote vessel dilatation of the skin, and then you can effectively cool.

DR. GUMP: I don't think there's really any argument about that. As I say, the heat is there. Whether it goes to raise the body temperature or raise the temperature of the room is something that could be determined.

DR. DEL GUERCIO: Does anyone in the audience have any evidence for oxidative uncoupling in clinical situations or even in states of hemorrhagic shock in an experimental situation? Has it even been demonstrated?

DR. KOVÁCH: In August, we had a symposium in Budapest on neurohumoral and metabolic aspects of injury, where Dr. Mela, Dr. Baue, and we presented results which suggested uncoupled oxidative phosphorylation in isolated rat liver and kidney mitochondria from hemorrhagic-shock animals. These findings were confirmed in mitochondria from the livers of patients in shock by workers in Baltimore. At the same symposium in Budapest, Dr. Kirby (New Castle-upon-Tyne) found an increased thyroid hormone release in early shock that may be related to the elevated oxygen consumption.

DR. DEL GUERCIO: You mean, the thyroid hormone produces uncoupling of oxidative phosphorylation, possibly?

DR. SCHUMER: In our endotoxic shock studies of cardiac muscle, skeletal muscle, and liver, we found that this uncoupling has been a very late phenomenon, occurring approximately 17 to 24 hours after endotoxin administration. When this occurs, shock appears to be irreversible.

DR. DEL GUERCIO: Dr. Spitzer, you have done metabolic studies on the myocardium. Have you ever seen any evidence to suggest uncoupling of oxidative phosphorylation?

DR. J.J. SPITZER *(Philadelphia, Pa.):* So far, our experimental design has not included a study of uncoupling under *in vivo* conditions.

DR. DEL GUERCIO: Is there any way you can measure the efficiency of utilization of the substrates under these two circumstances? In other words, what percent of the total available energy of either the free fatty acids or lactate is utilized in repletion of ATP? Can there be a concept of percent deficiency under these circumstances?

DR. SPITZER: We can calculate myocardial efficiency from our data, but the calculation involves a number of assumptions, which, in the absence of ATP measurements, make the conclusions rather uncertain, especially during shock.

DR. SCHUMER: Dr. Horwitz, you reported an increase of fatty acids in septic shock. I am interested in whether or not you also found an increase in the ketone bodies, acetoacetic acid, and beta-hydroxybutyric acid.

DR. HORWITZ: We really haven't looked for it, so I can't say if it's there or not. I think the whole question of the elevation of free fatty acids is very controversial, as we have seen from the conflicting data presented today. To change the subject a little bit away from ketones, I think that the data reflect on a great many experimental conditions, of which shock is only one. Stress to the animal from environment or anesthesia is another major factor. Although we're not supposed to be discussing models today, a lot of these answers will have to be withheld until we can come up with a model in which everything else has been eliminated. Perhaps the conditions employed for studying growth hormone in humans, where we have a subject in a dark room behind a screen and we draw blood from an indwelling catheter, may have to be used before we can really answer the question of whether fatty acids do indeed go up in shock.

DR. SPITZER: I wish to comment on the statement made by Dr. Horwitz concerning free fatty acid concentrations during shock. As he very correctly pointed out, this depends a great deal on the experimental conditions. In anesthetized dogs, for instance, after severe hemorrhage, there is no increase in FFA (Spitzer, J.A., and J.J. Spitzer. Plasma lipid changes during hemorrhagic shock. J. Trauma, in press). If anything, there is a decrease. However, the same treatment results in an increase in arterial FFA concentration in nonanesthetized animals (Spitzer, J.J., R. Wiener, and E.H. Wolf. In: *Neurohumoral and Metabolic Aspects of Injury*, edited by A.G.B. Kovách, B. Stoner, and J.J. Spitzer, Plenum Press, 1972). The different response in anesthetized *vs.* conscious dogs is not unreasonable to attribute to better perfusion of the adipose tissue in the conscious animals. In this regard, it is relevant to mention some work that has been done in our laboratory by Dr. Judy Spitzer (Spitzer, J.A., *et al.* In: *Neurohumoral and Metabolic Aspects of*

Injury, edited by A.G.B. Kovách, B. Stoner, and J.J. Spitzer, Plenum Press, 1972). The experiments were performed in dogs, under Nembutal anesthesia. Adipose tissue samples were removed from the subcutaneous (SC) and omental (O) regions both before and after endotoxin administration. Isolated fat cells were prepared from all the tissues, and norepinephrine-stimulated release of FFA and glycerol was determined under *in vitro* conditions. Figure 1 represents data from one of these experiments. In the lower panel, the release of FFA (open bars) and glycerol (dark or black bars) is shown in the presence of norepinephrine (0.2 g/ml) both before and after the administration of endotoxin (+glucose and -glucose indicate the presence or absence of 1 mg/ml of glucose in the incubation medium). In the upper panel, the ratio of FFA to glycerol release is indicated under the same conditions. It can be seen that, in each instance, the norepinephrine-stimulated FFA release or glycerol release is enhanced by endotoxin administration. This is true for adipocytes of both subcutaneous or omental origin. While this phenomenon may contribute to the elevated FFA release when adipose tissue perfusion is not severely impaired, the underlying mechanism responsible for it is the subject for further studies.

DR. SMITH: Could I ask you the nature of the free fatty acids that you find to be increased?

DR. SPITZER: We have studied the changes in both FFA concentration and in fatty acid composition of FFA after severe hemorrhage in anesthetized dogs. Our findings indicated that saturated fatty acids (mainly palmitic) made up a larger fraction, and unsaturated acids (mainly oleic) constituted a smaller fraction of the plasma FFA pool after hemorrhage than before (Spitzer, J.A., and J.J. Spitzer. Plasma lipid changes during hemorrhagic shock. J. Trauma, in press). These changes occurred in the face of a slightly lower total arterial FFA concentration after hemorrhage. Triglyceride fatty acids also became more saturated. The composition of phospholipid fatty acids did not change consistently. Thus, these data resemble the qualitative fatty acid changes described by Dr. Smith, even though the species and experimental conditions were different.

DR. DEL GUERCIO: I am amazed that cyclic AMP has been mentioned only twice in this entire conference, thus far. I would have been willing to bet that we all would have been talking about it consistently. The people who deal in substrates are particularly reluctant to talk about teleology and concepts. Dr. Cryer, would you be willing to stick your neck out in regard to what part, ultimately, substrate manipulation will play in the treatment of both forms of shock on the basis of the evidence we've had today?

DR. P. CRYER *(St. Louis, Mo.):* I would doubt that substrate

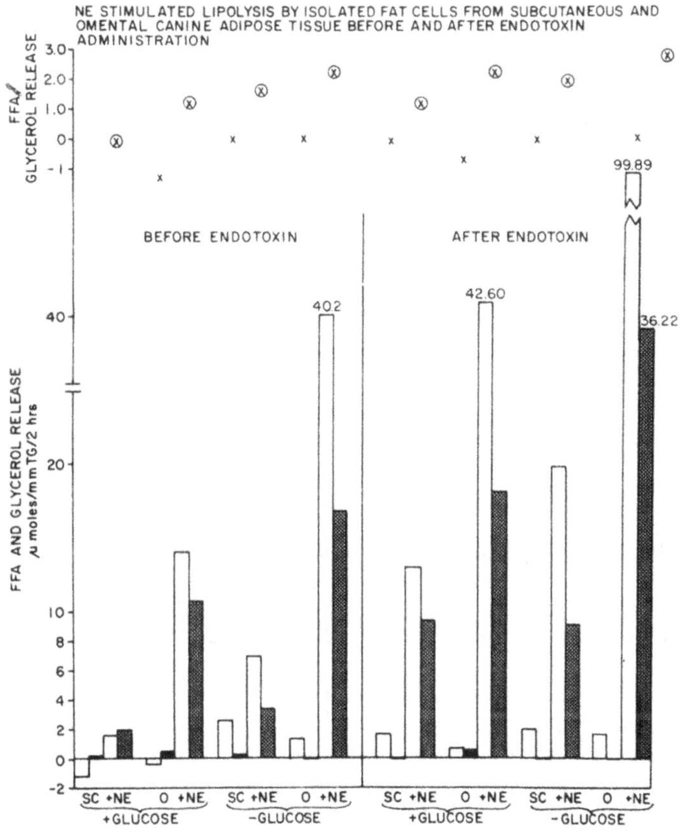

FIGURE 1

manipulation would have any beneficial effect.

DR. DEL GUERCIO: Well, that's sticking your neck out, all right. Thank you.

DR. JACOBSON: We now have direct evidence (this will be the third time "cyclic" is mentioned) that endotoxin activates adenyl cyclase in hepatic tissue of the guinea pig in fatal endotoxin shock. This would support Dr. Spitzer's speculation that cyclic AMP may indeed be involved here.

DR. DEL GUERCIO: Do we have any further questions from the audience?

DR. SWAN: I would like to ask Dr. Cryer a question. He has

indicated that the hypoinsulinemia and hyperglycemia associated with endotoxin shock is blocked by phentolamine. I presume, then, that this is a mechanism which is mediated through alpha-adrenergic receptors. If this is so, can you duplicate this phenomenon by exogenous administration of alpha-adrenergic agonists (and, in particular, phenylephrine), and can you block it by splanchnic nerve division?

DR. CRYER: We have done neither of those manipulations, so I cannot answer your question directly. I think that, as the data that I have presented indicate, alpha-adrenergic blockade did prevent the development of hyperglycemia and hypoinsulinemia in our animals. We have shown, in preliminary experiments, that this dosage of phentolamine also prevented the hyperglycemic and hypoinsulinemic response to intravenous epinephrine, but that is the only catecholamine we have worked out.

DR. DEL GUERCIO: Any further questions from the audience?

DR. SCHUMER: As long as we are conceptualizing, perhaps I can ask Dr. Cryer about the gluconeogenetic scheme occurring in stress. Proteins, amino acids, and fatty acids are catabolized, yielding carbon skeletons to keep the cycles functioning. In diabetes, which is in some ways very similar to the metabolic processes in the shock cell, glucose can inhibit the gluconeogenetic process, decreasing the catabolism of fatty acids. If fatty acids are as detrimental as we have heard today, why would administration of substrates, containing large amounts of glucose with insulin and potassium, not be therapeutically effective?

DR. CRYER: I'm very hesitant about that. I'm not aware of the fact that induced hyperglycemia will turn off gluconeogenesis in diabetic ketoacidosis. Certainly, the measurements I am aware of (which go back to Bondy's work in the late 40's) were that the liver is pouring out glucose despite really tremendous hyperglycemia in diabetic ketoacidosis. The provision of glucose with insulin would be expected to turn off gluconeogenesis as well as lipolysis.

DR. SMITH: Could I bring up a point, here? You're talking about diabetic ketoacidosis. As clinicians, we can treat patients in septic shock with antibiotics, but it takes us approximately 4 days to get the right antibiotic and the situation under control. We're looking for a situation somewhat parallel to the fact that, while insulin helps diabetic coma, insulin and potassium do better. We're looking for supportive mechanisms in order to keep these patients going long enough, but still we get back to the bacteria (at least, in septic shock), and antibiotics are the prime treatment. I would like to emphasize that. I would like to make another point. Underlying all of this discussion has been a slight suggestion that endotoxin shock and gram-negative rod shock are the same. Maybe they are not, and so we should refer exactly to what we are talking about. If we do mean gram-negative rod septicemic shock, we should say so and not necessarily call it endotoxin shock.

DR. SHANBOUR: This is a point that I would also like to make. When we talk about shock, it encompasses so many areas. Then we start talking about mechanisms, and whether there is overlap or not. One thing that bothers all of us is the irreversibility of shock. Again, if you look at cardiovascular effects or specific metabolic effects, we don't have any universal therapy. There has to be some basic effect that the therapy is just not taking care of. We have referred to the cyclic AMP system a couple of times. I would also like to point out that adenyl cyclase, which is responsible for the formation of cyclic AMP, is a membrane-bound enzyme.

DR. DEL GUERCIO: Any further questions from the audience? Any of the panelists wish to make any parting shots? Dr. Cryer.

DR. CRYER: I might clarify my answer to the question about substrate manipulation. My answer was in reference to direct manipulation of substrates. Hormonal manipulation, which would indirectly involve changes in substrate utilization, is a different matter. Our data would suggest that this might be a therapeutic possibility.

DR. HORWITZ: I want to reinforce what Dr. Cryer just said and take issue a little bit with what Dr. Schumer said in relation to using glucose to depress gluconeogenesis. I think many of the feedback cycles that are normally operative do not work in shock. A good example is the glucose-fatty acid cycle which Randle described many years ago, saying that if glucose goes up, fatty acids go down, and *vice versa*. This regulatory mechanism is out of commission probably because, as Dr. Cryer suggested, of excessive adrenergic stimulation of the pancreas depressing insulin secretion, which is what mediates the feedback. This is probably true throughout the body. As Dr. Cryer says, it's probably caused more by hormonal influences than substrate influences.

DR. SPITZER: As a further extension of what has just been dicusssed, I wish to mention that after acute hemorrhage in the conscious dog, we found that more lactate was recycled into glucose than during control conditions (Wiener, R., E.H. Wolf, and J.J. Spitzer. FFA and lactate turnover following severe hemorrhage in the conscious dog. Fed. Proc. 1972).

DR. CRYER: I think that's perfectly consistent with insulin lack.

DR. DEL GUERCIO: If there are no further comments, we want to thank the audience, and I'd like to personally thank the panel for a most interesting afternoon.

SESSION III

TOXIC FACTORS IN SHOCK

Panel Moderator:

Lloyd D. MacLean, M.D., Ph.D.
Department of Surgery
McGill University
Montreal, Quebec, Canada

SESSION III: INTRODUCTORY REMARKS

Lloyd D. MacLean, M.D., Ph.D., *Panel Moderator*

Department of Surgery, McGill University, Montreal, Quebec, Canada

For many years, interest in toxic factors in shock has waxed and waned. This area of research has gotten off to a rather slow start compared to hemodynamic studies, which have made tremendous inroads in the treatment of shock patients. The early workers, Cannon and Bayless, were stimulated by the fact that wounded soldiers pinned under fallen timbers in World War I appeared to deteriorate rapidly when their limbs were freed. This suggested to observers at that time that some toxic material was being released from the limb. Similar findings were also noted after sudden release of a tourniquet; and it was known that, if one proceeded with an amputation before removing the tourniquet, death was less likely to occur. Cannon and Bayless were stimulated to answer the following question: Is death, following a pressure injury, caused by toxic agents liberated from damaged tissues or is it due to loss of fluid at the site of injury? They concluded that it was probably due to release of toxic materials, despite the observations of Keith, Robertson, and others who clearly documented that all patients in shock with this sort of injury always had a decreased blood volume. Also, Dale and Richards had described histamine and its overt effects very shortly before that.

I look upon the work of Blalock and Phemister as one of the most important developments in shock research in this century. They recognized the relationship between traumatic shock and hypovolemia. Challenging the studies of Cannon and Bayless, they showed clearly that the amount of fluid and blood loss into the injured area was enough to account for the shock encountered. This may still be worth re-examining. Unfortunately, many patients, snatched from death's door by heroic hemodynamic measures, succumb at a later date to infection. Sepsis and toxic factors play an important role, and this, I think, is the challenge facing investigators who work in the field of shock.

RELEASE OF TOXIC AGENTS IN SEPTIC SHOCK

Alan P. Thal, M.D.

Department of Surgery, University of Kansas Medical Center, Kansas City, Kansas

Informal Presentation[1]

The presence of toxic factors in various forms of injury must have been obvious to prehistoric man when he first experienced the relief following spontaneous drainage of an abscess. Within a few hours, the tachycardia, sweating, feeling of weakness, and malaise disappeared, and he could not help but speculate on the toxic effects of pus, the subject that concerns us now. This dramatic systemic response to the drainage of an abscess is, I think, one of the most solid indicators of the possibility that a toxic agent emanating from an area of injured tissue is responsible for many of the systemic effects of sepsis. To this day, the most striking response seen in septic patients follows the drainage of an abscess, the removal of a septic uterus, or the amputation of a septic gangrenous leg.

Our particular interest in such toxic factors began in 1962 when we were studying the hemodynamic changes in various forms of shock. The patients in septic shock showed a clinical picture which often diametrically opposed that seen in cardiogenic and hypovolemic shock. In these patients alone, cardiac output was often normal or even high, unless there was associated hypovolemia or cardiac failure. While several possibilities may account for this lowered vascular resistance and comparably raised cardiac

---

[1]This manuscript appears here as presented at the symposium, with minor editorial revisions.

output, we chose to investigate the possibility that a septic vasodilator substance was involved. At that time, we began to detect protease activity in the blood of some of these patients. In the light of Roche e Silva's work, we looked at bradykinin as a possible septic vasodilator. Superficially, it bears a relationship to the substance we were seeking. A single injection produces hypotension, with a rise in cardiac output. However, the effect is very transitory. Using bioassay methods in the terminal phases of hemorrhagic or endotoxic shock, we found raised levels of histamine, release of serotonin, and increased protease activity. There was evidence of inadequate tissue perfusion as shown by increased lactate. The level of precursor bradykininogen fell, and there was a rise in bradykininase. These events were seen in the terminal phases of shock, and we wondered whether we were studying an agonal event or some basic phenomenon. Pursuing the release of toxic agents further, we found that when endotoxin was incubated with various tissues, a proteolytic reaction took place (as shown by a rise in TAME esterase), with a release of bradykinin and histamine. Similarly, in some cases of clinical septic shock we were able to detect minor increases in these agents. However, the methodology at that time consisted largely of bioassay, leaving much to be desired.

Since we had now established the hemodynamic characteristics of sepsis and septic shock in man, we were able to examine more critically what was then the accepted experimental model, endotoxin shock in the dog. It was immediately clear that this preparation bore little or no resemblance to the phenomenon we had measured in man. While the literature describing the pathophysiologic changes and the responses to therapy in the canine endotoxin shock model has become enormous, one must seriously question its relationship to sepsis and septic shock in man.

To study septic shock in the dog, we felt it was necessary to establish an appropriate anatomical site for sepsis. Initially, we used intraperitoneal sepsis (ligation of the cecal appendage). However, we soon found that the accompanying ileus, anorexia, and fluid loss masked the effects we were seeking. A more satisfactory model was obtained by inducing sepsis in one hind leg. The animal was able to tolerate this reasonably well, and the preparation could be studied for up to 4 days. About 50% of these animals responded with a significant rise in cardiac output, a fall in vascular resistance, pyrexia, and an increase in oxygen consumption. The cardiac output rose approximately 70%, while the oxygen consumption increased 12%. In summary, there was obviously an excess flow to the septic leg and extensive redistribution of flow. For example, on the septic side, the flow increased from 50% to 100%, whereas the blood flow declined in the contralateral normal leg. Some have assumed that the rise in cardiac output simply reflects the excessive flow through the area of sepsis. On the other hand, our studies show that flow through the area of sepsis accounts for only a small proportion of the total increase in cardiac output. Consequently, we could not account for this increase in cardiac output, amounting to an average of about 1,200 ml per minute, simply on the basis of increased flow through the septic leg. Flow had to be increased elsewhere, as well. In subsequent canine experiments, we demonstrated that at least some of this excess flow passed through the splanchnic viscera and the kidneys, and probably also through other areas not yet studied. (Kinney and Gump confirmed this in man.) It seemed clear, then, that shunting or vasodilation in the septic area did not entirely explain this unique hemodynamic response, but that systemic redistribution of flow in regions distant from the area of sepsis was occurring. Accordingly, it seemed likely that some agent released from the septic area was responsible for this. To test this hypothesis, we infused small aliquots of septic venous blood into the normal leg. Femoral artery flow increased dramatically on that side, and the arteriovenous oxygen difference narrowed markedly. When non-septic venous blood in precisely the same amount was added to the arterial inflow of the test leg, the values returned to normal. Thus, we felt that these studies, together with the extensive control experiments that were carried out, demonstrated the release of a septic vasodilator substance. Moreover, they pointed to the fact that the vascular responses in sepsis are not uniform, *i.e.*, that some vascular beds contract while others dilate. Certainly, this is observed in man during body chilling, when marked vasoconstriction of the skin blood vessels may occur in the face of a large increase in cardiac output.

To obtain further evidence for the presence of a septic vasodilator with systemic effects, the following experiment was carried out. In one group of animals, sepsis was induced in the leg in routine fashion. The other group served as control. Cardiac output, arterial blood pressure, and heart rate were measured continuously and total peripheral resistance was calculated. After 48 hours of sepsis, a rubber-coated wire tourniquet was placed around the septic limb for 2 hours and then released. A similar experiment was done in the control animal. In the septic animal, the previously lowered peripheral resistance rose when the tourniquet was applied and cardiac output fell to normal levels (Fig. 1). In the control animal, cardiac output and vascular resistance changed very little until the tourniquet was removed and fluid became trapped in the damaged limb. When the tourniquet was removed from the septic animal, the cardiac output again rose.

This study would seem to support the concept of a septic vasodilator substance being released from an area of sepsis and exerting systemic effects. In several patients with sepsis we

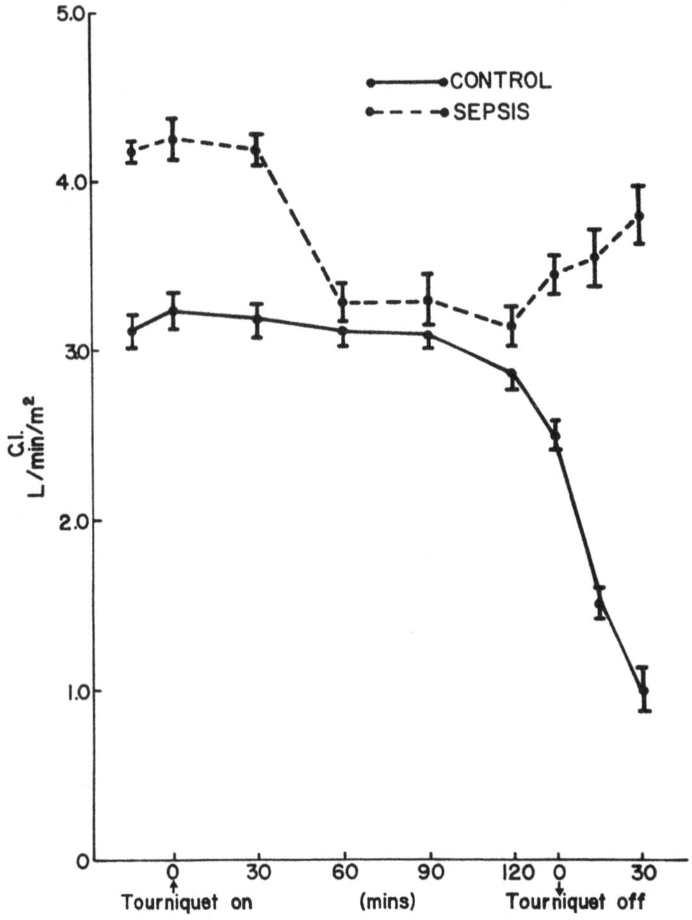

FIG. 1. Effect of tourniquet application upon cardiac index in dogs with leg sepsis and in control animals.

and others have noticed evidence of heart failure, even in younger individuals. The septic leg preparation offered us a means to study the response of the heart to sepsis of long duration. When the heart of the septic animal is stressed by volume load, by beta-adrenergic stimulation with isoproterenol, or by increased afterload caused by angiotensin, cardiac performance is clearly impaired. (The experimental details of this study have been described elsewhere.) These studies showed that the heart in the septic animal is under considerable sympathetic drive and depends upon it to maintain cardiac output. Attempts to abrograte this sympathetic drive with the beta-adrenergic blocking drug, propranolol, disastrously reduce cardiac performance and often cause death of the animal. Whether the cardiac deterioration in sepsis results from the action of a toxic agent such as myocardial depressant factor or simply represents fatigue in a laboring heart is not yet clear.

In order to place the evidence for the release of toxic agents in sepsis in proper perspective, we should not be seeking an agent which produces sudden hypotension and rapid death. This is not the picture we see in clinical sepsis or septic shock in man. Whether the patient survives does not depend primarily on our ability to manipulate blood pressure, cardiac output, and vascular resistance. Rather, survival is determined by a number of factors which are difficult to mimic in the experimental preparation. They include the initial degree of reduced vital organ function, as in the aged patient, the duration and severity of the insult, and the damage that occurs to vital organs—especially the lungs, heart, kidneys, and reticuloendothelial system during and immediately after the onset of shock. These toxic agents produce damage, and hence determine survival or death, either by altering the distribution of blood flow or by directly affecting vital organs.

THE RELATIONSHIP BETWEEN OXYGEN UPTAKE AND A TOXIC FACTOR IN SEPTIC SHOCK

John H. Duff, M.D.

Department of Surgery, Royal Victoria Hospital and
McGill University, Montreal, Quebec, Canada

Informal Presentation[1]

When one speaks about the toxic factor in clinical shock, one is generally referring to a shock state refractory to all present methods of therapy. I would like to talk about two aspects of the toxic factor. The first is related to those patients who die in shock due to sepsis, despite all present methods of management. The second aspect concerns an animal study using dogs rendered septic by ligation of the cecum. Interestingly enough, these animals show a toxic factor which may be related to refractory septic shock in human beings.

We have studied 20 patients who received all currently available methods of therapy but responded poorly. In fact, only two survived. We plotted oxygen uptake against arterial blood lactate in these patients and found that the higher the lactate, the lower the oxygen uptake. Since it is generally agreed that arterial blood lactate, measured serially, is an index of tissue hypoxia, it is possible to compare the hypoxia of sepsis with that of exercise. However, one basic assumption is necessary, *i.e.*, that patients in septic shock have increased oxygen demands. If they do, the question of oxygen debt, raised by Dr. Gump, would seem to be very important. If a number of normal subjects are studied in whom oxygen debt is created by exercise, we find that they respond by a rise in both lactate production and oxygen uptake. Whereas

---

[1]This manuscript appears here as presented at the symposium, with minor editorial revisions.

lactate is high in the hypoxia of both exercise and sepsis, oxygen uptake rises only in exercise.

Yet, clinically, these patients show ample evidence of increased demand for oxygen. Most would agree that fever, tachypnea, tachycardia, and restlessness are seen in most patients with severe sepsis. At the same time, oxygen transport is impaired compared to that of normal individuals. A septic lung lesion may decrease arterial oxygen saturation. The hemoglobin is seldom over 11 g, and often lower. We cannot be sure, in every case, that the patient in sepsis will be able to adequately compensate for decreased pO_2 and hemoglobin by raising his cardiac output. Finally, it appears that these particular patients are unable to broaden their arteriovenous difference to increase oxygen uptake.

Plotting the arteriovenous difference against the cardiac index in septic patients reveals a response opposite to that of a normal human being who has increased demands with exercise. In the septic patients, the higher the cardiac index rises the lower the arteriovenous difference becomes. In normal individuals during exercise, both the cardiac index and arteriovenous difference go up. The former phenomenon points to a peripheral cellular defect—either due to toxicity or some other effect of the sepsis. No proven specific therapy has yet been developed for this. Cortisone, as an agent that potentially affects the cell, may prove useful in this regard.

Animal studies raise a similar problem. Dogs were rendered septic by ligation of the cecum. Measurements were made before infection and 5 days after, when they were in sepsis but not yet in septic shock. They had intraperitoneal infection, abscess, and peritonitis. Their blood pressure was decreased and they were febrile, but not in what we would call shock. Muscle capillary blood flow in the leg and cardiac output were measured in these dogs. Capillary blood flow was determined by the xenon technique, which measures only capillary blood flow and not shunted blood flow.

Although it is difficult to increase blood flow in dogs made septic, we did have a group of about 10 dogs in which cardiac output rose. These dogs are the closest we can come experimentally to the hyperdynamic circulation in human septic shock. We found that capillary muscle blood flow in the leg varied according to the cardiac index. In point of fact, the muscle blood flow and the femoral arteriovenous difference varied exactly as the cardiac index and the over-all arteriovenous difference. So it appeared that the capillary blood flow in the leg mirrored, to some extent, the total picture of cardiac output and arteriovenous difference. Thus, the high flow situation in septic dogs was at least partly attributable to capillary blood flow.

We compared the group of dogs in sepsis with high cardiac output and high capillary blood flow to another group of dogs in which leg exercise was carried out by stimulation of the muscles. In exercise, the capillary muscle blood flow increases, as one would expect. At the same time, the femoral arteriovenous difference increases markedly. In other words, oxygen extraction becomes much greater. In the septic animal, we found the opposite. Although flow increased, there was narrowing of the arteriovenous difference, a response exactly opposite that observed during exercise. These results point out, I think, an altered response to oxygen demand in sepsis. In humans, this response appears to be lethal and I think is evidence of a toxic factor. It is this factor we will have to investigate further before we can improve the present survival rates in patients with septic shock.

DISCUSSION[1]

DR. I. M. SMITH *(Iowa City, Iowa)*: Dr. Thal, is cardiac output increased by digitalis?

DR. THAL: Yes, we found that ouabain was the only agent of those that we tried that could increase stroke volume and V max in the septic animal. With other drugs, such as isoproterenol, the animal reacted by an increase in heart rate which seemed to be its only mechanism for increasing output. Slowing the heart with propranolol failed to produce any improvement, but ouabain did shift the cardiac function curve toward normal.

DR. W. SCHUMER *(Chicago, Ill.)*: Dr. Thal, in the septic limb study, have you measured circulating vasoactive factors?

DR. THAL: Yes, we've measured a large number of factors, and one can find evidences of serotonin, small amounts of histamine, and very small amounts of bradykinin. We're in the process of setting up a radioimmunoassay because of the difficulties in assaying bradykinin. We have not consistently found endotoxin (using the limulus lysate method), only occasionally. We have not yet been able to correlate it with the changes we've seen; nor can we produce these effects on the contralateral leg using these agents (serotonin, histamine, *etc.*). The agent we have found that most closely reproduces this is endogenous leukocyte pyrogen. So, it's possible that we're dealing with a protease breakdown of

---

[1]This discussion also covers the presentation of Dr. Thal (see preceding paper).

the white cell that is producing, either directly or indirectly, an effect on the opposite limb. This is still preliminary, though.

DR. L. D. MACLEAN, *Panel Moderator (Montreal, Canada):* Inherent in Dr. Duff's study and at variance with some of the work reported yesterday is the fact that the large cardiac output is not due to A-V shunting, because one would have expected, with an increased cardiac output, the muscle blood flow not to keep up with it, using this technique. I wonder if anybody would like to comment on that aspect.

DR. A. M. LEFER *(Jerusalem, Israel):* I would like to comment, not on that particular point, but on the use of digitalis glycosides in shock. While it's perfectly true that digitalis glycosides will improve myocardial performance, at least transiently, they do not enhance survival. We've shown that one of the key factors, perhaps, in its lack of ultimate survival value is the fact that it constricts the splanchnic circulation markedly. So, as we will indicate later, lysosomal enzymes pour out and toxic factors are formed. After the initial burst of improved myocardial performance, you actually get an impairment of myocardial performance. So, I would like to raise a slight question about the utilization of digitalis glycosides, at least in hemorrhagic shock.

DR. THAL: We are not talking about hemorrhagic shock here, and I think that one should recognize the difference. In these particular septic preparations, the splanchnic blood flow is actually increased, although we do not know the pancreatic blood flow. Secondly, I think, in managing the septic shock patient, one of the most important areas of therapeutic gain is support of the lung, often with a ventilator, and support of the heart with fluids and digitalis. I think that, certainly in the septic shock patient, we have seen quite salutary effects from the use of digitalis and other standard methods to support cardiopulmonary function.

DR. DUFF: I'd like to bring up one point and ask Dr. Thal to amplify it. Our results are a little different in that his work seems to show the toxic factor to be in the blood, whereas we would suggest that the factor is in the periphery. At least, it appears this way in patients. Now, do I take it that you believe that the toxic factor is circulating in the blood in your dog work and the periphery is still normal? In patient studies, do you think this would apply as well?

DR. THAL: Dr. Duff, what do you mean by the "periphery still normal"? Is this in terms of flow or cytotoxic effects?

DR. DUFF: No, I mean the ability of the cells to take up oxygen.

DR. THAL: Well, I think this depends on the stage of the illness. Certainly in the pre-agonal stage, the cells may not have the ability to take up oxygen, and one can flow blood through them without producing any effect on oxygen uptake. But, in the early stage, I think the cells are still in a viable state and can take up oxygen. Now, I think one of the most clear-cut ways of demonstrating this is in the massively septic leg, where one has a greater degree of condensed sepsis than one could possibly have in the body as a whole. If one reduces flow mechanically to the septic leg, there is a prompt widening of the A-V oxygen difference, indicating that the blood is perfusing nutritional channels and that the normal mechanisms for oxygen extraction are still functioning. The oxygen consumption remains within the normal range.

DR. MACLEAN: I think others are going to answer this, but we have the distinct feeling that in the agonal stage, one might actually see an increased oxygen uptake—maybe not utilization, but certainly in many patients the decreased oxygen uptake becomes apparent long before you've worried about the patient dying.

DR. C. M. HERMAN *(Bethesda, Md.):* An alternative explanation for some of these observations might lie in the oxyhemoglobin dissociation curve of the red cell. I just wondered if you had a chance to look at this.

DR. DUFF: You are quite right. You have picked the one flaw in the argument. I think we will have to show by *in vitro* experiments whether the blood really can give up oxygen.

DR. THAL: I think, Dr. MacLean, I might add another point. If you take these animals that are septic and in very brittle state, and withdraw relatively small amounts of blood, they rapidly deteriorate into a form of hypovolemic shock. The animal is then able to widen its A-V oxygen difference, if you measure this continuously. So, I think this is still a moot question.

DR. K. G. SWAN *(Washington, D.C.):* I would like to ask Dr. Thal if he has measured circulating catecholamines in the septic leg condition?

DR. THAL: Yes, catecholamine concentrations are raised in the septic model. We have infused catecholamines into the septic limb and found that the treated vasodilated limb is very responsive and will constrict. It is very difficult to produce additional vasodilation with an alpha blocking agent. But they are responsive to vasoconstriction, and I think this is a point where we would disagree with Dr. Duff and Dr. MacLean in believing that muscle blood flow has a direct relationship to what is happening in the internal viscera. In our preparation, there is a diversion of blood flow from the muscle and skin. The increase in blood flow occurs predominantly in the area of sepsis and in the viscera such as the kidney and the splanchnic viscera. One sees this in some patients who appear to be vasoconstricted according to clinical judgment (cardiac observations, the skin, coldness of the extremities) and whose cardiac output is still within the normal or raised range. So, I think that the muscle and the skin are much more subservient to sympathomimetic influence.

DR. E. D. JACOBSON *(Houston, Texas):* I'd like to back up what Dr. Lefer said about glycosides. We have found in dogs and in monkeys, whether normal or in hemorrhagic or endotoxin shock, that mesenteric vasoconstriction takes place. If we couple that with the finding that over 90% of patients dying of hemorrhagic necrosis of the gut have received digitalis, I think one can raise a serious question about the prophylactic usage of the glycoside in the shock patient.

ROLE OF THE PANCREAS IN THE PATHOGENESIS OF CIRCULATORY SHOCK[1]

Allan M. Lefer, Ph.D.[2], and Thomas M. Glenn, Ph.D.[3]

Department of Physiology, University of Virginia School of Medicine, Charlottesville, Virginia

Several toxic factors have been proposed as mediators of irreversibility in circulatory shock (6,17,29,48,57). Most, however, have not been enthusiastically received because their participation in the pathophysiology of the shock state remains unsupported by convincing evidence and no factor has been isolated. Recently, a myocardial depressant factor (MDF) has been isolated from the plasma of both experimental animals (30) and man (42) in a variety of shock states, including hemorrhagic (9,32,54), endotoxic (55), cardiogenic (23), bowel ischemic (20,37), burn (2), and pancreatitis (35) shock.

MDF has been identified as a peptide with a molecular weight of 800-1,000 (36,38). It is capable of inducing circulatory shock when injected intravenously into normal animals in concentrations comparable to those found in the peripheral plasma during circulatory shock (22). Thus, MDF fulfills the basic requirements of a shock factor: (a) it is produced in circulatory shock of several types but is absent in nonshocked animals; (b) it is a chemical entity which can be isolated from shocked animals and studied in

[1]Supported by grants-in-aid from the American Heart Association and the Virginia Heart Association, and by Research Grant HE-14277 from the National Heart and Lung Institute, NIH.

[2]Established Investigator of the American Heart Association.

[3]National Heart and Lung Institute Postdoctoral Fellow. Present address: Department of Pharmacology, Medical College of Pennsylvania, Philadelphia, Pa. 19129.

detail; (c) it is capable of inducing shock when injected into nonshocked recipients; (d) its primary action (*i.e.*, depression of the heart) is associated with a serious pathologic disturbance; and (e) it is present in man as well as laboratory animals during circulatory shock.

The major purpose of this communication is to review the current status of the formation and action of MDF and to describe its relation to the pancreas during a variety of shock states.

PROCESSES IN THE FORMATION OF MDF

Pancreatic Blood Flow

In most forms of circulatory shock sustained or transient hypotension appears early in the development of the shock state. Invariably, this markedly reduces splanchnic blood flow (41), due to several factors: (a) diminished intravascular driving force which passively decreases vessel diameter, thereby lowering blood flow; (b) release of vasoconstrictor substances (*i.e.*, adrenal medullary catecholamines, vasopressin, angiotensin II, serotonin, *etc.*); (c) microthrombi in the splanchnic vessels impeding blood flow; and (d) active neurogenically induced sympathetic vasoconstriction. These mechanisms do not completely depend upon the presence of a systemic arterial hypotension since, in pancreatitis, pancreatic blood flow is reduced to below 10% of normal in the presence of a normotensive state (26).

Because total splanchnic flow constitutes a large fraction of the cardiac output and supplies many organs with blood, the redistribution of splanchnic blood flow in shock is of prime importance. When regional splanchnic blood flow was measured during experimental shock, pancreatic blood flow was found to decrease markedly, remaining low throughout the shock state (16,58). In conscious monkeys, however, liver and intestinal blood flow decreased less than pancreatic and splenic flow. These findings emphasize that (a) pancreatic blood flow markedly decreases in the unanesthetized primate during shock; (b) pancreatic blood flow decreases more than intestinal or hepatic flow in shock, and (c) pancreatic ischemia is not readily reversible in shock, remaining depressed throughout the course of shock. These data may help to explain the finding of Brobmann and Jacobson (10) that superior mesenteric blood flow did not significantly decrease in endotoxin shock in the monkey. Thus, pancreatic blood flow decreases markedly in various forms of circulatory shock, regardless of whether intestinal flow decreases, and apparently represents an important event early in the animal's response to injury or trauma.

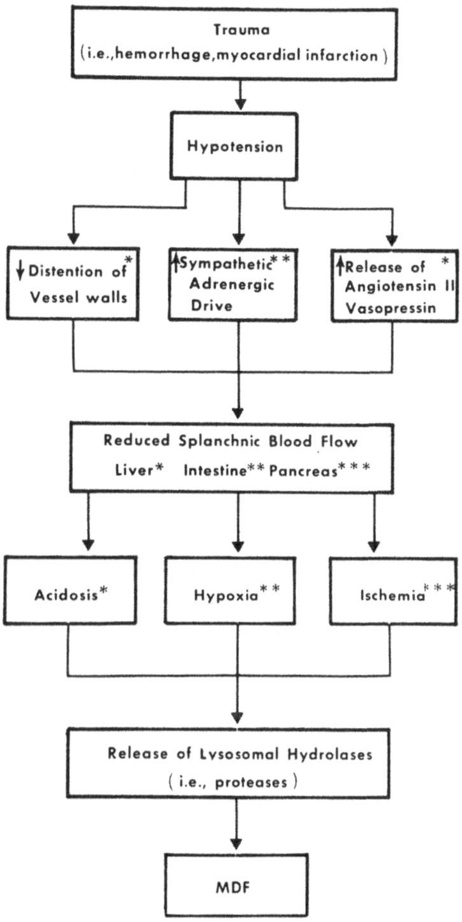

FIG. 1. Physical and humoral events leading to the formation of MDF in various types of circulatory shock. Number of asterisks indicate the degree of contribution of a given factor: * = slight to moderate; ** = moderate to severe; *** = very severe.

Figure 1 summarizes the current working hypothesis on the formation of MDF in circulatory shock. Pancreatic hypoperfusion is the crucial step in this pathway. The evidence supporting this point is as follows:

(a) Plasma MDF activity is inversely related to splanchnic blood flow (*i.e.*, superior mesenteric artery flow) in endotoxin (55) and hemorrhagic shock (34).

(b) A 2-4 hour lag occurs between the decrease in superior mesenteric artery flow and MDF production in hemorrhagic (34), endotoxic (55), cardiogenic (23), and pancreatitis (35) shock.

(c) Pharmacologic blockade of the celiac ganglia with lidocaine (a local anesthetic) before the induction of endotoxic shock prevents the decrease in superior mesenteric artery flow and the increase in plasma MDF activity (55).

(d) Occlusion of the celiac artery and both mesenteric arteries for 2 hours followed by release of the clamps yields high plasma MDF activities (22,37).

(e) Occlusion of the pancreatic arteries alone results in MDF activities comparable to those observed in shock (37).

(f) Pancreatectomy before occlusion of the splanchnic arteries or induction of hemorrhagic shock almost completely abolishes MDF production (37).

(g) Producing either ischemia (*i.e.*, reducing flow) or hypoxia (*i.e.*, reducing pO_2 at a constant flow) in the isolated perfused cat pancreas (14) results in the production of large amounts of MDF.

Stimuli for Lysosomal Disruption

These data show that hypoperfusion of the splanchnic region in general, and of the pancreas in particular, is an important link in the pathogenesis of circulatory shock. Hypoperfusion establishes three conditions: hypoxia, ischemia, and acidosis. These three stimuli cause lysosomal disruption by altering the permeability characteristics of the lysosomal membrane, thereby producing leakage of lysosomal hydrolases into the cytoplasm (51). These phenomena occur during hypotension and shock, particularly in the splanchnic region (3,40,46). The relative influences of these three factors on lysosomal stability were studied in experiments on the isolated perfused pancreas, under conditions which allowed these stimuli to be individually varied. In addition to measuring the tissue and effluent concentration of lysosomal hydrolases (*e.g.*, β-glucuronidase, cathepsin D), sections of the pancreas were examined for changes in lysosomal ultrastructure. Hypoxia or ischemia for 90-minute periods constituted an effective stimulus for releasing pancreatic lysosomal hydrolases (Fig. 2), whereas acidosis to a pH of 7.0 *per se* did not. Furthermore, large doses of methylprednisolone, a lysosomal-stabilizing agent (20), prevented this decrease in total tissue β-glucuronidase. The decrease in tissue β-glucuronidase activity during hypoxia or

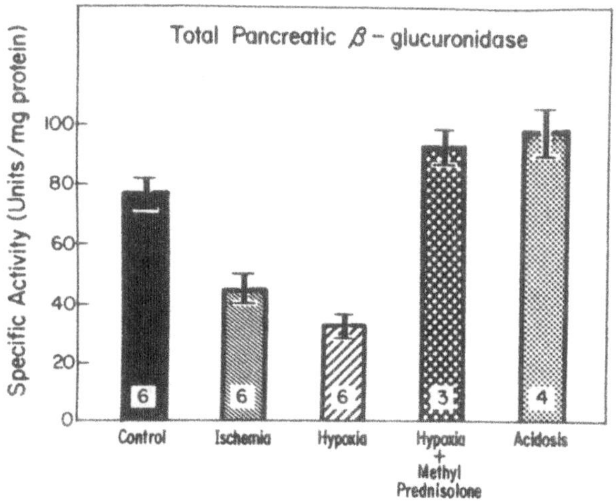

FIG. 2. Total pancreatic tissue specific activity of the lysosomal hydrolase β-glucuronidase in a variety of conditions in the isolated perfused cat pancreas. Height of the bars indicates the mean; brackets indicate the standard error of the mean; and numbers at the bottom of the bars indicate the number of pancreata analyzed. (Courtesy of Am. J. Physiol., in press.)

ischemia is not due to reduced protein synthesis, since the lost enzyme could be recovered in the pancreatic transudate (*i.e.*, largely lymphatic drainage) (see Table 1). In addition to these biochemical observations, ischemia or hypoxia induced the formation of large vacuoles within the lysosomes of the acinar cells of the pancreas, and the over-all size of these phagolysosomes (or secondary lysosomes) was larger than that of the primary lysosomes in control preparations. Also, the mitochondria and endoplasmic reticulum showed signs of damage. Methylprednisolone administration effectively prevented the ultrastructural alterations in the lysosomes but not in the other cytoplasmic organelles, indicating a degree of specificity of the methylprednisolone effect for lysosomes.

Taken collectively, these data indicate the following:

(a) Hypoxia and ischemia comparable to that observed in shock are potent stimuli for increased permeability of pancreatic lysosomes.

(b) Acidosis *per se* is not a potent lysosomal-labilizing stimulus, although it may potentiate the other stimuli.

TABLE 1

LYSOSOMAL ENZYME ACTIVITY IN TRANSUDATES FROM PERFUSED PANCREATA[a]

Group	No. organs	β-glucuronidase activity (units[b]/ml)	Cathepsin D activity (units[c]/ml)
Control	10	283± 66	32± 7
Ischemia	6	579±122[d]	53± 7[d]
Hypoxia	8	721±185[d]	59±12[d]
Hypoxia + methylprednisolone	5	224± 54	32± 6
Acidosis	4	320± 48	40± 5

[a]All values are means ±SE.

[b]Expressed as μg of phenolphthalein released/ml/hr at 37°C x transudate volume (ml).

[c]Expressed as mEq of tyrosine released x 10^{-4}/ml/hr at 37°C x transudate volume (ml).

[d]*P* < 0.01 compared to control.

(Courtesy of Am. J. Physiol., in press.)

(c) Lysosomal-stabilizing agents such as methylprednisolone can almost entirely prevent these changes in the face of severe lysosomal-labilizing stimuli (*e.g.*, hypoxia).

(d) Lysosomal disruption occurs rather than decreased synthesis of lysosomal hydrolases.

(e) Lysosomal disruption in the pancreas is associated with MDF production (to be discussed in detail later).

These findings point to the lysosomes as key subcellular structures in the mediation of tissue damage in circulatory shock.

Lysosomal Involvement in Shock

Lysosomes have been suggested to play a role in shock (4,8, 18-22,28,36,49,56). That lysosomal hydrolases contribute to the pathogenesis of circulatory shock is supported by the following evidence:

(a) The activity of plasma lysosomal enzymes rises dramatically early in many forms of shock (3,20,22,34,49).

(b) The total tissue activity of pancreas and liver are markedly reduced in postoligemic (22) and splanchnic ischemia shock (20), whereas the spleen and intestine are only moderately influenced and the heart is not significantly involved (see Table 2).

(c) The percent of lysosomal enzymes in the "free" or unbound form increases during shock, indicating increased lysosomal fragility (20,56).

(d) The activity of almost all the known lysosomal enzymes is optimal at acid pH (*e.g.*, pH 3-6), favoring their action during shock (22).

(e) Some of the degradative enzymes of lysosomal hydrolases and/or their products, as well as the reticuloendothelial system which clears the plasma of much of their activity, do not function effectively in shock (24).

(f) The morphology of lysosomes in splanchnic tissues changes dramatically in shock (becoming larger, developing more and bigger vacuoles), indicating increased fragility (5,12,22,47).

(g) Lysosomal enzymes exert deleterious effects on the circulation (24)(to be discussed in detail elsewhere).

(h) Lysosomal enzymes appear to be related to the formation of MDF and perhaps other toxic agents (to be discussed later).

(i) Agents which prevent the release of lysosomal enzymes (*e.g.*, glucocorticoids) protect in shock, increasing survival time as well as rate (21,36,53,56).

Current evidence thus implicates the lysosomal enzymes as contributors to the pathogenesis of circulatory shock, but fails to clarify whether their role is direct or indirect or whether it is crucial to the underlying lethal mechanisms in shock. Particularly important are the changes in the sensitive splanchnic tissues, *i.e.*, the liver and pancreas. Since the liver is much larger than the pancreas and pancreatic sensitivity does not much exceed that of the liver, the liver contributes more total lysosomal enzyme activity to the circulation. However, the pancreas plays a unique role in the development of the shock state,

TABLE 2

PLASMA CATHEPSIN D ACTIVITY DURING VARIOUS TYPES OF CIRCULATORY SHOCK[a]

Stage of Shock	Cathepsin D activity[b]			
	Hemorrhagic (4 cats)	Splanchnic ischemia (6 cats)	Endotoxic (4 dogs)	Cardiogenic (5 dogs)
Preshock control	5.0±0.6	5.9±0.8	3.5±0.7	3.0±0.8
Oligemic, occlusive, or 2-3 hours post-trauma	14.1±1.5	9.5±1.2	6.5±1.5	3.6±0.6
Early postoligemic, postocclusive, or 4-5 hours post-trauma	17.9±2.8	11.8±2.1	—	7.0±1.2
Late postoligemic, postocclusive, or 6-7 hours post-trauma	22.7±2.5	21.1±3.7	11.8±3.2	—

[a]All values are means ±SE.

[b]Cathepsin D units are expressed as the number of milliequivalents of tyrosine released/mg protein/hr at 37°C.

(Courtesy of Exerpta Medica, in press.)

and its lysosomal hydrolases appear to be key agents in this process.

The Pancreas in Shock

The blood flow to the pancreas is dramatically reduced during various forms of shock, as previously discussed. This hypoperfusion rapidly leads to alterations in pancreatic ultrastructure, biochemistry, and physiology. Recently, Seifert (50) has been so impressed with the alterations in pancreatic function during shock and the possibility that it releases a toxic factor that he termed the pancreas a major shock organ. These major alterations in the pancreas occur during shock:

(a) Insulin secretion is suppressed in early shock, at least partially because of the inhibitory effect of angiotension II and/or catecholamines, the reduced blood flow, and the elevated blood glucose concentrations resulting from glycogenolysis and gluconeogenesis (13,45).

(b) The plasma concentration of glucagon is increased (27), enhancing the disruption of splanchnic lysosomes (11,34).

(c) Pancreatic duct transport of digestive enzymes from acinar cell zymogen granules continues during shock. Whether this secretory activity increases during shock is unknown. Regardless, however, the rate of ductal transport of digestive enzymes is sufficient to irritate the duodenal mucosa to release its lysosomal enzymes (7,8). This effectively triggers a secondary release of lysosomal enzymes into the circulation. Moreover, within pancreatic acinar cells, zymogen granules may further disrupt and secondarily release lysosomal hydrolases from adjacent lysosomes, by the process of crinophagy. Figure 3 depicts a zymogen granule emptying part of its contents onto an adjacent lysosome which appears to be in the process of releasing its contents into the cytoplasm. This is the only known report of crinophagy in the pancreas. If it occurs to a significant degree, it may partially account for the extreme sensitivity of pancreatic lysosomes to trauma and shock. This may also help to explain the protective action of aprotinin (Trasylol) in hemorrhagic shock, a polypeptide which acts as a very potent trypsin inhibitor (38).

(d) Ultrastructural damage to pancreatic acinar cells occurs early in shock, including increased lysosomal vacuolization and size and damage to both the endoplasmic reticulum and mitochondria (12,22).

(e) The content of pancreatic lysosomal hydrolases, particu-

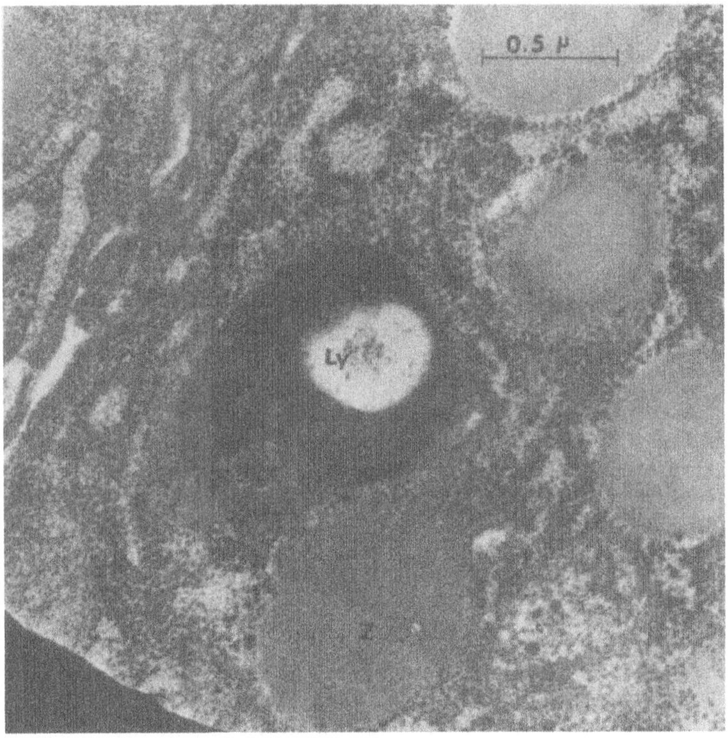

FIG. 3. Electron micrograph of a portion of a cat pancreatic acinar cell (X61,142). A zymogen granule (clear oval body) and a lysosome (vacuolated granular body) lie close to each other. Part of the zymogen granular contents have leaked out of the zymogen granule and appear to be over or in the lysosome, illustrating the phenomenon of crinophagy. The black particles in the lysosome are acid-phosphatase-positive lead phosphate precipitates.

larly the proteolytic enzymes (*e.g.*, the cathepsins), markedly decreases in hemorrhagic (22) and splanchnic ischemic shock (20).

(f) The pancreas is the primary source of the cardiotoxic peptide, MDF. Several lines of evidence point to this conclusion: First, selective occlusion of the pancreaticoduodenal arteries for 2 hours followed by restoration of patency results in high plasma MDF activity. Occlusion of the iliac arteries produces no MDF (37). Second, pancreatectomy performed before induction of hemorrhagic shock prevents plasma accumulation of MDF and increases survival in postoligemic shock (37). Third, induction of acute pancreatitis in dogs by injection of a trypsin-bile salt mixture directly into

TABLE 3

IN VITRO PRODUCTION OF MDF BY HOMOGENATES OF SPLANCHNIC TISSUES[a]

Splanchnic tissues	No. organs	Nonincubated homogenate	Incubated Homogenate (2 1/2 hrs)	
			Krebs-Henseleit solution	Plasma
Duodenum	3	20±2.8	20±3.3	16±3.8
Liver	2	19±2.7	25±3.4	28±4.3
Pancreas	5	15±4.1	59±3.2[b]	61±3.8[b]
Spleen	3	15±2.7	23±9.8	5±1.0

[a]All values are expressed as mean MDF units ±SE.
[b]$P < 0.001$. (Courtesy of Circ. Res. 29:338-349, 1971.)

the major pancreatic duct produces a state of shock with high plasma MDF activity (35). Fourth, perfusion of the isolated pancreas free of duodenal influence under either ischemic or hypoxic conditions produces amounts of MDF comparable to those observed in shock (14). Fifth, in addition to large amounts of MDF released into the blood during shock, considerable amounts of residual MDF remain within the pancreas; this may indicate the continued pancreatic production of MDF during shock (22). Sixth, chronic ligation of the pancreatic ducts confers complete protection against an otherwise uniformly lethal splanchnic ischemic shock. The mechanism appears to operate via induction of a more stable form of pancreatic lysosomes and perhaps by alteration of the zymogen granules. In any event, no significant amounts of MDF are produced in these duct-ligated animals (18).

Finally, perhaps the strongest evidence supporting the pancreatic origin of MDF is its production by incubating homogenates of splanchnic tissues (22) (Table 3). Pancreatic homogenates produce MDF, whereas duodenal, hepatic, and splenic homogenates fail to generate significant quantities. Unincubated homogenates of any of these tissues produce no MDF, suggesting that an enzymatic process is involved in MDF formation. The other point of interest is that incubation with plasma does not increase the amount of MDF produced above that formed in Krebs-Henseleit solution, indicating that plasma substrates are unnecessary for MDF production and that all the components of the MDF-forming reaction (*i.e.*, substrate,

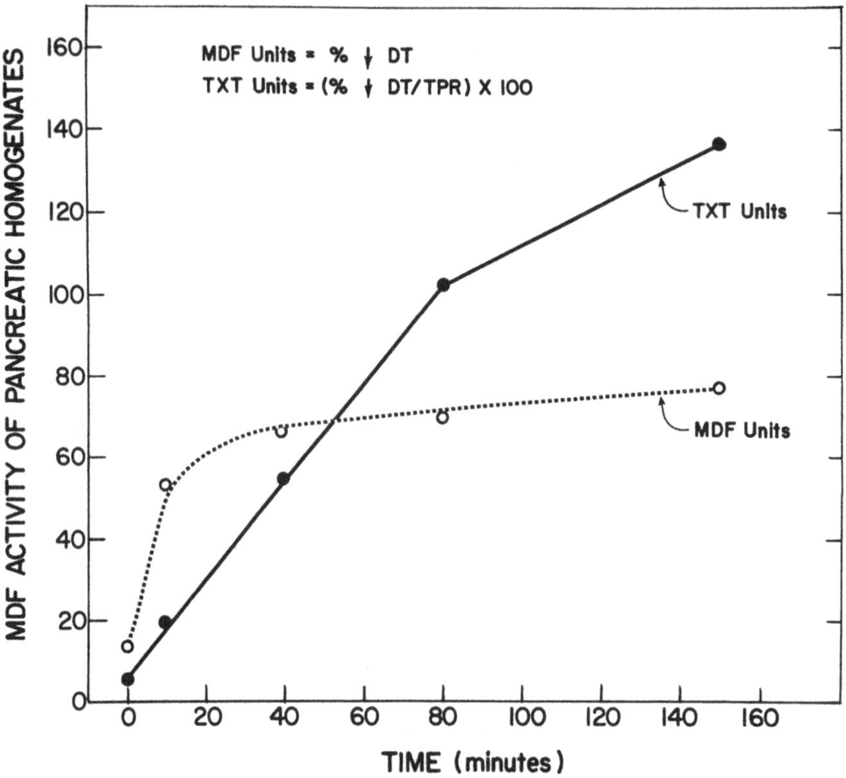

FIG. 4. Time course of the *in vitro* production of MDF by pancreatic homogenates incubated at 37°C in Krebs-Henseleit solution. Dashed line represents MDF activity in conventional MDF units. Solid line represents the activity of the same samples computed in tension x time (TXT) units, which accounts for the velocity as well as the amplitude of the negative inotropic effect.

enzymes, cofactors, *etc.*) are present within the pancreas. Figure 4 illustrates the relatively linear rate of production of MDF by incubated pancreatic homogenates, at least up to about 60-80 minutes. These data indicate that, beyond this time, substrate may become depleted or the enzymes inhibited. These data also indicate the high activities of MDF that can be generated by pancreatic tissue.

In summary, the pancreas appears to be the major, if not the sole, site of MDF production. Presumably this means that the hydrolytic enzymes, the protein substrate, and the cofactors necessary for the formation of MDF are all present within the

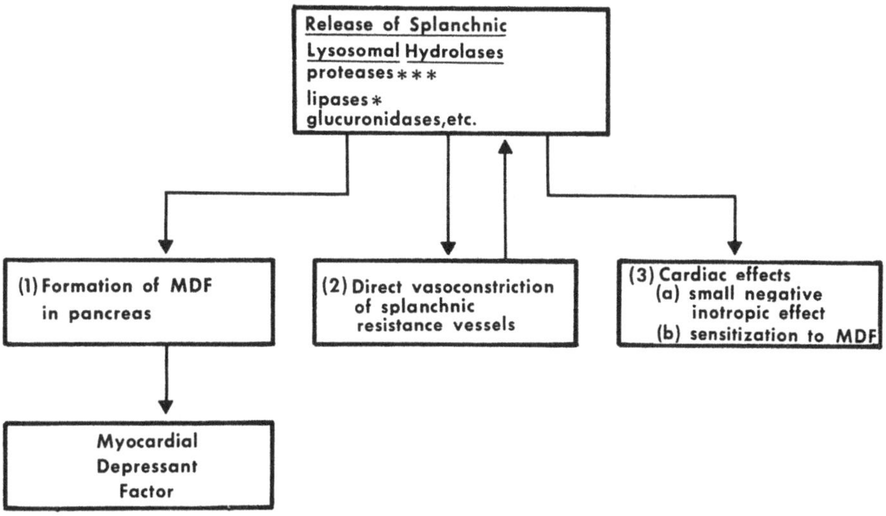

FIG. 5. The major proposed actions of lysosomal hydrolases in the pathogenesis of circulatory shock.

pancreas (*i.e.*, cellular contents and/or extracellular fluid). MDF is produced by selective pancreatic ischemia as well as by splanchnic artery occlusion and by acute hemorrhagic pancreatitis. Pancreatectomy or pancreatic duct ligation prevents the formation of MDF. Furthermore, MDF can be produced *in vitro* only by the pancreas. MDF is found within the pancreas during circulatory shock at activities comparable to those existing in plasma, indicating perhaps the continued pancreatic production of MDF.

DELETERIOUS ACTIONS OF LYSOSOMAL HYDROLASES

It is now becoming clear that lysosomal hydrolases can exert direct effects upon various organ systems, particularly the circulatory system, to alter its function and/or to sensitize it to the effects of other agents. Since these various enzymes arise from many sources during shock (*e.g.*, liver, pancreas, kidneys, *etc.*), this clearly represents a major mechanism in the pathogenesis of circulatory shock.

Figure 5 summarizes the effects of lysosomal hydrolases on circulatory function and outlines the actions of these enzymes in circulatory shock. Lysosomal enzyme preparations obtained from liver and splenic extracts were studied in order to determine the

TABLE 4

HEMODYNAMIC ACTIONS OF LYSOSOMAL ENZYMES IN DOGS WITH NONFUNCTIONING SPLANCHNIC RETICULOENDOTHELIAL SYSTEMS[a]

Group	Time (min)	Arterial blood pressure (mm Hg)	Cardiac output (ml/min/kg)	Central venous pressure (cm H_2O)
Controls (RE exclusion only)	0	102± 5	128±19	0.3±0.6
	10	101± 5	118±22	0.0±0.8
	60	105± 5	95± 7	0.0±1.0
	180	102±10	120±18	0.5±1.3
RE exclusion + lysosomal enzymes	0	90± 3	88±13	0.7±0.7
	10	61± 6[b]	83±16	0.5±0.6
	60	85± 7[c]	48± 5[b]	0.0±1.1
	180	69± 6[c]	43± 6[b]	-0.5±1.7

[a] All values are means ±SE for six dogs in each group.

[b] $P < 0.001$.

[c] $P < 0.02$.

(Courtesy of Exerpta Medica, in press.)

direct actions of lysosomal hydrolases upon circulatory dynamics. These extracts significantly lowered cardiac output and splanchnic blood flow when injected intravenously in dogs. However, the enzymes cleared from the plasma within 1 hour, and most of the effects then dissipated. In an attempt to sustain the plasma enzyme activity at shock levels, splenectomy and liver bypass (*i.e.*, portacaval shunt) were instituted before injection of the lysosomal enzyme preparation in dogs (24). Table 4 summarizes these data and compares the results to those observed in controls (*i.e.*, splenectomy plus portacaval shunt, but no enzyme infusion). Arterial blood pressure significantly declined within 10 minutes after enzyme infusion, remaining low for the entire 3-hour observation period. Cardiac output progressively decreased to about half of control values at 60 minutes and then declined further over the next 2 hours. Central venous pressure did not change significantly over this time. No significant circulatory effects occurred in the untreated dogs or in those which received denatured lysosomal extract. Thus, administration of lysosomal enzymes results in deleterious cardiovascular effects which are reflected by a significant cardiac depression and a splanchnic vasoconstriction. Plasma MDF activities were 59±6 MDF units in the extract-treated liver-bypass group and only 22±3 units in the untreated liver-bypass group. Since MDF itself depresses cardiac function and induces splanchnic vasoconstriction, it is unclear how much of the circulatory effects of the enzyme injection is due to a secondary release of endogenous MDF and how much is due to direct enzyme effects.

In an attempt to answer this question, lysosomal enzymes obtained from cat livers were added to the perfusate of isolated perfused cat hearts (*i.e.*, Langendorff preparation). These hearts were perfused at a constant coronary perfusion pressure of 35 mm Hg and electrically paced at a rate just above their spontaneous rate in the isolated state (*e.g.*, 150-170 beats/minute) (24). Within 2 minutes after addition of the enzymes, coronary flow and contractile force decreased by about 30%. Thus, some of the negative inotropic effects can be explained by coronary vasoconstriction. However, the same enzyme preparations depressed the developed tension of isolated cat papillary muscles 24%, indicating that a significant portion of the cardiac depressant actions of the enzymes were due to a direct negative inotropic effect.

Lysosomal enzyme preparations were also injected into the inflow circuit of isolated perfused pancreata. The specific activity of these lysosomal enzymes rose threefold in the perfusate, to levels approximating those in the plasma during circulatory shock. Within 1 minute after addition of the enzymes, a rapid increase in perfusion pressure usually occurred (to 180-190 mm Hg), indicating a sixfold increase in vascular resistance. This large increase in perfusion pressure may reflect damage to the microcirculation and blockade of some of the vascular channels, or it may represent a direct effect on vascular smooth muscle. In any event, lysosomal enzymes exert a prominent vasoconstrictor action on the pancreatic vasculature, and these findings support the *in vivo* results in the intact dog. By virtue of these circulatory effects, exogenous lysosomal hydrolases can lead to endogenous MDF formation in the whole animal as well as in the isolated perfused pancreas.

Recently, liver lysosomal enzymes have been shown to damage liver mitochondria during shock (43,44), indicating yet another adverse effect of lysosomal enzymes during shock. In fact, this mitochondrial poisoning effect of lysosomal hydrolases (*i.e.*, depression of mitochondrial oxygen consumption, ion transport, ATPase activity, and oxidative phosphorylation) could be the mechanism which sensitizes the heart to MDF, if this occurs in heart mitochondria as well as in liver. Lysosomally induced mitochondrial poisoning in the liver may also contribute to the reticuloendothelial depression usually observed in circulatory shock (1,6).

In summary, lysosomal enzymes directly disturb circulatory homeostasis when released into the blood at activity levels as high as those observed in circulatory shock. These effects, namely a negative inotropic and a splanchnic vasoconstrictor action (and perhaps even a systemic vasoconstrictor action), may initially weaken the heart and further promote MDF production, which markedly depresses cardiac function later. Depression of mitochondrial function may be a key mechanism in these effects. Thus, the lysosomal hydrolases may sensitize the circulatory system to the effects of MDF as well as contribute to the positive feedback loops that occur in circulatory shock.

PATHOPHYSIOLOGICAL EFFECTS OF MDF

The full spectrum of the circulatory actions of MDF is depicted in Figure 6. The three major actions of MDF are: (a) myocardial depression, (b) splanchnic vasoconstriction, and possibly (c) reticuloendothelial depression.

The first major effect of MDF to be studied was its negative inotropic or myocardial depressant effect, a finding which prompted its discovery (9). MDF exerted a pronounced negative inotropic effect in the isolated papillary muscle sensitized by prior exposure to hemorrhagic shock (9) or in the nonsensitized cat papillary muscle (32). Williams *et al.* (57) confirmed these findings in isolated nonsensitized rat papillary muscle strips. These workers

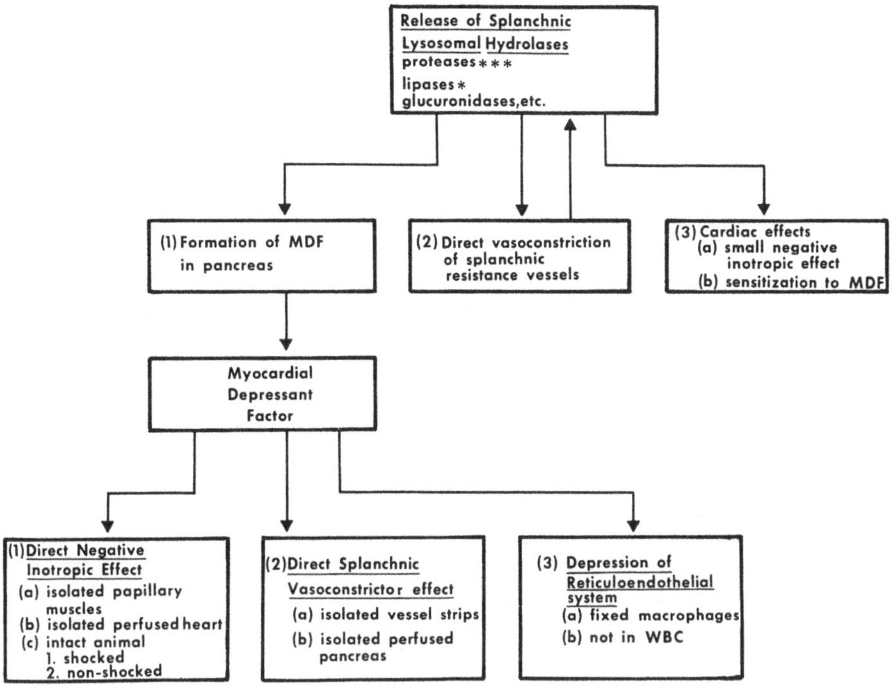

FIG. 6. The deleterious actions of the entire lysosomal protease-MDF system in shock. This diagram illustrates the interrelationships among the lysosomal hydrolases (particularly the proteases) and MDF.

also showed that the negative inotropic effect was characterized primarily by a reduction in developed tension and not by a change in the time to peak tension. We have confirmed these findings in isolated cat papillary muscles (33). These observations suggest that MDF exerts its cardiodepressant action by lowering the responsiveness of the contractile elements in cardiac muscle cells. Also, Lefer and Rovetto (39) showed that the negative inotropic effect of MDF is not accompanied by any significant alteration in the cardiac transmembrane potentials (*i.e.*, resting membrane potential, action potential), and thus MDF does not exert its negative inotropic effect via alterations in membrane excitability.

MDF also exerts prominent cardiodepressant effects in the isolated cat heart perfused at a constant coronary perfusion pressure and electrically paced at a fixed rate. Under these conditions, addition of a purified MDF preparation resulted in a prominent negative inotropic effect within 40 seconds. This cardiodepressant effect occurred before the onset of any arrhythmia and without a significant decrease in coronary flow (52). Cardiac arrest occurred after the peak depressant effect, but the heart resumed beating within 20 seconds. The major point is that MDF added to the whole heart depressed the contractile mechanism without exerting significant dromotropic, chronotropic or coronary vasoconstrictor effects.

Now that MDF has been produced *in vitro*, sufficient quantities have become available to inject into intact animals so that its inotropic effects may be tested in the nonshocked, nonsensitized intact animal. Injection of the MDF produced from 3 g of cat or dog pancreas (approximately that amount present in the plasma of cats in postoligemic shock) into a normal cat produced profound shock. Within 60-70 minutes after injection, mean arterial blood pressure had dropped to 60 mm Hg, cardiac output was only about 40% of initial values, and central venous pressure had decreased significantly (19). Furthermore, when left ventricular function curves were computed after challenging the heart with a volume infusion, cardiac function was markedly depressed (*i.e.*, mean decrease in cardiac power of 54±4%). Figure 7 depicts a typical set of ventricular function curves in a cat just before and 60 minutes after MDF injection. This cat exhibited a decrease in peak cardiac power of 66% at 60 minutes. The results demonstrate for the first time that MDF is capable of depressing the completely normal heart in the intact animal to the extent found in the late states of circulatory shock (22,54).

In addition to its cardiac depressant action, MDF exerts a vasoconstrictor effect on isolated strips of vascular smooth muscle (25). MDF significantly increased the tension of the strips in both the absence and the presence of angiotensin II or norepinephrine. However, MDF did not alter the responsiveness of the strips to either vasoactive agent. These data suggest that MDF acts to reinforce the already-existing splanchnic ischemia in shock, presumably allowing additional MDF to be produced, which further depresses the myocardium. Thus, MDF may trigger a positive feedback loop to threaten the circulatory equilibrium existing in shock and to contribute to the onset of irreversible shock.

Another possible MDF-generated positive feedback loop may be depression of the reticuloendothelial system (RES). The RES is markedly depressed in circulatory shock (1,6). A reticuloendothelial depressant substance (RDS) has been described by Blattberg and Levy (6) which contributes to this depression. MDF and RDS share many properties (31). Thus, MDF, which may or may not be identical to RDS, may act as a reticuloendothelial defense mechanism, which probably is a major route of clearance of lysosomal hydrolases and perhaps of MDF from the plasma. This double action

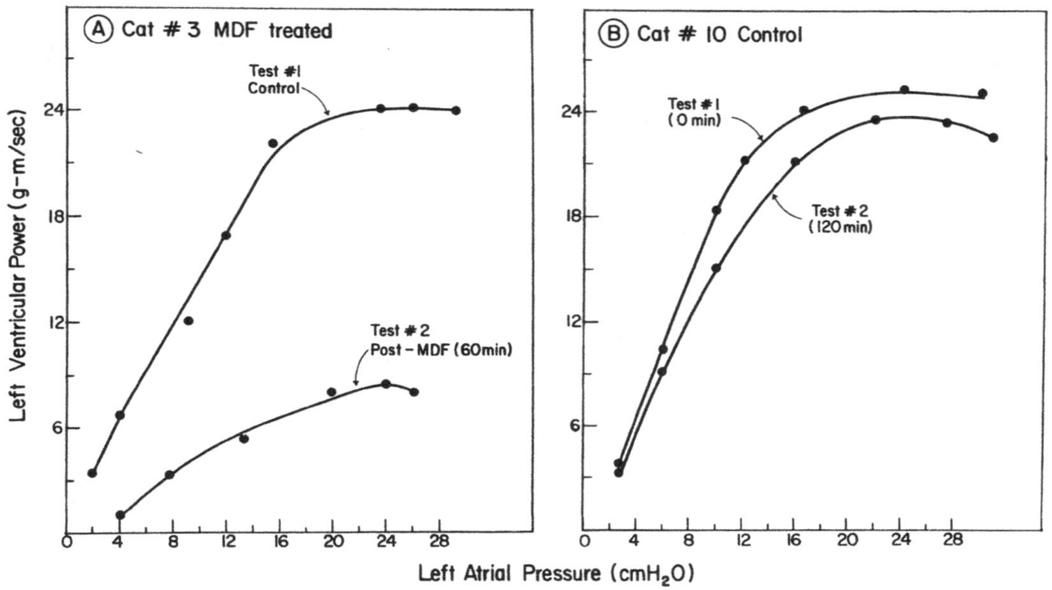

FIG. 7. Typical left ventricular function curves in normal cats treated with MDF (panel A) and in untreated cats (panel B). Two curves were obtained in each cat at the times indicated. Peak left ventricular power had decreased 66% in the cat receiving MDF but only 6% in the control.

(Courtesy of Circ. Res. 29:338-349, 1971.)

constitutes another positive feedback loop. Regardless of whether MDF *per se* significantly contributes to RES depression, the prominence of RES depression in shock is probably a major reason for the accumulation of MDF in the plasma during circulatory shock.

Finally, MDF alters the mechanical activity of intestinal smooth muscle (*i.e.*, isolated strips of cat jejunum). It appeared to abolish tonic contractions of the gut strips (33). Generally this activity was restored after 2-3 minutes, followed by slow forceful waves of contraction. Although the physiological implications of these effects remain unclear, these data indicate that the target organs of MDF may be widespread and not confined to the cardiovascular system. This finding also serves to differentiate MDF from other peptides, particularly kinins, which are known to stimulate cat jejunal strips (15).

SUMMARY

A myocardial depressant factor (MDF) has been found in the plasma of cats, dogs, baboons, and man in various forms of circulatory shock, including hemorrhagic, endotoxic, cardiogenic, bowel ischemic, burn, and pancreatitis shock. MDF is a peptide with a molecular weight of 800-1,000 which originates in the ischemic, hypoxic pancreas. This peptide appears to be formed from an endogenous protein substrate within the pancreas by the action of acid proteases released from lysosomes during shock. The lysosomal hydrolases, in addition to forming MDF, may act to sensitize the organism to the subsequent effects of MDF. These enzymes also enhance the splanchnic vasoconstriction present in shock and thus favor the continued production of MDF. Moreover, they depress myocardial contractility, thus consuming some of the remaining cardiac reserve and rendering the heart vulnerable to other depressant influences.

MDF has been produced *in vitro* in pancreatic tissue but not in splenic, hepatic, or intestinal tissue. Thus, a certain specificity is conferred upon pancreatic tissue in this process. MDF exerts a marked negative inotropic effect in the intact animal and in isolated cardiac tissue, constricts splanchnic resistance vessels, alters intestinal motility, and probably contributes to the reticuloendothelial blockade observed in shock. Thus, MDF is a potent toxic factor which exerts several positive feedback actions contributing to the lethality of circulatory shock.

REFERENCES

1. Altura, B.M., and S.G. Hershey. RES phagocytic function in

trauma and adaptation to experimental shock. Am. J. Physiol. 215:1414-1419, 1968.

2. Baxter, C.R., W.A. Cook, and G.T. Shires. Serum myocardial depressant factor of burn shock. Surg. Forum 17:1-2, 1966.

3. Berman, I.R., R.V. Mosely, P.B. Lamborn, and H.K. Sleeman. Thoracic duct lymph in shock: Gas exchange and base balance and lysosomal enzymes in hemorrhagic and endotoxic shock. Ann. Surg. 169:202-209, 1969.

4. Bitensky, L., J. Chayen, J.G. Cunningham, and J. Fine. Behaviour of lysosomes in hemorrhagic shock. Nature 199: 493-494, 1963.

5. Blair, O.M., R.J. Stenger, R.W. Hopkins, and F.A. Simeone. Hepatocellular ultrastructure in dogs with hypovolemic shock. Lab. Invest. 18:172-178, 1968.

6. Blattberg, B., and M.N. Levy. A humoral reticuloendothelial-depressing substance in shock. Am. J. Physiol. 203:409-411, 1962.

7. Bounous, G. "Tryptic enteritis": Its role in the pathogenesis of stress ulcer and shock. Can. J. Surg. 12:397-409, 1969.

8. Bounos, G., and A.H. McArdle. Release of intestinal enzymes in acute mesenteric ischemia. J. Surg. Res. 9:339-346, 1969.

9. Brand, E.D., and A.M. Lefer. Myocardial depressant factor in plasma from cats in irreversible post-oligemic shock. Proc. Soc. Exptl. Biol. Med. 122:200-203, 1963.

10. Brobmann, G.F., and E.D. Jacobson. Vergleichends Untersuchungen zur Endotoxinwirkung auf die Darmdurchblutung bei Hund und Affe. Beitrag zur Pathophysiologie des Endoxinshocks. Bruns. Betr. Klin. Chir. 218:368-375, 1970.

11. Deter, R.L., and C. deDuve. Influence of glucagon, an inducer of cellular autophagy, on some physical properties of rat liver lysosomes. J. Cell. Biol. 33:437-449, 1967.

12. Donath, K., H. Mitschke, and G. Seifert. Ultrastrukturelle Veränderungen am Rattenpankreas beim Hamorrhagischen Schock. Beitr. Path. 141:33-51, 1970.

13. Drucker, W.R. Insulin secretion during hemorrhagic shock in dogs. Symposium on Neurohumoral and Metabolic Aspects of

Injury, Budapest, Aug. 3-7, 1971.

14. Ferguson, W.W., T.M. Glenn, and A.M. Lefer. Mechanism of production of humoral shock factors in the isolated perfused pancreas. Am. J. Physiol, in press.

15. Ferreira, S.H., and J. Vane. The detection and estimation of bradykinin in the circulating blood. Brit. J. Pharmacol. 29: 367-375, 1967.

16. Forsyth, R.P., B.I. Hoffbrand, and K.L. Melmon. Redistribution of cardiac output during hemorrhage in the unanesthetized monkey. Circ. Res. 27:311-320, 1970.

17. Fukuda, T. Endogenous shock-inducing factor in canine hemorrhagic shock. Nature 205:392-393, 1965.

18. Glenn, T.M., B.L. Herlihy, W.W. Ferguson, and A.M. Lefer. Protective effect of pancreatic duct ligation in splanchnic ischemia shock. Am. J. Physiol, in press.

19. Glenn, T.M., and A.M. Lefer. Protective effect of thoracic lymph diversion in hemorrhagic shock. Am. J. Physiol. 219: 1305-1310, 1970.

20. Glenn, T.M., and A.M. Lefer. Role of lysosomes in the pathogenesis of splanchnic ischemia shock in cats. Circ. Res. 27:783-797, 1970.

21. Glenn, T.M., and A.M. Lefer. Anti-toxic action of methylprednisolone in hemorrhagic shock. Eur. J. Pharmacol. 13: 230-238, 1971.

22. Glenn, T.M., and A.M. Lefer. Significance of splanchnic lysosomal proteases in the pathogenesis of hemorrhagic shock. Circ. Res., in press.

23. Glenn, T.M., A.M. Lefer, J.B. Martin, W.L. Lovett, J.N. Morris, and S.L. Wangensteen. Production of a myocardial depressant factor in cardiogenic shock. Am. Heart J. 82: 78-85, 1971.

24. Glenn, T.M., J.R. Morris III, A.M. Lefer, A.M. Lopez-Rasi, T.S. Serati, W.W. Ferguson, and S.L. Wangensteen. Circulatory responses to infusion of splanchnic lysosomal hydrolases in the dog. To be published.

25. Glucksman, E.E., and A.M. Lefer. Effects of a myocardial depresant factor on isolated vascular smooth muscle. Am. J.

Physiol. 220:1581-1585, 1971.

26. Goodhead, B. Acute pancreatitis and pancreatic blood flow. Surg. Gynecol. Obstet. 129:331-336, 1969.

27. Halmagyi, D.F.J., I.R. Neering, L. Lazarus, J.D. Young, and J. Pullin. Plasma glucagon in experimental posthemorrhagic shock. J. Trauma 9:320-326, 1969.

28. Janoff, A., G. Weissman, B. Zweifach, and L. Thomas. Pathogenesis of experimental shock. IV. Studies on lysosomes in normal and tolerant animals subjected to lethal trauma and endotoxemia. J. Exptl. Med. 116:451-463, 1962.

29. Kobold, E.E., and A.P. Thal. Quantitation and identification of vasoactive substances liberated during various types of experimental and clinical intestinal ischemia. Surg. Gynecol. Obstet. 117:315-325, 1963.

30. Lefer, A.M. Role of a myocardial depressant factor in the pathogenesis of circulatory shock.

31. Lefer, A.M., and B. Blattberg. Comparison of the effects of two factors present in plasma of shocked animals. J. Reticuloendothel. Soc. 5:54-60, 1968.

32. Lefer, A.M., R. Cowgill, F.F. Marshall, L.M. Hall, and E.D. Brand. Characterization of a myocardial depressant factor present in hemorrhagic shock. Am. J. Physiol. 213:492-498, 1967.

33. Lefer, A.M., and T.M. Glenn. The interrelationship between splanchnic blood flow and a myocardial depressant factor in circulatory shock. In: *The Splanchnic Circulation in Shock*, edited by D.G. Reynolds and K.D. Swan. New York: Prentice-Hall, in press.

34. Lefer, A.M., T.M. Glenn, A.M. Lopez-Rasi, S.F. Kiechel, W.W. Ferguson, and S.L. Wangensteen. Mechanism of the lack of a beneficial response to inotropic drugs in hemorrhagic shock. Clin. Pharmacol. Ther. 12:506-516, 1971.

35. Lefer, A.M., T.M. Glenn, T.J. O'Neill, W.L. Lovett, W.T. Geissinger, and S.L. Wangensteen. Inotropic influence of endogenous peptides in experimental hemorrhagic pancreatitis. Surgery 69:220-228, 1971.

36. Lefer, A.M., and J. Martin. Mechanism of the protective effect of corticosteroids in hemorrhagic shock. Am. J.

Physiol. 216:314-320, 1969.

37. Lefer, A.M., and J. Martin. Origin of a myocardial depressant factor in shock. Am. J. Physiol. 218:1423-1427, 1970.

38. Lefer, A.M., and J. Martin. Relationship of plasma peptides to the myocardial depressant factor in hemorrhagic shock in cats. Circ. Res. 26:59-69, 1970.

39. Lefer, A.M., and M.J. Rovetto. Influence of a myocardial depressant factor on physiologic properties of cardiac muscle. Proc. Soc. Exptl. Biol. Med. 134:269-273, 1970.

40. Lewis, G.P. Intracellular enzymes in local lymph as a measure of cellular injury. J. Physiol. (London) 191: 591-604, 1967.

41. Lillehei, R.C., J.K. Longerbeam, J. Bloch, and W.G. Manax. Nature of irreversible shock: Experimental and clinical observations. Ann. Surg. 160:682-736, 1964.

42. Lovett, W.L., S.L. Wangensteen, T.M. Glenn, and A.M. Lefer. Presence of a myocardial depressant factor in patients in circulatory shock. Surgery 70:223-231, 1971.

43. Mela, L., L.V. Bacalzo, Jr., and L.D. Miller. Defective oxidative metabolism of rat liver mitochondria in hemorrhagic and endotoxin shock. Am. J. Physiol. 220:571-577, 1971.

44. Mellors, A., A.L. Tappel, P.L. Sawant, and I.D. Desai. Mitochondrial swelling and uncoupling of oxidative phosphorylation by lysosomes. Biochim. Biophys. Acta 143:299-309, 1967.

45. Moss, G.S., G.M. Cerchio, D.C. Siegel, P.A. Popovich, and E. Butler. Serum insulin response in hemorrhagic shock in baboons. Surgery 68:34-39, 1970.

46. Nagy, S., T. Barankay, and K. Tárnoky. Effect of hemorrhagic shock on oxygen tension of thoracic duct lymph. Acta Physiol. Acad. Sci. Hung. 35:87-92, 1969.

47. Rangel, D.M., J.E. Byfield, G.E. Adomian, G.H. Stavens, and E.W. Fonkalsrud. Hepatic ultrastructural response to endotoxin shock. Surgery 68:503-511, 1970.

48. Ravin, H.A., F.B. Schweinburg, and J. Fine. Host resistance in hemorrhagic shock. XV. Isolation of toxic factors from hemorrhagic shock plasma. Proc. Soc. Exptl. Biol. Med. 99: 426-431, 1958.

49. Reich, T., B.M. Dierolf, and B.M. Reynolds. Plasma cathepsin-like acid proteinase activity during hemorrhagic shock. J. Surg. Res. 5:116-119, 1965.

50. Seifert, V.G. Das Pankreas als Schockorgem. In: *Leber-und Pankreas-schaden durch Schock und Narkose*, edited by H. Horatz. Stuttgart: Geog Thieme Verlag, 1970, pp. 17-30.

51. Slater, T.F. Lysosomes and experimentally induced tissue injury. In: *Lysosomes in Biology and Pathology*, edited by J.T. Dingle and H.B. Fell. New York: Elsevier, 1969, pp. 469-492.

52. Thalinger, A.R., and A.M. Lefer. Cardiac actions of a myocardial depressant factor isolated from shock plasma. Proc. Soc. Exptl. Biol. Med. 136:354-358, 1971.

53. Wangensteen, S.L., R.S. Crampton, W.L. Lovett, J.N. Morris, Jr., R.H. Harris, R. Weitzmann, T.M. Glenn, and A.M. Lefer. Methylprednisolone treatment in cardiogenic shock following acute myocardial infarction. To be published.

54. Wangensteen, S.L., J.D. deHoll, S.F. Kiechel, J. Martin, and A.M. Lefer. Influence of hemodialysis on a myocardial depressant factor in hemorrhagic shock. Surgery 67:935-943, 1970.

55. Wangensteen, S.L., W.T. Geissinger, W.L. Lovett, T.M. Glenn, and A. M. Lefer. Relationship between splanchnic blood flow and a myocardial depressant factor in endotoxin shock. Surgery 69:410-418, 1971.

56. Weissman, G., and L. Thomas. Studies on lysosomes. I. Effects of endotoxin tolerance and cortisone on the release of acid hydrolases from a granular fraction of rabbit liver. J. Exptl. Med. 116:433-443, 1962.

57. Williams, L.F., Jr., A.H. Goldberg, B.J. Polansky, and J.J. Byrne. Myocardial effects of acute intestinal ischemia. Surgery 66:138-145, 1969.

58. Wyler, F., R.P. Forsyth, A.S. Nies, J.M. Neutze, and K.L. Melmon. Endotoxin-induced regional circulatory changes in the unanesthetized monkey. Circ. Res. 24:777-786, 1969.

VASCULAR LESIONS IN ENDOTOXEMIA[1]

Evelyn Gaynor, M.D.

Department of Hematology, Medical Division, Montefiore Hospital and Medical Center, Bronx, New York

In the past, vascular lesions in animals injected with endotoxin have been considered to result from anoxia secondary to occlusive thrombotic deposits in vessels. The thrombosis was thought to be caused by activation of clotting factors and platelet procoagulant activity in the flowing blood, with subsequent trapping of fibrin and platelet emboli in small vessels (19). This view was supported by the observation that infusion of thrombin or thromboplastin produced pathologically similar lesions, particularly renal cortical necrosis (16,17); treatment of animals with anticoagulants before endotoxin injection (12,24) prevented the development of such pathological changes.

Because of the striking hemodynamic alterations noted after injection of endotoxin, a vascular reaction of one sort or another has been pathogenetically implicated by numerous investigators. In 1961, Stetson (31) reviewed the vascular effects of endotoxin and concluded that these were secondary to some undefined primary event. Rubenstein and co-workers noted localization of endotoxin in vascular walls (23). They inferred that the endotoxin may have directly produced peripheral vascular collapse, perhaps after being delivered by the polymorphonuclear leukocyte (PMN). Zweifach (35), inquiring into possible cytotoxic mechanisms that allow endotoxin to penetrate from the vascular to the extravascular compartment, stated that no evidence existed that bacterial endotoxins have a generalized effect on the capillary wall. However, Gray described

[1]This work was supported by Grant HE 05415-11 from the National Heart Institutes, National Institutes of Health, United States Public Health Service.

damage to the endothelium of the general vasculature, and particularly to the pulmonary vessels, within 4 minutes of the intravenous injection of Shear's polysaccharide (11). An early endothelial lesion in response to endotoxin was anticipated by Spaet and Lejnieks (28), who proposed that mitotic activity be used as an index of prior endothelial injury. Boler and Bibighaus (1) demonstrated desquamation of sinusoidal endothelium in the livers of dogs undergoing endotoxin shock, within 15 minutes of injection, and in the absence of fibrin formation at this time. Subsequent studies in various laboratories have revealed more concrete evidence of such damage. This topic is the subject of the following presentation.

In our laboratory, investigations designed to demonstrate an endothelial lesion underlying and initiating thrombosis in endotoxemia were prompted by three major considerations:

First, evidence was inconclusive for the development of significant coagulant activity in the blood of animals treated with endotoxin. Even if such activity were generated *in vivo*, adequate homeostatic mechanisms had been shown capable of effecting its clearance (4,14,25,26,33).

Second, injury to the vessel wall had been demonstrated by numerous investigators to initiate what has become accepted as the sequence of events in the normal hemostatic response (27). Exposure of subendothelial surfaces starts the coagulation cascade. Platelets adhere to the denuded surface and release adenosine diphosphate, attracting more platelets to form an aggregate *in situ*. With degranulation, there is release of platelet factor 3, enhancing coagulation, and of serotonin and histamine, causing vasospasm in large vessels and increased permeability in the microvasculature. With the formation of fibrin, consolidation of the newly formed hemostatic plug occurs.

Third, although evidence of endothelial damage had been described incident to the presence of occlusive thrombi in a number of studies on endotoxemia (1,19) no experiments had been performed in animals treated with anticoagulants, and thus the possibility of an endothelial lesion unassociated with fibrin formation had been unexplored. In addition, large arteries, where flow characteristics would not allow occlusive masses of platelets to form, had not been systematically examined for the presence of endothelial injury.

The studies reported herein present evidence that early widespread damage occurs to the vascular endothelium in both large and small vessels, and in the absence of fibrin formation. Heparinized rabbits intravenously injected with endotoxin are found to have circulating endothelial cells (7), aortic endothelial injury and sloughing as shown by electron microscopy (8), and increased mitotic activity of endothelium in large and small vessels (10).

Adult New Zealand rabbits were given intravenous injections either of a small dose of endotoxin in saline, or of saline alone. Control rabbits received intravenously injected heparin before the endotoxin or saline treatment, in doses which rendered their blood incoagulable. The animals were bled at various intervals after treatment, by free flow from the abdominal aorta through an 18-gauge needle. After collection of specimens for circulating endothelium and blood counts, the aorta was fixed for electron microscopy by perfusion with glutaraldehyde.

An additional group of rabbits was given a single pulse of tritiated thymidine 72 hours after heparinization and endotoxin or saline treatment. This had been shown in other studies to be the time of maximal mitotic activity in endothelium after injury. In this group of rabbits, sections of lung and kidney and häutchen preparations of aortic endothelium were processed for autoradiography.

Of the rabbits given endotoxin, 80% showed evidence of circulating endothelial cells (Fig. 1). These were seen, singly or in clumps, as soon as 5 minutes after injection. They were identified as endothelium by light and electron microscopic comparison with endothelium which had been scraped from normal rabbit aorta, added to normal rabbit blood, and processed identically (9,29). None of the blood samples from rabbits which had received saline alone or heparin and saline was positive for endothelium. Heparin pretreatment did not alter the incidence of circulating endothelium, since specimens from 82% of the rabbits treated with anticoagulant before endotoxin injection were positive in this respect.

Electron microscopic examination of randomly selected areas from the aortas of the rabbits treated with endotoxin and those treated with heparin plus endotoxin showed significant endothelial cell damage or desquamation in 50% of the former group and 40% of the latter. No significant abnormalities were noted in the aortas of the control animals treated with saline or heparin plus saline. These findings were supported by the demonstration of a ninefold increase of aortic endothelial cell labeling with tritiated thymidine in the endotoxin-treated rabbits, compared to saline-treated controls. In addition, the endotoxin-treated rabbits had a mean threefold increase in the labeling of pulmonary capillaries, and a 7.7-fold rise in the renal capillaries over the saline-treated controls. Since the animals in this part of the study were all pretreated with heparin, the evidence of increased regenerative

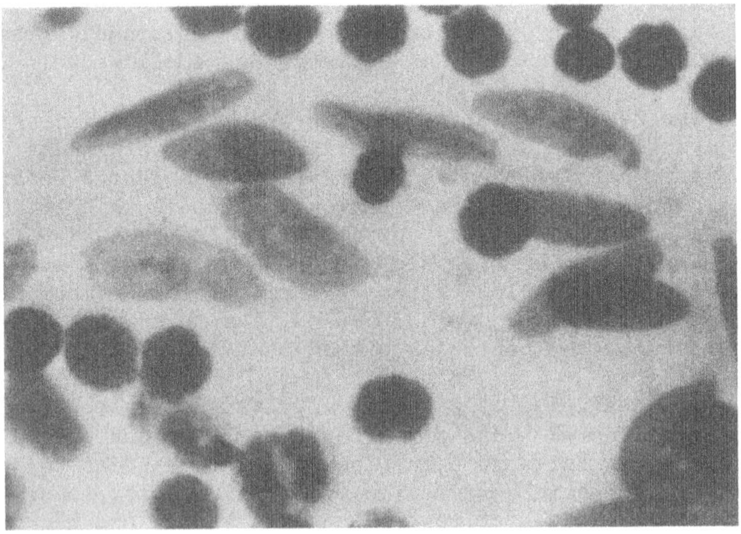

FIG. 1. A cluster of endothelial cells (elongated nuclei) in blood obtained from a rabbit 40 minutes after intravenous injection of heparin (1000 USP units) and endotoxin (40 µg/kg). Original magnification X1000.

activity reflects endothelial damage occurring in the absence of thrombin formation. In the aorta, the damage occurred in a vessel too large to be occluded by platelet masses.

Our data give evidence of an early, multifocal, and disseminated lesion of vascular endothelium in the rabbit pretreated with anticoagulant and then given a single small intravenous dose of endotoxin. Endothelial lesions induced with lethal doses of endotoxin, in the absence of prior heparinization, had been previously described in the organs of experimental animals, but these generally had been ascribed to the effects of occlusive platelet or fibrin emboli. Desquamation of large sheets of continuous endothelium in the mesenteric arteries of rabbits had been demonstrated by McGrath (18) and Stewart (32) at 24 hours after endotoxin administration. In their studies, the rabbits examined at 1 hour after treatment showed evidence of endothelial cell nuclear vacuolization and adherence of blood cells, particularly platelets. It would be reasonable to assume that these cells were adherent to exposed subendothelial structures, since our studies have indicated that endothelial desquamation may appear as soon as 5 minutes after treatment (8).

Our data are derived from studies with single doses of endotoxin, but these lesions would probably be extended in the generalized Shwartzman reaction (gSr) seen after the second dose, where similar although more pronounced blood and tissue changes are present. Damage to vascular endothelium results in its detachment and appearance in the circulating blood. Subendothelial thrombogenic surfaces are then exposed, and platelet accretions form at these sites. Subsequent fibrin deposition results from the initiation of coagulation in the unheparinized animal.

The mechanism whereby endotoxin effects endothelial damage is unknown. Vesiculation, lytic cytoplasmic areas, and even desquamation of these cells have been described after various chemical, thermal, anoxic, mechanical, and immune types of injury. Theories have thus been generated involving a final common chemical mediator, such as histamine, serotonin, epinephrine, or kinins (3,6,22).

Other investigators have proposed lysosomal or chemical mediators released from platelets or polymorphonuclear leukocytes (13,20) as the pathogenetic mechanism underlying the profound vascular effects of endotoxin. However, degranulation of PMNs sequestered in the lungs of primates undergoing septic shock was not associated with significant changes in endothelium or fibrin formation (2). In this study, Coalson and co-workers described indistinct endothelial plasma membranes at the sites of PMN adhesion to the capillary wall; even 4 hours after endotoxin administration, however, only a few rare vesicles were noted in the endothelium.

Undoubtedly, PMNs are essential for the development of the full-blown gSr, since this state cannot be induced in granulocytopenic animals. Viable granulocytes, as well as endotoxin, have been shown necessary for the development of renal cortical necrosis, the hallmark of the gSr (5,34). Recent studies by Lerner and co-workers (15) have demonstrated the *in vitro* development of a potent tissue-factor-like activity in PMN which phagocytoses endotoxin in the presence of a serum factor. Moreover, Niemetz (21) has produced renal cortical necrosis in rabbits infused intra-arterially with washed PMNs derived from exudates of donor animals given endotoxin intraperitoneally. Unfortunately, that study did not exclude the possibility that undetoxified endotoxin might be present in the infusion. Recent work in our laboratory would indicate that PMNs are not essential for the development of the endothelial lesion induced by endotoxin (Gaynor, unpublished data). Of 11 rabbits rendered neutropenic with nitrogen mustard (HN_2) 72 hours before injection with endotoxin, nine had endothelial cells in their circulating blood. At this time, platelet counts were normal in the neutropenic animals. This incidence of endothelial injury resembles that seen in control animals given endotoxin without HN_2 pretreatment. Blood specimens from only two of 11 rabbits given HN_2 72 hours earlier were positive for endothelial cells without subsequent treatment. Although this may have been due to a cytotoxic effect of HN_2 on endothelium, it is more likely that these rabbits suffered from autogenous infection with coliform organisms, since both had severe diarrhea.

It is conceivable that PMN and endothelial cell changes, as well as platelet alterations, are concurrent but pathogenetically unrelated events, and that the development of the full-blown gSr is not caused by a sequential chain of reactions, but by the summation of a series of isolated simultaneous effects. For example, each of the aforementioned cells (and perhaps others as well) may be involved as "innocent bystanders" in an antigen-antibody-complement interaction such as immune adherence. Indeed, such a reaction has been demonstrated by Spielvogel (30) in rabbit platelets exposed to endotoxin. Historically, an immune mechanism underlying the effects of endotoxin has been suggested by countless investigators, and the role of complement and antibody has been intensively studied. Similar studies are necessary, as well, to understand the mechanism whereby endotoxin induces endothelial damage.

SUMMARY

An early lesion of vascular endothelium is associated with endotoxemia in rabbits and may initiate the sequence of events leading to thrombosis in the generalized Shwartzman reaction. The lesion is not caused by occlusive thrombi, since it occurs in the animal treated with anticoagulant and in vessels too large to be occluded by platelet thrombi.

The injury is manifested by evidence of (a) aortic endothelial desquamation, as shown by electron microscopy, (b) endothelial cells in the circulating blood, and (c) increased endothelial cell turnover. PMNs do not appear to be essential for the development of this endothelial lesion.

REFERENCES

1. Boler, R.K., and A.J. Bibighaus, III. Ultrastructural alterations of dog livers during endotoxin shock. Lab. Invest. 17:537-561, 1967.

2. Coalson, J.J., L.B. Hinshaw, and C.A. Guenter. The pulmonary

ultrastructure in septic shock. Exptl. Mol. Pathol. 12:84-103, 1970.

3. Constantinides, P., and M. Robinson. Ultrastructural injury of arterial endothelium. II. Effects of vasoactive amines. Arch. Pathol. 88:106-112, 1969.

4. Deykin, D. The role of the liver in serum-induced hypercoagulability. J. Clin. Invest. 45:256-263, 1966.

5. Forman, E.N., C.F. Abildgaard, J. Bolger, C.A. Johnson, and I. Schulman. Generalized Shwartzman reaction: Role of the granulocyte in intravascular coagulation and renal cortical necrosis. Brit. J. Haematol. 16:507-515, 1969.

6. Gabbiani, G., M.C. Badonnel, and G. Majno. Intra-arterial injections of histamine, serotonin, or bradykinin: A topographic study of vascular leakage. Proc. Soc. Exptl. Biol. Med. 135:447-452, 1970.

7. Gaynor, E., C.A. Bouvier, and T.H. Spaet. Circulating endothelial cells in endotoxin-treated rabbits. Clin. Res. 16:535, 1968.

8. Gaynor, E., C.A. Bouvier, and T.H. Spaet. Vascular lesions: Possible pathogenetic basis of the generalized Shwartzman reaction. Science 170:986-988, 1970.

9. Gaynor, E., C.A. Bouvier, and T.H. Spaet. A technique for locating rare cells in circulation for ultramicroscopy. Proc. Soc. Exptl. Biol. Med. 133:520-523, 1970.

10. Gaynor, E. Increased mitotic activity in rabbit endothelium after endotoxin: An autoradiographic study. Lab. Invest. 24:318-320, 1971.

11. Gray, M. Discussion: Part VI. In: *Bacterial Endotoxins*, edited by M. Landy and W. Braun. New Brunswick: Rutgers University Press, 1964, p. 627.

12. Hardaway, R.M., and D. Johnson. Clotting mechanisms in endotoxin shock. Arch. Intern. Med. 112:775-782, 1963.

13. Horn, R.G., and R.D. Collins. Fragmentation of granulocytes in pulmonary capillaries during development of the generalized Shwartzman reaction. Lab. Invest. 19:451-459, 1968.

14. Lee, L. Reticuloendothelial clearance of circulating fibrin in the pathogenesis of the generalized Shwartzman reaction.

J. Exptl. Med. 115:1065-1082, 1962.

15. Lerner, R., R. Goldstein, and G. Cummings. Endotoxin stimulation of thromboplastic activity generated by leukocytes. Clin. Res. 19:461, 1971.

16. Lewis, J.H., and I.L.F. Szeto. Effects of intravenous tissue thromboplastin in dogs: Development of an anticoagulant. J. Lab. Clin. Med. 60:261-273, 1962.

17. Margaretten, W., H.O. Zunker, and D.G. McKay. Production of the generalized Shwartzman reaction in pregnant rats by intravenous infusion of thrombin. Lab. Invest. 13:552-559, 1964.

18. McGrath, J.M., and G.J. Stewart. The effects of endotoxin on vascular endothelium. J. Exptl. Med. 129:833-848, 1969.

19. McKay, D.G., W. Margaretten, I. Csayossy. An electron microscope study of the effects of bacterial endotoxin on the blood-vascular system. Lab. Invest. 15:1815-1829, 1966.

20. Mustard, J.R., L. Jørgenson, and M. Packham. Formed elements as a source of vascular injury. Thromb. diath. Haemorrh. Suppl. 40:137, 1970.

21. Niemetz, J., and I. Fani. Procoagulant activity of leukocytes: Role in the generalized Shwartzman reaction. Blood 36:835, 1970.

22. Northover, A.M., and B.J. Northover. The effect of vasoactive substances on rat mesenteric blood vessels. J. Pathol. 101:99-108, 1970.

23. Rubenstein, H.S., J. Fine, and A.H. Coons. Localization of endotoxin in the walls of the peripheral vascular system during lethal endotoxemia. Proc. Soc. Exptl. Biol. Med. 111:458-467, 1962.

24. Shapiro, S.S., and D.G. McKay. The prevention of the generalized Shwartzman reaction with sodium warfarin. J. Exptl. Med. 107:377-381, 1958.

25. Spaet, T.H., H.I. Horowitz, D. Zucker-Franklin, J. Cintron, and J.J. Biezenski. Reticuloendothelial clearance of blood thromboplastin by rats. Blood 17:196-205, 1961.

26. Spaet, T.H. Studies on the *in vivo* behavior of blood coagulant product I in rats. Thromb. diath. Haemorrh. 8:276-285,

1962.

27. Spaet, T.H. Hemostatic homeostasis. Blood 28:112-123, 1966.

28. Spaet, T.H., and I. Lejnieks. Mitotic activity of rabbit blood vessels. Proc. Soc. Exptl. Biol. Med. 125:1197-1201, 1967.

29. Spaet, T.H., and E. Gaynor. Vascular endothelial damage and thrombosis. Advan. Cardiol. 4:47-66, 1970.

30. Spielvogel, A.R. An ultrastructural study of the mechanism of platelet-endotoxin interaction. J. Exptl. Med. 126:235-250, 1967.

31. Stetson, C.A., Jr. Vascular effects of endotoxins. Bull. N. Y. Acad. Med. 37:486-492, 1961.

32. Stewart, G.J., and M.J. Anderson. An ultrastructural study of endotoxin-induced damage in rabbit mesenteric arteries. Brit. J. Exptl. Pathol. 52:75-80, 1971.

33. Stormorken, H., and P.A. Owren. Physiopathology of hemostasis. Seminars in Hematology 8:3-29, 1971.

34. Weissmann, G., and L. Thomas. On a mechanism of tissue damage by bacterial endotoxins. In: *Bacterial Endotoxins*, edited by M. Landy and W. Braun. New Brunswick: Rutgers University Press, 1964, pp. 602-609.

35. Zweifach, B. Vascular effects of endotoxin. In: *Bacterial Endotoxins*, edited by M. Landy and W. Braun. New Brunswick: Rutgers University Press, 1964, pp. 110-117.

THE ROLE OF TARGETS AND MEDIATORS IN ENDOTOXIN SHOCK

Tibor G. Kovàts, M.D.

Institute of Experimental Surgery, Medical University,
Szeged, Hungary

TOXIC EFFECTS OF ENDOTOXIN UPON ORGAN SYSTEMS IN GENERAL AND THE MICROCIRCULATION IN PARTICULAR

Endotoxin may be characterized by its primary toxic and secondary toxic actions. If we assume that the first effect of endotoxin is the release of different mediators from different sites, then this action, together with the effects of mediators on different tissues, would be a direct effect. The primary toxic action is exerted on adrenergic nervous structures and on certain cellular targets, but these structures are affected without involvement of immune factors. The secondary toxic effect is exerted on cellular targets by means of immunologic mechanisms; both immediate and delayed hypersensitivity are elicited by means of opsonin and complement. Endotoxin is less toxic to cells in the absence of immune factors.

By the expression "direct" action of endotoxin, one implies that the effect is directly due to endotoxin insult. On the other hand, "indirect" implies that the effect is induced by some earlier alterations caused by endotoxin. The term "indirect", then, is only relative. It is important to recognize, however, that endotoxin has a direct effect in binding to receptors and in acting on the targets. What follows later is presumably a gradually deteriorating chain reaction with complex interactions. It might be more appropriate to distinguish only between early and late effects of endotoxin. Figure 1 represents an approach to this problem.

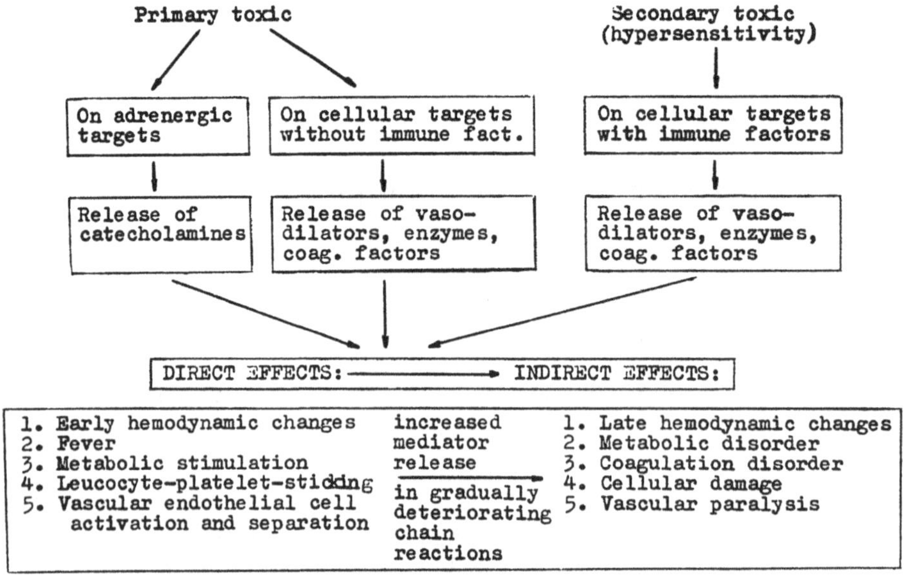

FIG. 1. Proposed scheme of direct and indirect effects of endotoxin.

THE PATHOPHYSIOLOGICAL ROLE OF VARIOUS MEDIATORS IN SHOCK STATES

Pharmacology defines toxins as substances which, in relatively small quantities, damage life functions. In this view, endotoxin should not be compared to smaller toxic molecules such as cyanide and mercuric ion compounds which have definite and well-known subcellular targets. Furthermore, small doses of endotoxin are not harmful and cause only "stimulation" of adrenergic nerves and cellular targets. The result of this stimulation is a moderate release of different mediators, which in themselves may not be considered to have toxic actions.

Larger doses of endotoxin produce an increased release of mediators such as vasoconstrictors, vasodilators, enzymes, and coagulation factors, which together with the progressing deterioration of metabolism, account for endotoxin toxicity. It is also possible that endotoxin has some subcellular targets which are as yet not clearly identified. Probably several enzymes of metabolism are involved which usher in a complex chain of events.

It is interesting that some mediators of endotoxin effect, *e.g.*, the catecholamines, can inhibit metabolic processes and produce hypoxia. During the altered and complex metabolic disorder,

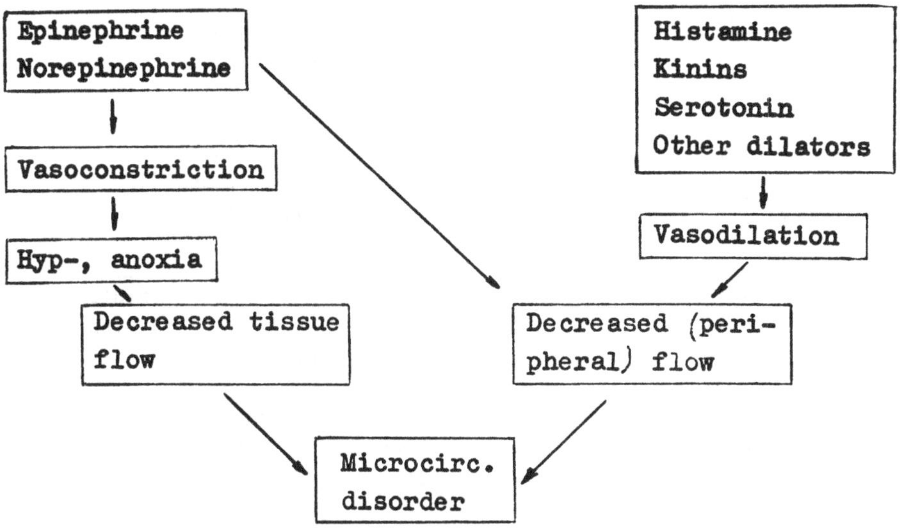

FIG. 2. Hemodynamic effects of certain vasoactive mediators.

metabolic by-products may be produced (*e.g.*, lactic acid) possessing pharmacodynamic activities.

The above generalizations approximate the pathophysiology of the shock state. The course of events in endotoxin shock is diagrammed in three schemata (Figs. 2, 3, and 4) to provide a better understanding of the shock state. Figure 2 outlines the hemodynamic effects of some vasoactive mediators. Figure 3 shows the effects of these mediators on certain target cells and on metabolic processes implicated in shock. It is evident that mediators *per se* can produce similar hemodynamic changes in different types of shock, including endotoxin shock. The first, or reversible, phase of endotoxin shock may be evoked by the release of catecholamines and vasodilators. The mediators in themselves produce effects similar to those induced by endotoxin. The mutual releasing effects of vasoconstrictors and dilators are fairly well demonstrated, as follows:

(a) Spink *et al.* (35) state that histamine stimulates the secretion of epinephrine from the adrenal medulla. Baur and Staub (2) found increased blood histamine levels after administration of epinephrine. Norepinephrine was five times less effective in this respect. The two agents have a mutual secreting action (41). It is not clear how histamine and epinephrine influence each other's secretion. Green (18) believes that histamine and methyl-

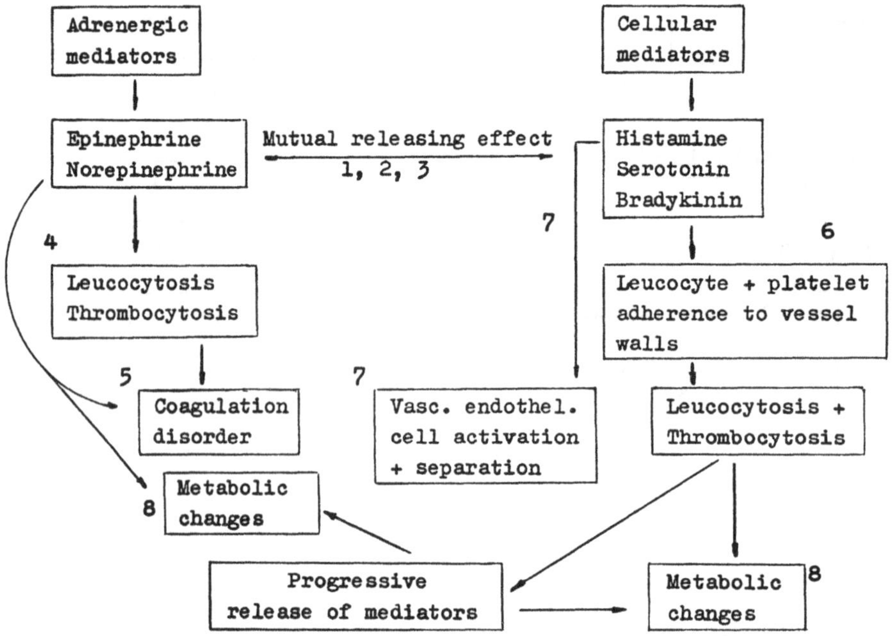

FIG. 3. The known cellular effects of some vasoactive mediators.

histamine may prove to be physiological neurotransmitters or neuromodulators through the synaptic transmission in the peripheral sympathetic centers.

(b) Feldberg and Lewis (11) have shown the release of epinephrine by bradykinin and angiotensin. Lecomte and Dresse (28) stated that kinins indirectly affect airway function through their ability to release catecholamines, either from the adrenal glands or by stimulation of sympathetic ganglia. This explains both the potentiation of kinins by some antagonists of epinephrine and some of the paradoxical self-antagonistic effects exerted by kinins. It was further demonstrated that angiotensin and histamine have a similar epinephrine-releasing capacity. The observed antagonistic and synergistic effects of the above mediators are probably responsible for the partial physiological recovery in the early phase of shock.

(c) Feldberg (10) claimed that low doses of bradykinin were readily antagonized by epinephrine and isoproterenol, while higher doses of bradykinin were unopposed. Similar effects of bradykinin, kallidin, and eledoisin were demonstrated by Gjuri and Westerman

(17). Zweifach (43) has shown that bradykinin and serotonin have a synergistic action of venular spasm followed by capillary stasis and extravasation of red cells through defects in the walls of postcapillary venules.

(d) Leukocytosis is known to occur after epinephrine and norepinephrine administration (40). Baur and Staub (2) studied epinephrine-induced leukocytosis and observed an increased level of histamine which could not be correlated with the epinephrine-induced leukocytosis. In this experiment, an increased number of platelets was also observed which may have been the source of the increase in histamine. Bierman *et al.* (see ref. 24) found an early granulocytosis and lymphopenia after the administration of epinephrine or small doses of endotoxin. Keresztes *et al.* (24) observed that ACTH and cortisone produced early granulocytosis. Sen *et al.* (34) found increased numbers of platelets after epinephrine administration, which they correlated with the observed decreased clotting time.

(e) Seegers (33) stated that the addition of relatively low concentrations of epinephrine or norepinephrine reduces the clotting time of whole blood *in vitro*. Epinephrine also shortens the bleeding time (27). The above data point to the possibility that the release of mediators stimulated by endotoxin influences both cell number and intravascular coagulation.

(f) Probably histamine and kinin-induced leukocytosis and thrombocytosis begin with the adherence of these elements to the vessel wall. Zweifach (42) was able to demonstrate the effect of histamine in rat mesentery. Dilatation of capillaries with a microlesion was seen, along with the adherence of leukocytes and platelets to capillary walls. Cardoso *et al.* (4) found that bradykinin also induces leukocytosis in man and in dogs, after initial adherence (10-30 minutes). It has been shown that histamine in itself can morphologically alter the leukocytes (16).

(g) Jancsó (23) has made a very interesting observation on the effect of histamine on vascular endothelial cells. He found that histamine "activates" these cells to become reticuloendothelial cells which are able to engulf carbon particles and invade neighboring tissues. Jancsó also demonstrated an activating effect of histamine on Kupffer cells. If this effect is induced by endotoxin and not just by histamine, then the direct cellular toxic effect of endotoxin may readily induce vascular endothelial cell damage (12,39).

The metabolic effects of epinephrine and norepinephrine are well reviewed by Ellis (9). Disturbance of citric acid cycle metabolism and increased rates of glycogenolysis and lactic acid production were reported. Plaut and Goldman (30) demonstrated the inhibition of oxidative metabolism in the Krebs cycle by endotoxin *in vitro*. (Because of their complexity, the role of hormones, the change in hormone levels, and the simultaneously occurring metabolic alterations must necessarily be excluded from the schema presented herein [25]). It was shown that the administration of a water-soluble glucocorticoid-type steroid to dogs in hemorrhagic shock results in considerable elevation of blood pressure during oligemia, improved survival, and a decrease of some metabolic changes characteristic of shock (29).

Figure 4 is a simplified schema of the main mechanisms to explain the course of endotoxin shock, including the development of the chain reaction.

(a) Endotoxin acts partly through the direct stimulation or damage of adrenergic nervous structures as targets. Considering the close connection between adrenergic and cholinergic mechanisms, the latter are probably also affected. However, the action of endotoxin on the autonomic nervous system seems to begin with a strong stimulating and later a paralyzing effect on the adrenergic (sympathetic) nervous system. These effects have been cited by Thomas (40), Fine (12), Fine and Minton (13), Fishel *et al.* (14), Kováts (26), Vick and Hinshaw, as cited by Hinshaw (21), and Bälint, Végh, and Kováts (1).

(b) Endotoxin also acts through the stimulation or damage of certain cells (cellular targets), exerting a direct (primary) toxic effect and also implicating immunologic mechanisms (*i.e.*, delayed or immediate hypersensitivity involving opsonin plus complement). The affected cellular elements are microphages, platelets, vascular endothelial cells (which are involved early in endotoxin shock), as well as mastocytes and macrophages. Influential factors include: the vasodilators histamine, acetylcholine, serotonin, and kinins; enzymes and platelet factors which cause vasodilation; metabolic and coagulation disorders; and, lastly, cellular damage. All of the mechanisms are induced by mediators (15,21, 26). It is an interesting possibility that the vasodilator prostaglandin E-c may also be liberated at adrenergic nerve endings or by catecholamines (36).

(c) When small doses of endotoxin are injected, the adrenergic and cellular targets are only stimulated and not damaged. They may also be stimulated, however, shortly after larger doses in the reversible phase of the hemodynamic changes. In this stage, the mediators and mechanisms become interdependent, and there is a definite tendency for restoration toward the normal state. This signifies that constrictor and dilator agents can mutually influence each other's secretion, and that a counter-regulation

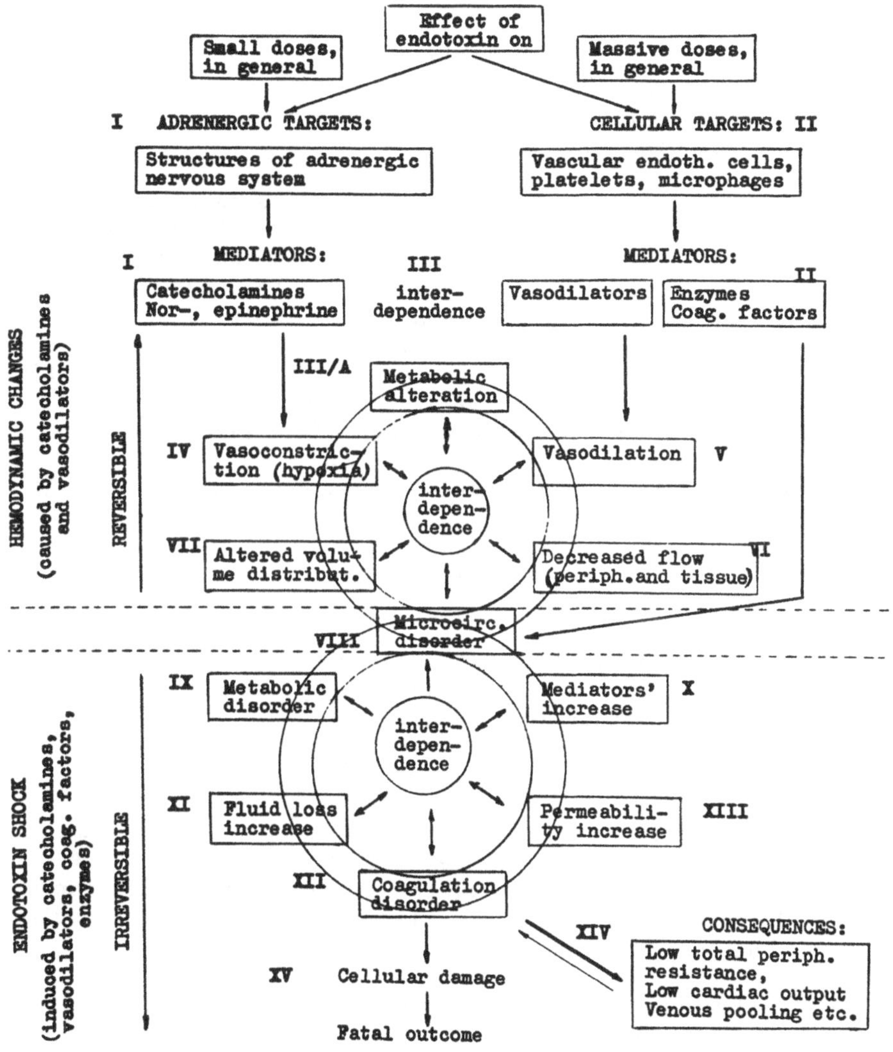

FIG. 4. The primary mechanisms in endotoxin shock.

begins to restore the hemodynamic equilibrium. For example, if the endotoxin-induced changes begin with constriction (catecholamine release), the liberation of histamine, kinin, acetylcholine, and perhaps other dilators follows as a compensatory response. By contrast, the state of vasodilation is compensated by the release of catecholamines. The mutual releasing effects of catecholamines and histamine were shown by Baur and Staub (2), Spink *et al.* (35), and Went and Varga (41). Those between bradykinin and epinephrine were shown by Feldberg and Lewis (11).

The above counter-regulation mechanisms are adequately compensatory if small endotoxin doses are given, or at the beginning of endotoxin shock. (Until this phase, the endotoxin-caused hemodynamic change is reversible, except if shock is induced by massive endotoxin doses.) The counter-regulation is limited, however, if endotoxin shock begins with vasodilation (*e.g.*, in primates). However, there is a tendency toward restoration if the epinephrine level is rising after 1-2 hours (21). The beginning metabolic alterations are progressive in development (see [i] below).

(d) In most species, an initial vasoconstriction occurs (5,6).

(e) The constriction is followed by dilation, or the process begins with a dilation, as Hinshaw (21) showed in the endotoxin shock of primates.

(f) Decreased peripheral flow may be the consequence of dilation, but decreased tissue flow is induced by catecholamine release which is preceded by (g), below.

(g) Volume distribution is altered.

All of the above mechanisms can be induced by catecholamines and vasodilators alone. This phase, illustrated in the first circle of Figure 4 is reversible. (Here, there are no severe disorders which would produce damage). The release of enzymes and coagulation factors may be insignificant in this phase.

(h) Following these effects comes the transit period, which may represent a gradual transition toward the irreversible phase, as illustrated in the lower circle by a *circulus vitiosus*, or fatal sphere, separated with two dotted lines. The starting position of the fatal circle is the microcirculatory disorder, suggesting this to be the transitory link between the reversible and irreversible states. This is probably correct, because the constrictor- and dilator-induced reversible phase begins to worsen when coagulation factors and enzymes intervene. Due to the further stimulation of targets, a progressive release of all mediators follows, with a progressive deviation of normal metabolism (lack of oxygen, acidosis, inhibition of Krebs cycle) and the emergence of coagulation disorders, leading to generalized intravascular coagulation. The compensatory mechanism is upset in this stage and, as a result, altered permeability and fluid loss readily occur. There is, to be sure, a close interdependence among the links of the "fatal circle". The progressive deterioration ultimately causes cellular damage, which is the irreversible and final outcome, as described below.

(i) Metabolic disorders are due primarily to progressive hypoxia, acidosis, and inhibition of the Krebs cycle. The role of hormones in these changes is evident (25).

(j) The increase in the outpouring of mediators is well documented in the progress of different kinds of shock (7,15,21,22,31, 32).

(k) The increase in fluid loss during shock is well known.

(l) The role of coagulation disorders in endotoxin shock and the formation of microthrombi in circulation have been shown by Hardaway and Johnson (20). The importance of disseminated intravascular coagulation in the irreversible shock state was further stressed by Hardaway (19).

(m) The permeability increase in shock states leads to fluid loss.

(n) Finally, cellular damage ensues, involving first leukocytes and platelets adhering to the vessel wall, releasing high quantities of vasodilators and coagulation factors (prerequisites of thrombus formation). Enzymatic release then occurs, followed by damage of the vascular endothelial lining and, ultimately, severe morphologic changes (state of irreversibility). Dietrich (8), Fine (12), Kováts (26), Berdis and Vick (3), and Christy (5) have described this chain of events.

(o) The striking hemodynamic changes include decrease in venous return, pooling of blood, lowered cardiac output, and general hypotension. However, these are merely consequences of the main mechanisms depicted in the diagram. Of course, they may, in turn, affect the progressing main mechanisms in variable degrees.

REFERENCES

1. Bálint, G., P. Végh, and T.G. Kováts. Untersuchungen zur Rolle des parasympatischen Nervensystems bei der hämodinamischen Wirkung von Endotoxin. Med. Pharmacol. exp. 16:385-389, 1957.

2. Baur, H., and H. Staub. Histamin und peripher Leucocytose nach Sympathomimetica. Helv. physiol. pharmacol. Acta 7: 482-492, 1949.

3. Berdis, C.C., and J.A. Vick. Endotoxin and traumatic shock. JAMA 204:191-194, 1968.

4. Cardoso, S.S., O.S. Amorin, A.D. Nogueira, J.A. Alencar, A.P. Corrado, and S.M. Rego. In: *Proceedings of the International Symposium on Vasoactive Polypeptides,* edited by M. Rocha e Silva and H.A. Rothschild. Riverside, N.J.: Hafner Publishing Co., 1967, p. 263.

5. Christy, J.H. Pathophysiology of gram-negative shock. Am. Heart J. 81:694-701, 1971.

6. Delaunay, A., J. Lebrun, M. Delaunay, and E. Fouquier. Lésions et réactions du tissue lymphoide: Troubles circulatoires et lésions lymphocytaires. Ann. Inst. Pasteur 76: 314-330, 1949.

7. Des Prez, R.M., N. Fallon, and E.W. Hook. Modification of lethal effect of bacterial endotoxin by substances altering the metabolism of 5-hydroxytryptamine. Proc. Soc. Exptl. Biol. Med. 107:529-532, 1961.

8. Dietrich, A. Reaktive Thrombose im Tierversuch. Virchows Arch. path. Anat. 307:281-296, 1941.

9. Ellis, S. The metabolic effect of epinephrine and related amines. Pharmacol. Rev. 6:485-562, 1956.

10. Feldberg, W. The role of mediators in the inflammatory tissue response. Intern. Arch. Allergy 8:15-31, 1956.

11. Feldberg, W., and P. Lewis. The action of peptides on the adrenal medulla: Release of adrenaline by bradykinin and angiotensin. J. Physiol. (London) 171:98-108, 1964.

12. Fine, J. Some observations on the mechanism of action of bacterial endotoxin. In: *Bacterial Endotoxins,* edited by M. Landy and W. Braun. New Brunswick, N.J.: Rutgers University Press, 1964, pp. 588-595.

13. Fine, J., and R. Minton. Mechanism of action of bacterial endotoxin. Nature (London) 219:97-98, 1966.

14. Fishel, C.W., A. Szentivanyi, and W. Talmage. Adrenergic factors in *Bordatella pertussis*-induced histamine and sero-

tonin hypersensitivity of mice. In: *Bacterial Endotoxins*, edited by M. Landy and W. Braun. New Brunswick, N.J.: Rutgers University Press, 1964, pp. 474-481.

15. Gilbert, R.P. Mechanism of the hemodynamic effects of endotoxin. Physiol. Rev. 40:245-279, 1960.

16. Gillissen, G. Histamine and its possible role in cytolysis of whole blood cells in guinea pig sensitized with tubercle bacilli. Nature (London) 196:1950, 1962.

17. Gjuri, S.V., and E. Westerman. Bronchoconstrictor action of bradykinin, kallidin, and eledoisin. Nature (London) 205: 402-404, 1965.

18. Green, J.P. Histamine and the nervous system. Fed. Proc. 23: 1095-1102, 1964.

19. Hardaway, R.M. Disseminated intravascular coagulation with special reference to shock and its treatment. Mil. Med. 130: 451, 1965.

20. Hardaway, R.M., and C.D. Johnson. Clotting mechanism in endotoxin shock. Arch. Int. Med. 112:775-782, 1963.

21. Hinshaw, L.B. Release of vasoactive agents and the vascular effects of endotoxin. In: *Microbial Toxins*. New York: Academic Press, 1971, vol. IV, chapt. 8.

22. Hinshaw, L.B., M.M. Jordan, and J.A. Vick. Histamine release and endotoxin shock in the primate. J. Clin. Invest. 40: 1631, 1961.

23. Jancsó, N. Histamine as a physiological activator of reticuloendothelial system. Nature (London) 160:227, 1947.

24. Keresztes, M., and P. Kertai. The role of hypophysis and adrenals in the endotoxin-caused leucocytosis. Kisérl. Orvostud. 18:347-352, 1966.

25. Kovách, A.G.B. In: *Proceedings of a Conference on Recent Progress in the Field of Shock*, edited by S.F. Seely and R.J. Weisiger, Fed. Proc. (Suppl. 9) 20:122-137, 1961.

26. Kováts, T.G. Endotoxin susceptibility and endotoxin hypersensitivity. Szeged: Studia Medica, 1967.

27. Kuschinsky, G., and H. Schimassek. Über die Rolle des Histamins bei der Verkürzung der Blutungszeit nach Adrenalin.

Arch. exp. Path. Pharmak. 226:5-8, 1955.

28. Lecomte, J., and A. Dresse. Stimulation de médullo-surrénalienne par la bradykinine. Arch. Int. Physiol. 69: 89-91, 1961.

29. Nagy, S., K. Tárnoky, and G. Petri. Effect of a water-soluble corticosteroid analogue in experimental haemorrhagic shock. J. Surg. Res. 4:62-69, 1964.

30. Plaut, M.E., and J.K. Goldman. Inhibition of substrate oxidation by endotoxin *in vitro*. Proc. Soc. Exptl. Biol. Med. 133:433-434, 1970.

31. Rosenberg, J.C., R.C. Lillehei, J.K. Longerbeam, and B. Zimmerman. Studies on hemorrhagic and endotoxin shock in relationship to vasomotor changes and endogenous circulating epinephrine, norepinephrine, and serotonin. Ann. Surg. 154: 611, 1961.

32. Schayer, R.W. Relationship of induced synthesis of histamine to some biological actions of endotoxin. In: *Bacterial Endotoxin,* edited by M. Landy and W. Braun. New Brunswick, N.J.: Rutgers University Press, 1964, pp. 182-186.

33. Seegers, W.H. The influence of certain drugs on blood coagulation and related phenomena. Pharmacol. Rev. 3: 278-344, 1951.

34. Sen, P.B.M., J.N. Mukherjes, and A. Maiti. Investigation on the mechanism of action on coagulation of blood. J. Physiol. 7:82-86, 1953.

35. Spink, W.W., R.B. Dawis, R. Porter, and S. Chartrand. The initial stage of canine endotoxin shock as an expression of anaphylactic shock: Studies on complement titers and plasma histamine concentrations. J. Clin. Invest. 43:696-704, 1964.

36. Shaw, J.E. Prostaglandin release from adipose tissue *in vitro* evoked by nerve stimulation or catecholamines. Fed. Proc. 25:770, 1966.

37. Simmons, R.L., R.W. Anderson, T.B. Ducker, K. Sleeman, J.A. Collins, and K.P. Boothman. The role of central nervous system in septic shock. II. Hemodynamic, respiratory and metabolic effect of intracisternal or intraventricular endotoxin. Ann. Surg. 167:158-167, 1968.

38. Simmons, R.L., T.B. Ducker, M.R. Martin, R.W. Anderson, and

H.E. Noyes. The role of the central nervous system in septic shock. I. Pathologic changes following intraventricular and intracisternal endotoxin in the dog. Ann. Surg. 167:145-157, 1968.

39. Tanaka, N., T. Nishimura, and T. Yoshiyuki. Histochemical studies on the cellular distribution of endotoxin of *Salmonella enteritidis* in mouse tissues. Japan J. Microbiol. 3:191-201, 1959.

40. Thomas, L. The role of epinephrine in the reactions produced by the endotoxins of gram-negative bacteria. I. Hemorrhagic necrosis produced by epinephrine in the skin of endotoxin-treated rabbits. J. Exptl. Med. 104:865-880, 1956.

41. Went, I., and E. Varga. Experimentelle Untersuchungen über die chemische Gegenregulation des Blutdruckes. Acta physiol. Acad. Sci. hung. 3:377-393, 1952.

42. Zweifach, B.W. Indirect methods for regional blood flow. I. Microscopic observations of circulation in rat meso-appendix and dog omentum: Use in study of vasotropic substances. Methods Med. Res. 1:131, 1948.

43. Zweifach, B.W. In: *Bacterial Endotoxins*, edited by M. Landy and W. Braun. New Brunswick, N.J.: Rutgers University Press, 1964, p. 629.

DISCUSSION[1]

DR. E. G. ERDÖS *(Oklahoma City, Okla.)*: Dr. Lefer, how long does your factor survive in the circulation?

DR. LEFER: During shock, it's virtually infinite because the animal dies before there is any evidence of clearance of MDF. The renal bed is shut down, so it can't get out through the kidneys; and the reticuloendothelial system is depressed, so it can't be removed by macrophages. And there's virtually no enzymatic hydrolysis because of the lower pH. So, the MDF stays around and continues to accumulate. It is not cleared.

DR. ERDÖS: This would mean that, after a single release from the pancreas, it stays in the circulation.

---

[1]This discussion also covers the presentations of Drs. Lefer and Gaynor (see preceding two papers).

DR. LEFER: No, in the early stages there is a dynamic balance between clearance and production because neither the kidneys nor the reticuloendothelial system is markedly depressed very early in shock. But as these systems are knocked out and as MDF is continuously produced, it keeps building up.

DR. ERDÖS: It would be easier for me to assume that the pancreas would continuously release a proteolytic activator. This would persist in the circulation, and the substrate and everything else would be available in the plasma.

DR. LEFER: Well, the pancreas does actually release hydrolases which perhaps continue to produce MDF in the plasma, but the initial event is in the pancreas.

DR. ERDÖS: Something analogs onto trypsin activation in the pancreas, which would then trigger some other reactions.

DR. LEFER: We have evidence that there is an interaction between zymogen granules and lysosomes such that the zymogen granules actually enhance lysosomal disruption.

DR. ERDÖS: Dr. Gaynor, do you find any damage in the vascular endothelium in the lung?

DR. GAYNOR: Yes. In the tritiated thymidine study, the animals that had received endotoxin had three times the number of labeled capillary endothelial cells in the lung over normal controls.

DR. ERDÖS: Because, if the vascular endothelium of the lung is damaged by the endotoxin, that may explain the findings of others, for example the presence of peptides such as bradykinin in the circulation, or the blocking of the release of angiotensin II, and maybe even the lack of disappearance of prostaglandins. Many of the enzymes involved in peptide metabolism are thought to be located here.

DR. GAYNOR: Right. I agree with you 100%.

DR. J. L. KITZMILLER *(San Diego, Calif.):* Dr. Gaynor, what degree of neutropenia did you obtain in your experiments with the nitrogen mustard?

DR. GAYNOR: The same degree of neutropenia as had been reported to prevent development of the generalized Shwartzman reaction by Forman *et al.* There was a mean total leukocyte count of 800 with a range of about 500-2,000 (the latter in only one animal). The total polymorphonuclear leukocyte count, in most animals, was pretty close to zero. The mean was around 20; the maximum was about 100.

DR. M. H. WEIL *(Los Angeles, Calif.)*: Dr. Lefer, Dr. Visscher and I were wondering whether there was an opportunity to study the tolerant animal, particularly referring to the reticuloendothelial effects of the myocardial depressant factor. Are there any data available? And if not, would you perhaps care to speculate?

DR. LEFER: To my knowledge, no definitive data are available on that very point. I would predict that if, in fact, the tolerance is manifested by both a stimulation of reticuloendothelial function and a stabilization of lysosomal membrane, this might be the mechanism by which the tolerance occurs—namely, the prevention of MDF formation, or at least a diminution of MDF formation and enhanced clearance of MDF when it is produced. I think that is a very good suggestion and a fruitful possibility.

DR. R. J. LAFFAN *(New Brunswick, N.J.)*: Dr. Lefer, how do you correlate the ubiquitous presence of MDF in all forms of shock with the reports that we've heard over and over again of increased cardiac output in shock? And, secondly, is the vasoconstriction which occurs in the splanchnic area restricted to that or does it occur in the femoral area?

DR. LEFER: In answer to the first question, the only situation I know of in which cardiac output is increased in shock is in septic shock. This is in a situation where pancreatic blood flow is still markedly reduced. So, it's essentially a compensatory mechanism and very well may be reflected by the vasodilator mechanisms that Dr. Thal described. However, it does not necessarily apply to the pancreatic vasculature, which either has cut-off mechanisms or the adrenergic mechanisms that constrict it. So it is not inconsistent to have, perhaps, an increased cardiac output and still have diminished splanchnic or pancreatic blood flow. Now, the second point was?

DR. LAFFAN: Does this constrict the femoral vessels?

DR. LEFER: No. To our knowledge, it does not. We've just used isolated strips, but it does not. So, it's somewhat specific for splanchnic vasculature.

DR. D. L. HORWITZ *(Chicago, Ill.)*: I'd like to ask Dr. Gaynor if she's had the opportunity to look at the time course of appearance of endothelial cells in the blood.

DR. GAYNOR: Well, we haven't quantitated it precisely, but we have looked as early as 5 minutes after these small doses of endotoxin and found the cells, but not in all animals. But, you know, there's individual variation, too. The lesion seems to appear very early.

DR. B. D. LOWERY *(Baltimore, Md.)*: Dr. Gaynor, did you not see the endothelial cells most frequently at 1 hour?

DR. GAYNOR: Yes, I think I mentioned in my talk that it was most easy to find these cells in the treated animals between 30-60 minutes after endotoxin, but they could be found in some rabbits as early as 5 minutes after injection, and in some as late after injection as 24 hours.

DR. H. WHIGHAM *(Los Angeles, Calif.)*: Dr. Lefer, would you just say a word about how you treated the sham preparation?

DR. LEFER: Which sham preparation are you referring to? There's a variety.

DR. WHIGHAM: The pancreatectomized.

DR. LEFER: There was a laparotomy with an exposure of the pancreatic vasculature, loose ligatures, but no pancreatectomy.

DR. L. D. MACLEAN, *Panel Moderator (Montreal, Canada)*: The second question that we are going to deal with in this session is what evidence exists to support a significant pathophysiological role in shock states for vasoactive substances. Dr. Haberland, would you make some comments on this?

DR. G. L. HABERLAND *(Wuppertal-Elberfeld, Germany)*: Let me try a pharmacologist's approach to this pandemonium of various shock parameters. When we look for the various possibilities which lead to a reduction in flow in the microcirculation, there is, through the release of catecholamines, an active vasoconstriction which is the primary cause of the defect. But, at the same time, there is immobilization of triglycerides which form fat globules, and by this mechanism the fat globules form thrombi directly in the lung. Eventually, through the reduction of flow in the microcirculation, resulting in oxygen deficiency, acidosis occurs. A variety of proteases are then activated which contribute further to thrombus formation. Through the elaboration of mediators such as MDF or kinins (kallidin, bradykinin), permeability is increased, leading to circulatory perivascular edema, which is another cause of the inadequate microcirculation.

I wish to comment on Dr. MacLean's opening remark about the soldiers' limbs in World War I. When one gets a release of a vascular obstruction, certain proteinase inhibitors are able to reduce edema. A tourniquet placed on the hind leg of the dog or rat for 5 1/2 hours, followed by release, will lead to an increase of the volume of the limb by some 70%. Administering a proteinase inhibitor when the tourniquet is released will elicit a dose-dependent reduction in edema production. Another inhibitor was tested in a model in which a single fracture of a limb was produced which causes shock to develop after 24 hours, with a 25% mortality rate. If these animals are treated with heparin or with streptokinase, 100% of the animals die within 6 hours. If they are treated with a proteinase inhibitor, none die within 24 hours. An application of this knowledge has already been transposed to the clinic. It has been shown in limb restorative arterial operations that treatment with inhibitors prevents both edema of the leg and the increase in the lactate level.

DR. MACLEAN: Dr. Gurd and his colleagues have shown that an elemental diet might influence the course of endotoxin shock in dogs and eliminate or greatly decrease the intestinal lesion. Would you comment on that? How do you think that is related?

DR. HABERLAND: With regard to intestinal lesions in the dog, the diet, of course, has influence. The main shock organ of the dog actually is the intestine. The intestine is very rich in proteases simply because the dog is a carnivore. But these proteases (trypsin, kallikrein) are all inhibited by the same substance. This last year, in studies on hypovolemic shock, it was shown that one could inhibit these lesions, too, by giving these inhibitors systemically.

LIBERATION OF VASOACTIVE MATERIALS FROM MAST CELLS IN ANAPHYLACTIC SHOCK

Alice R. Johnson, Ph.D.

Department of Pharmacology, Emory University, Atlanta, Georgia

Anaphylactic shock is a sudden and often fatal syndrome that can occur when antigen combines with antibodies in a sensitized individual. The reaction involves at least two steps, *i.e.*, fixation of bivalent immunoglobulin and activation of processes leading to release of vasoactive mediators from the cell. The effects of this acute allergic reaction include hypotension, hypovolemia, bronchoconstriction, increased capillary permeability, and stasis and hemorrhage in visceral vascular beds. The actions of various mediators, and thus the prominence of these manifestations of shock, vary from one animal species to another. For example, in dogs, the more pronounced effects of anaphylactic shock are hypotension, portal venous constriction, and hemorrhage of the gastrointestinal tract. In guinea pigs, bronchoconstriction is most prominent, and anaphylaxis in man may be manifest by a combination of urticaria, hypotension, and bronchoconstriction.

Histamine was the first substance recognized as a mediator of shock (15). In most species, histamine release plays an important role in anaphylaxis (40). Histamine cannot account for all manifestations of anaphylactic shock, however. Undoubtedly other mediators are involved. Other amines, such as serotonin or catecholamines, polypeptides such as bradykinin or anaphylatoxin, or the lipid "slow-reacting substance" (SRS), probably also contribute to the development of anaphylactic shock (Table 1).

PHARMACOLOGICALLY ACTIVE SUBSTANCES IN MAST CELLS

Some pharmacologically active agents that are stored in tissue

TABLE 1

PHARMACOLOGIC ACTIONS OF MEDIATORS OF ANAPHYLACTIC SHOCK

Agent	Hypotension	Increased capillary permeability	Broncho-constriction
Histamine	+	+	+
Serotonin	+ or -	+	+ or -
Slow-reacting substance (SRS)	-	+	+
Bradykinin	+	+	+

Note: + = present; - = absent.

mast cells have been implicated in anaphylactic shock. The association of histamine and heparin with mast cells is well established (52). In some species, mast cells also contain serotonin (10) or dopamine (2,20). Mast cells contain proteolytic enzymes (11,34,36) and have the capacity to form or liberate "slow-reacting substance" (SRS) (Table 2).

The amines are bound in inactive form to a complex of heparin and protein in mast cell granules (1,35). As a result of an antigen-antibody reaction or injury to the mast cell, the granules are expelled and the amines are released to react with tissue receptors in smooth muscles and glands.

Which of the other granule constituents are released in an anaphylactic reaction probably depends upon the solubility of the granule matrix. In at least one species, histamine and heparin are released simultaneously. Anaphylaxis in dogs is accompanied by delayed coagulation of the blood, probably indicating release of soluble heparin from mast cells (49,54). In the rat, antigen-antibody reactions induce simultaneous release of two amines bound in mast cell granules—histamine and serotonin (23)—but heparin is not readily released from rat mast cells (4). Rat mast cell granules are insoluble except in alkaline solutions or in solutions of high salt concentrations (35,36). Thus, under conditions where amines are readily liberated, heparin probably remains bound to granule protein.

TABLE 2

BIOLOGICALLY ACTIVE SUBSTANCES IN MAST CELLS[a]

Granules	Particulate	Cytoplasm	Cell membrane
Histamine	Acid phosphatase	Lactic dehydrogenase	ATP
Serotonin (rat, mouse)	Alkaline phosphatase		
Dopamine (hamster, ungulates)		Dopa decarboxylase	ATPase
	Succinic dehydrogenase	Histidine decarboxylase	
	Amine oxidase	5-Hydroxytryptophan decarboxylase	Phospholipase A
Heparin	Fumarase		
	ATP		SRS (?)
Chymotrypsin (rat)		Sulfurylase	
Trypsin (man, dog)		Sulfokinase	
Leucineaminopeptidase (man, rat)			
Esteroprotease (mouse)			

[a] Modified from Uvnäs, B. Ann. N. Y. Acad. Sci. 116:880-890, 1964.

Although mast cell granules are known to contain proteolytic enzymes (36), release of an active protease as a concomitant of amine release has not been established. Proteolytic enzymes from mast cells might induce release of vasoactive mediators from platelets or white blood cells, or they might liberate or destroy kinins. However, protein of rat mast cell granules, like heparin, is insoluble under conditions in which amines are released (35), and evidence for protein release from mast cells of other species is lacking.

The formation of a lipid spasmogen, "slow-reacting substance" (SRS), may be associated with anaphylactic histamine release (3,29). SRS has not been completely characterized, but it is distinct from prostaglandins (45). Although SRS can be formed in cells other than mast cells, it is released, with histamine, from lung fragments of sensitized monkeys (29) or humans (47) or from rat peritoneal cells (46) after contact with antigen. This suggests that both mediators may originate from mast cells in an anaphylactic reaction.

AGENTS THAT RELEASE SUBSTANCES FROM MAST CELLS

Release of histamine and other substances from mast cells can be induced by antigen-antibody reactions, by injury, or by various chemical agents (Table 3). The reaction of an antigen with specific antibodies associated with the mast cell membrane stimulates the release reaction in anaphylaxis (42). This interaction requires fixation of "anaphylactic" (IgE) antibodies (28) but does not require complement (7). The reaction is selective in that constituents of the granules can be released without apparent damage to the cell membrane or without release of other constituents of the cell (32). The release reaction can be blocked by low temperatures, by anoxia, and by a variety of other inhibitors of cell metabolism (13,40). This has been taken as evidence for an enzymatic process, but specific enzymatic pathways remain unidentified, and it is impossible to differentiate energy requirements for release from requirements for maintenance of metabolically intact cells.

Agents derived from other target cells or from injured tissues may also release substances from mast cells. Cationic proteins from leukocytes (5,31) cause histamine release from mast cells, presumably by a selective multistep process (51). Proteolytic enzymes or products of tissue injury probably release substances from mast cells nonselectively by lysing the cells. Peptides such as bradykinin (26) or anaphylatoxins that are produced during the complement cascade (14,18) release histamine from mast cells by undetermined mechanisms. The actions of these agents on mast

TABLE 3

AGENTS THAT RELEASE SUBSTANCES FROM MAST CELLS

Selective	Nonselective	Undetermined
Antigen-antibody	Tissue injury	Anaphylatoxin
Cationic proteins	Proteolytic enzymes	Bradykinin
Amines *d*-Tubocurarine Stilbamidine Morphine Polymyxin B Compound 48/80	Venoms	Endotoxin (?)

cells might be an important factor in production of inflammation, septic shock, or traumatic shock.

A number of drugs cause release of active substances from mast cells (53). The prototype of these chemical releasing agents, compound 48/80, has been used to study the release reaction similar to that of anaphylaxis. After a latent period of 30-60 seconds, a fall in blood pressure occurs, accompanied by rising concentrations of plasma histamine and delayed coagulation of the blood (48). The reaction to 48/80 in the rat is similar to an antigen-antibody reaction in several ways. Antigen and 48/80 induce similar morphologic changes in rat mast cells, *i.e.*, an explosive "degranulation" associated with histamine release (43,60). The effect of 48/80 on rat peritoneal mast cells is shown in Figure 1. Histamine and serotonin are released simultaneously from rat mast cells by either antigen or 48/80 (22,23) within seconds after addition of the releasing agent (32,41). Finally, the actions of either antigen or 48/80 on mast cells are blocked by various inhibitors of cell metabolism (Table 4).

MECHANISMS OF RELEASE OF AMINES FROM MAST CELLS

Release of amines from mast cells involves at least two distinct steps, *i.e.*, exocytosis of the granules and displacement of amines from the heparin-protein matrix (57,58). Electron microscopic studies of mast cells suggest that exocytosis involves structural changes in the intracellular membranes similar to those occurring in pancreatic cells during active secretion of zymogen granules (21). In the reaction of mast cells with antigen, peri-

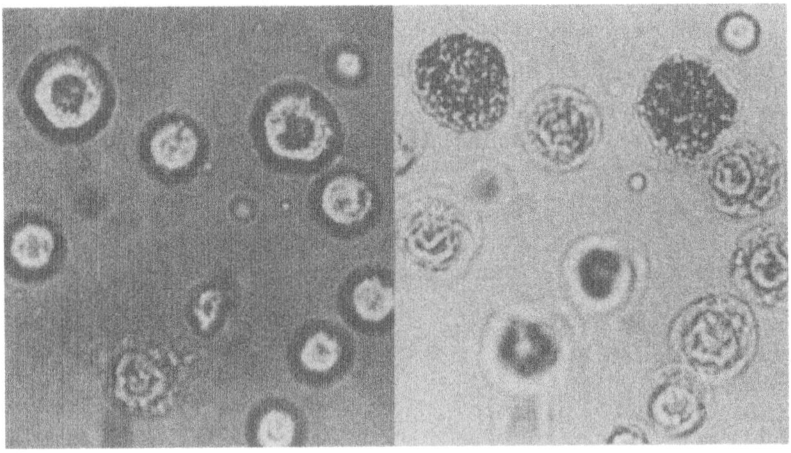

FIG. 1. Effect of compound 48/80 on rat mast cells. Mast cells isolated from serous fluids of rats were photographed through the light microscope before and after addition of compound 48/80 (5 μg/ml) (photograph by Dr. C.R. Kinsolving) (Courtesy of Acta Physiol. Scand. 78:415, 1970).

TABLE 4

AGENTS THAT INHIBIT HISTAMINE RELEASE AND MAST CELL DEGRANULATION INDUCED BY ANTIGEN AND 48/80[a]

SH group inhibitors	NH_2 group inhibitors	Inhibitors of oxidative metabolism	Temperature
Iodoacetate	Ninhydrin	Anoxia	Cold (0-20°C)
p-Chloromercuribenzoate	Dinitrofluorobenzene	Cyanide	Heat (45°C)
N-ethylmaleimide	Phenylisocyanate	Dinitrophenol	
o-Iodosobenzoate			

[a]Adapted from Mota, I., and T. Ishii, Brit. J. Pharmacol. 15: 82-87, 1960; Uvnäs, B., Ann. N. Y. Acad. Sci. 116:880-890, 1964.

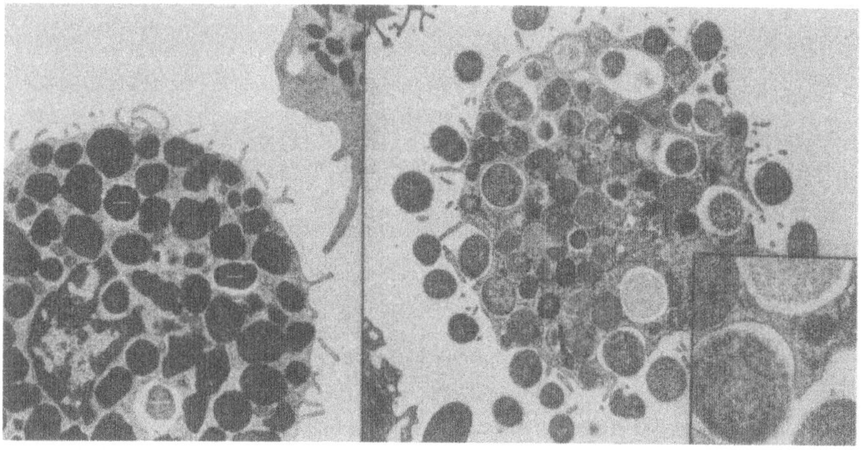

FIG. 2. The effect of antigen on sensitized rat mast cells. Electron photomicrographs were taken from Bloom and Chakravarty (1970). *Left*, untreated rat mast cells. *Right*, mast cells 60 seconds after addition of antigen (0.1 mg). (Courtesy of Bloom, G.D., and N. Chakravarty. Acta Physiol. Scand. 78:410-419, 1970).

granular membranes become fused with each other and with the cell membrane so that the granule matrix is excluded from the interior of the cell (12) (Fig. 2). Once the granules are exposed to the external medium through channels formed by fused membranes or by extrusion to the surface of the cells, the amines are rapidly displaced by cations from the extracellular fluid (57,58) (Fig. 3).

The fundamental biochemical changes that induce this reaction are still obscure. Although displacement of amines from granules is proportional to the concentration of cations in the medium (57,58), the role of cations in exocytosis is not known. Release of histamine from tissues by antigen (40) or white blood cells (39) occurs only when calcium is present in the medium. Similarly, the action of 48/80 on tissue (13) or mesentery mast cells in the rat (27) requires calcium, but 48/80-induced release from isolated peritoneal mast cells is not inhibited by EDTA (60), and degranulation can be induced in a cation-free (sucrose) medium (58). Since calcium plays an important part in the coupling of stimulus and secretion in various secretory cells (19), it may be involved in the release reaction in mast cells.

Evidence exists for a membrane ATPase in rat mast cells (16), but whether this enzyme stimulates release of histamine is unknown. Other enzymes in mast cells might be implicated in the release

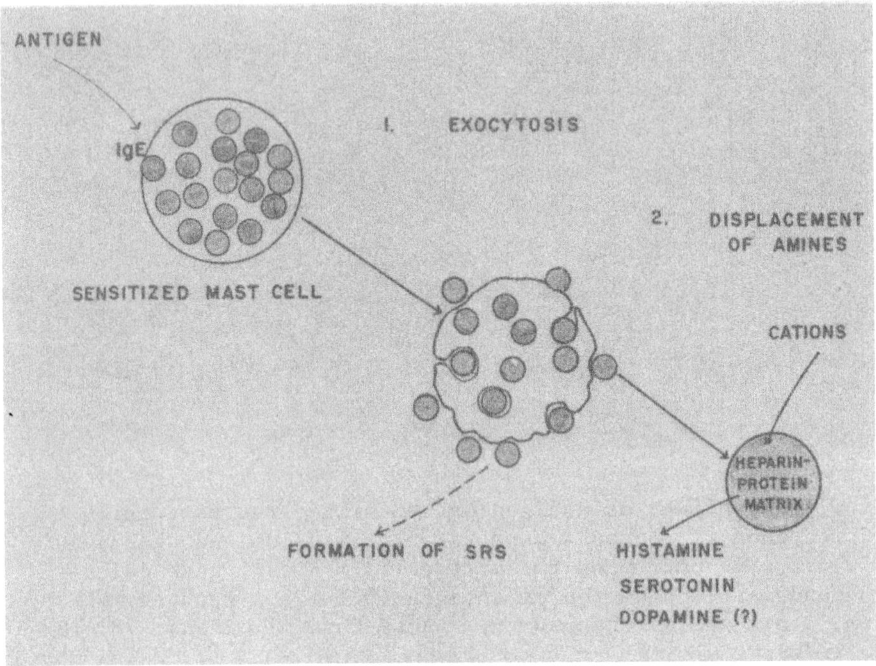

FIG. 3. General mechanism of histamine release from mast cells. Antigen interacts with specific immunoglobulins associated with mast cell membranes. Exocytosis (Step 1) exposes the mast cell granules to the external medium and results in formation of SRS. Amines are displaced from the granule matrix (Step 2) by cations in extracellular fluid.

---

reaction. Phospholipase-A causes degranulation of mast cells (59). Because isolated rat mast cells have phospholipase activity (24), it was suggested that this enzyme might trigger the release reaction and that cleavage of a lipid substrate might produce SRS (3). However, no definitive evidence has yet appeared for the action of this enzyme in the release process.

Amine release may require activation of an esterase that resembles chymotrypsin (8,9). Exposure of mast cells to chymotrypsin causes degranulation (59), and a chymotrypsin-like enzyme is localized in mast cell granules (36). However, Perera and Mongar (50) found that cleavage of chymotrypsin substrates by mast cells could be dissociated from release of histamine, indicating that this enzyme is probably not an integral part of the release mechanism.

Exocytosis of granules may involve contractile proteins in

membranes or other subcellular elements. Colchicine and other agents that "disorganize" microtubules inhibit histamine release in rat mast cells (25) and in human white blood cells (37). High concentrations of colchicine (5 x 10^{-4}M) only partially inhibit release in mast cells, however, and electron microscopic evidence for microtubules in mast cells is lacking.

The rapidity of the release reaction and its dependence upon metabolically intact cells suggests that exocytosis might be triggered by depolarization of the mast cell membrane. Tasaka and associates (56) measured changes in membrane potentials in individual rat mast cells during stimulation by ATP or 48/80, but these changes did not correlate precisely with degranulation. Diamant and Krüger (17) found that electrical stimulation of individual mast cells did not induce degranulation. We found that mast cells labeled with ^{42}K responded to antigen or 48/80 with a small efflux of isotope that occurred within the time course of histamine release (32). Others observed uptake of ^{22}Na after treatment with 48/80, but sodium uptake did not coincide precisely with the release of histamine (55). Therefore, no obvious correlation of ion fluxes or changes in membrane potential can be made with the release reaction. Probably deformation of the mast cell membrane by reaction of antigen with fixed antibody induces physical changes in the cell that stimulate rearrangement of intracellular membranes through one or more enzymatic steps, *e.g.*, cleavage of ATP by membrane ATPase and liberation of calcium or other "intracellular messengers."

Recently cyclic adenosine monophosphate (cAMP) has been suggested to be an "intracellular messenger" in the release mechanism. Although drugs that affect tissue levels of cAMP, such as catecholamines and phosphodiesterase inhibitors, inhibit antigen-induced release of mediators from white blood cells (38) or monkey lung (30), no direct evidence yet exists for an action of cAMP on the release process in mast cells. That is, no studies have demonstrated simultaneous changes in cAMP levels or changes in activities of adenyl cyclase and phosphodiesterase which correlate with release.

We found that high levels of catecholamines (10^{-4} to 10^{-3}M) block histamine release from rat mast cells in response to either antigen or 48/80 (33), but others found that isoproterenol and salbutamol in much lower concentrations (10^{-4} to 10^{-3}M) prevented histamine release from human lung tissue *in vitro*. Although these differences indicate that the sensitivity of the release mechanisms may differ from one type of preparation to another, they provide no clue to the biochemical processes underlying the release reaction.

SUMMARY

Although the phenomenon of anaphylaxis may involve different target cells and release of various chemical mediators, release of histamine from mast cells probably accounts for manifestations such as hypotension, bronchospasm, and increased capillary permeability evoked by challenge of a sensitized individual with antigen. The mechanism of histamine release from mast cells is not fully understood, but it is presumably a multistep process requiring metabolically intact cells.

The role of histamine release in hemorrhagic, traumatic, or septic shock is less well established. Mast cells are usually in close proximity to blood vessels, and toxic agents from blood or tissue fluids could release substances from mast cells that might contribute to the development of shock. The role of mast cells in shock other than anaphylaxis could be defined with proper experimental techniques.

Although the mast cell is a target cell for the antigen-antibody reactions in anaphylactic shock, substances from mast cells might affect other cells or other mediators of shock. For example, enzymes from mast cell granules or charged macromolecules, such as heparin, might activate or inactivate components of the kinin or complement systems. Mast cells might participate indirectly in the production of inflammation by liberating chemotactic substances or by causing release of mediators from other target cells.

REFERENCES

1. Åborg, C.H., J. Novotny, and V. Uvnäs. Ionic binding of histamine in mast cell granules. Acta physiol. scand. 69: 276-283, 1967.

2. Adams-Ray, J., A. Dahlstrom, and C. Sachs. Uptake of 3,4-dihydroxyphenylalanine and 5-hydroxytryptophan by catecholamine-forming mast cells in the hamster. Acta physiol. scand. 67:295-299, 1966.

3. Änggård, E., B. Bergqvist, B. Högberg, K. Johansson, I.L. Thon, and B. Uvnäs. Biologically active principles occurring in histamine release from cat paw, guinea pig lung, and isolated rat mast cells. Acta physiol. scand. 59:97-110, 1963.

4. Archer, G.T. Release of heparin from the mast cells of the rat. Nature (London) 191:90, 1961.

5. Archer, G.T., and M. Jackas. Disruption of mast cells by a component of eosinophil granules. Nature (London) 205: 599-600, 1965.

6. Assem, E.S.K., and H.O. Schild. Inhibition by sympathomimetic amines of histamine release by antigen in passively sensitized human lung. Nature (London) 224:1028-1029, 1969.

7. Austen, K.F., and Bloch, K.J. Differentiation *in vitro* of antigen-induced histamine release from complement-dependent immune injury. In Boston: *Ciba Foundation Symposium on Complement*, edited by G.W. Wolstenholme and J. Knight. Little, Brown & Co., 1965.

8. Becker, E.L., and K.F. Austen. A comparison of the specificity of inhibition by phosphonate esters of the first component of complement and the antigen-induced release of histamine from guinea pig lung. J. Exptl. Med. 120:491-506, 1964.

9. Becker, E.L., and Austen, K.F. Mechanisms of immunologic injury of rat peritoneal mast cells. I. The effect of phosphonate inhibitors on the homocytotropic antibody-mediated histamine release and the first component of rat complement. J. Exptl. Med. 124:379-395, 1966.

10. Benditt, E.P., R.L. Wong, M. Arase, and E. Roeper. 5-Hydroxytryptamine in mast cells. Proc. Soc. Exptl. Biol. Med. 90:303-304, 1955.

11. Benditt, E.P., and M. Arase. An enzyme in mast cells with properties like chymotrypsin. J. Exptl. Med. 110:451-460, 1959.

12. Bloom, G.D., and N. Chakravarty. Time course of anaphylactic histamine release and morphological changes in rat peritoneal mast cells. Acta physiol. scand. 78:410-419, 1970.

13. Chakravarty, N. The mechanism of histamine release in anaphylactic reaction in guinea pig and rat. Acta physiol. scand. 48:146-166, 1960.

14. Cochrane, C.G., and H.J. Muller-Eberdard. The derivation of two distinct anaphylatoxin activities from the third and fifth components of human complement. J. Exptl. Med. 127:371-385, 1968.

15. Dale, H.H., and P.P. Laidlaw. Histamine shock. J. Physiol. 52:355-390, 1918-19.

16. Diamant, B., and P.G. Krüger. Histamine release from isolated rat peritoneal mast cells induced by adenosine 5-triphosphate. Acta physiol. scand. 71:291-302, 1967.

17. Diamant, B., and P.G. Krüger. Structural changes of isolated rat peritoneal mast cells induced by adenosine triphosphate and adenosine diphosphate. J. Histochem. Cytochem. 16: 707-716, 1968.

18. Dias da Silva, W., and I.H. Lepow. Complement as a mediator of inflammation. II. Biological properties of anaphylatoxin prepared with purified components of human complement. J. Exptl. Med. 125:921-946, 1967.

19. Douglas, W.W. Stimulus secretion coupling: The concept and clues from chromaffin and other cells. Brit. J. Pharmacol. 34:451-474, 1968.

20. Falk, B., T. Nystedt, E. Rosengren, and J. Stenflo. Dopamine and mast cells in ruminants. Acta pharmacol. toxicol. 21: 51-58, 1964.

21. Fawcett, D.W. Physiologically significant specializations of the cell surface. Circulation 26:1105-1126, 1962.

22. Garcia-Arocha, H. Release of histamine and 5-hydroxytryptamine from cells of the peritoneal fluid of rats. Can. J. Biochem. Physiol. 39:395-403, 1961.

23. Garcia-Arocha, H. Liberation of 5-hydroxytryptamine and histamine in the anaphylactic reaction of the rat. Can. J. Biochem. Physiol. 39:403-416, 1961.

24. Giacobini, E., G. Sedvall, and B. Uvnäs. Phosphatidase A activity of isolated rat mast cells and of red blood cells, white blood cells, and spinal ganglion cells. Exptl. Cell Res. 37:368-375, 1965.

25. Gillespie, E., R.J. Levine, and S.E. Malawista. Histamine release from rat peritoneal mast cells: Inhibition by colchicine and potentiation by deuterium oxide. J. Pharmacol. Exptl. Therap. 164:158-165, 1968.

26. Goth, A. Effect of drugs on mast cells. Advan. Pharmacol. 5:47-78, 1967.

27. Hogberg, B., and B. Uvnäs. Further observations on the disruption of rat mesentery mast cells caused by compound 48/80, antigen-antibody reaction, lecithinase A, and decylamine.

Acta physiol. scand. 48:133-145, 1960.

28. Ishizaka, K. Human reaginic antibodies. Ann. Rev. Med. 21: 187-200, 1970.

29. Ishizaka, T., K. Ishizaka, R.P. Orange, and K.F. Austen. The capacity of human immunoglobulin E to mediate the release of histamine and slow-reacting substance of anaphylaxis from monkey lung. J. Immunol. 104:335-343, 1970.

30. Ishizaka, T., K. Ishizaka, R.P. Orange, and K.F. Austen. Pharmacologic inhibition of the antigen-induced release of histamine and slow-reacting substance of anaphylaxis (SRS-A) from monkey lung tissues mediated by human IgE. J. Immunol. 106:1267-1273, 1971.

31. Janoff, A., S. Schaefer, J. Scherer, and M. Bean. Mediators of inflammation in leukocyte lysosomes. II. Mechanisms of action of lysosomal cationic protein upon vascular permeability in the rat. J. Exptl. Med. 122:841-851, 1965.

32. Johnson, A.R., and N.C. Moran. The selective release of histamine from rat mast cells by compound 48/80 and antigen. Am. J. Physiol. 216:453-459, 1969.

33. Johnson, A.R., and N.C. Moran. Inhibition of the release of histamine from rat mast cells: The effect of cold and adrenergic drugs on release of histamine by compound 48/80 and antigen. J. Pharmacol. Exptl. Therap. 175:632-640, 1970.

34. Katayama, Y., J.V. Auditore, and N. Ende. Purification and characterization of a mouse mast cell esteroprotease. Exptl. Mol. Pathol. 14:228-242, 1971.

35. Lagunoff, D. Structural aspects of histamine binding: The mast cell granule. In: *Mechanisms of Release of Biogenic Amines*, edited by U.S. Von Euler, S. Rosell, and B. Uvnäs. New York: Pergammon Press, 1966, pp. 79-94.

36. Lagunoff, D. The properties of mast cell proteases. Biochem. Pharmacol. (Suppl.) 17:221-227, 1968.

37. Levy, D.A., and J.A. Carlton. Influence of temperature on the inhibition by colchicine of allergic histamine release. Proc. Soc. Exptl. Biol. Med. 130:1333-1336, 1969.

38. Lichtenstein, L.M., and S. Margolis. Histamine release *in vitro:* Inhibition by catecholamines and methylxanthines. Science 161:902-904, 1968.

39. Lichtenstein, L.M., and A.G. Osler. Studies on the mechanisms of hypersensitivity phenomena. IX. Histamine release from human leukocytes by ragweed pollen antigen. J. Exptl. Med. 120:507-530, 1964.

40. Mongar, J. L., and H.O. Schild. Cellular mechanisms in anaphylaxis. Physiol. Rev. 42:226-270, 1962.

41. Moran, N.C., B. Uvnäs, and B. Westerholm. Release of 5-hydroxytryptamine and histamine from rat mast cells. Acta physiol. scand. 56:26-41, 1962.

42. Mota, I. The mechanism of anaphylaxis. I. Production and biological properties of "mast cell sensitizing" antibody. Immunology 7:681-699, 1964.

43. Mota, I., and W. Dias da Silva. Antigen-induced damage to isolated sensitized mast cells. Nature (London) 186: 245-246, 1960.

44. Mota, I., and T. Ishii. Inhibition of mast cell disruption and histamine release in rat anaphylaxis *in vitro*: Comparison with compound 48/80. Brit. J. Pharmacol. 15: 82-87, 1960.

45. Orange, R.P., and K.F. Austen. Slow-reacting substances of anaphylaxis. Advan. Immunol. 10:106-145, 1969.

46. Orange, R.P., D.J. Stechschulte, and K.F. Austen. Immunochemical and biologic properties of rat IgE. II. Capacity to mediate the immunologic release of histamine and slow-reacting substance of anaphylaxis (SRS-A). J. Immunol. 105:1087-1095, 1970.

47. Orange, R.P., G.W. Austen, and K.F. Austen. Immunological release of histamine and slow-reacting substance of anaphylaxis from human lung. I. Modulation by agents influencing cellular levels of cyclic 3'5'-adenosine monphosphate. J. Exptl. Med. 134:136s-148s, 1971.

48. Paton, W.D.M. Compound 48/80: A potent histamine liberator Brit. J. Pharmacol. 6:499-508, 1951.

49. Patterson, R., and Sparks, D.B. The passive transfer to normal dogs of skin reactivity, asthma and anaphylaxis from a dog with spontaneous ragweed pollen hypersensitivity. J. Immunol. 88:262-268, 1962.

50. Perera, B.A.V., and J.L. Mongar. The role in anaphylaxis

of a chymotrypsin-like enzyme in rat mast cells. Immunology 6:478-483, 1963.

51. Ranadive, N.S., and C.G. Cochrane. Mechanisms of histamine release from mast cells by cationic protein (band 2) from neutrophil lysosomes. J. Immunol. 106:506-516, 1971.

52. Riley, J.F. *The Mast Cells*. Edinburgh and London: E. & S. Livingstone, 1959.

53. Rothschild, A.M. Histamine release by basic compounds. In: *Handbook of Experimental Pharmacology*, edited by O. Eichler and A. Farar, vol. 18; *Histamine and Antihistaminics*, edited by M. Rocha e Silva, New York: Springer-Verlag, 1966, Part 1, pp. 386-430.

54. Scroggie, A.E., and L.B. Jaques. The release of histamine and heparin by antigen from the isolated perfused liver of the sensitized dog. J. Immunol. 62:103-116, 1949.

55. Slorach, S.A., and B. Uvnäs. Dissociation of histamine release and Na uptake in rat mast cells exposed to compound 48/80 *in vitro*. Acta physiol. scand. 76:201-212, 1969.

56. Tasaka, K., K. Sugiyama, S. Komoto, and H. Yamasaki. Dissociation of degranulation and depolarization of the rat mesentery mast cell exposed to compound 48/80 and ATP. Proc. Japan Acad. 46:826-830, 1970.

57. Thon, I.L., and B. Uvnäs. Degranulation and histamine release: Two consecutive steps in the response of rat mast cells to compound 48/80. Acta physiol. scand. 71: 303-315, 1967.

58. Uvnäs, B. Release processes in mast cells and their activation by injury. Ann. N.Y. Acad. Sci. 116:880-890, 1964.

59. Uvnäs, B., and J. Antonsson. Triggering action of phosphotidase A and chymotrypsins on degranulation of rat mesentery mast cells. Biochem. Pharmacol. 12:867-873, 1963.

60. Uvnäs, B., and I.L. Thon. Evidence for enzymatic histamine release from isolated rat mast cells. Exptl. Cell Res. 23:45-57, 1961.

PROTEASES AND ANTIPROTEASES IN EXPERIMENTAL LOW-FLOW STATES

Walter H. Massion, M.D.[1], Leo Peschl, M.D., and Günther Blümel, M.D.

Department of Anesthesiology, University of Oklahoma Medical Center, Oklahoma City, Oklahoma, and Department of Experimental Surgery, University of Vienna, Vienna Austria

Refractory hypotension due to hemorrhage, septicemia, or myocardial infarction continues to be a major cause of death. The mechanism responsible for the development of the so-called "irreversible phase" in low-flow states has been under investigation for a number of years. Many theories (1,13,15) have been advanced to explain why vigorous therapy aimed at volume replacement, reduction of peripheral resistance, and correction of acidosis often fails to save the patient. While it appears unlikely that any single factor in the pathophysiology of shock can account for the irreversibility mechanism, good evidence exists that hypercoagulability of the blood and capillary leakage play a prominent role. In addition, emphasis on myocardial depression (10) has been renewed as a major contributory factor to the mortality from shock. Recent studies (18) have suggested that a group of humoral agents called kinins are released or activated as a result of tissue trauma and intestinal ischemia. These agents have been shown to exert a damaging effect on the microcirculation (12) and have also been implicated in the myocardial depression following hemorrhage. In this paper, we will review what is known about the circulatory effects of kinins in shock and present some preliminary evidence on the possible benefits of a proteolytic enzyme inhibitor to prevent kinin release.

---

[1]Recipient, NIH Research Career Development Award 5-K3-GM-17, 651.

Kinins are vasoactive polypeptides which lower the blood pressure, increase capillary permeability, and produce pain. They are formed from inactive precursors, the kininogens, which are present in the plasma of most warm-blooded animals and are bound to the alpha-2-globulin fraction of plasma proteins. Inactive kininogen is transformed into the active kinin in the presence of proteolytic enzymes released from leukocytes or injured tissue. The structure, physiology, and pharmacology of a few kinins, such as bradykinin and kallidin, have been well characterized (3,21), but the presence of various other kinin-like peptides during low-flow states must be assumed. Lefer (10) has reported the presence of a myocardial depressant factor (MDF) in the plasma during hemorrhagic shock which appears to be a peptide with a molecular weight of 800-1,000. High plasma MDF activity is associated with short survival times in shock. While MDF and bradykinin are probably not identical, their release can be prevented by the proteolytic enzyme inhibitor aprotinin (11). Among the proteolytic enzymes which can catalyze the formation of kinins from inactive plasma kininogens, kallikrein and trypsin have received considerable attention. Both are present in the pancreas (Greek: *kallikreas*), but kallikrein is also widely distributed in other glandular tissues, in the intestinal wall, and in the kidneys, where it is excreted in the urine. The kinin-releasing enzymes may enter into the circulation as a consequence of local tissue injury, intestinal ischemia, or lysosomal destruction—all conditions which are manifest during the late phase of shock. A simplified version of the release and inactivation of kinins is shown in Figure 1.

Our own interest in the possible role of vasoactive kinins in shock was stimulated by a study conducted jointly with Erdös (16), which showed that inhibition of proteolytic enzymes had a protective effect in endotoxin shock. Aprotinin, an inhibitor of a variety of proteases including kallikrein and trypsin, significantly reduced the mortality of dogs injected with *Escherichia coli* endotoxin, compared with the mortality in untreated control animals. Of 11 dogs treated with aprotinin (2,000 kallikrein inactivator units/kg), seven survived for 1 week, while only one of the 11 untreated controls survived this period. However, no measurements of plasma kinins or their precursors were obtained. In the present study, animals were subjected to a well-defined model of hemorrhagic shock (23) in an attempt to correlate changes in the plasma kininogen level with concurrent changes of hematocrit and plasma protein.

METHODS

Fourteen rabbits, matched in seven pairs of two animals each,

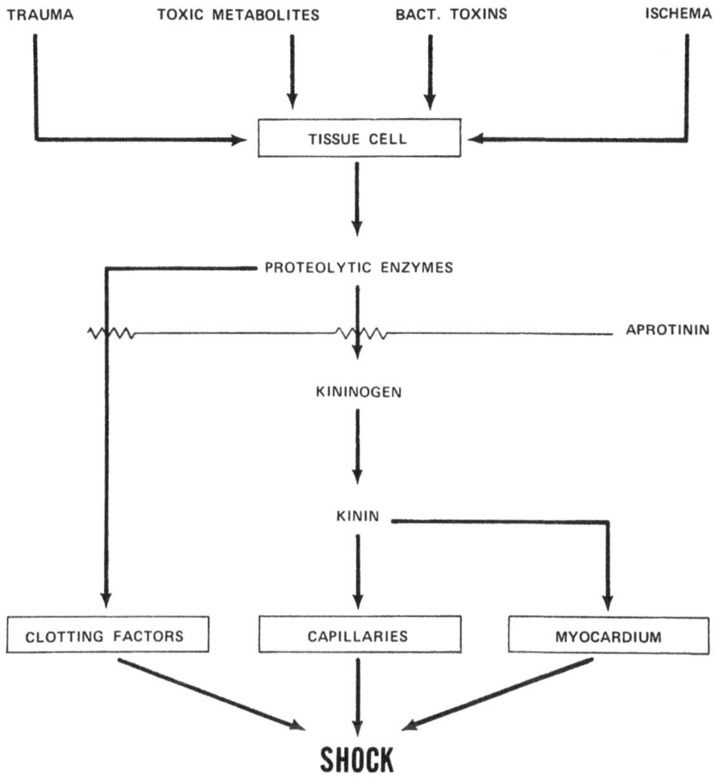

FIG. 1. Simplified hypothesis of the effects of kinin and kinin-like peptides during shock. (Modified from Werle, B. Arztl. Forsch. 18:281-292, 1964.)

were used. They were anesthetized with ether and heparin was administered. One femoral artery was connected to a silicon-treated reservoir which could be raised or lowered to maintain the blood pressure at a predetermined level. The mean arterial blood pressure was recorded from the opposite femoral artery via a pressure transducer. Ten minutes before bleeding, one animal of each pair received 10,000 kallikrein inactivator units (KIU) of aprotinin per kilogram of body weight; the other animal received an equal volume of saline. The animals were then bled a sufficient volume to lower the blood pressure to 35 mm Hg. Rectal temperature was measured by a telethermometer and maintained at 37±1°C by intermittent use of a heating pad placed under the trunk of the animal. Blood samples were obtained 5 minutes before bleeding, 60 minutes after bleeding, and 15 minutes after retransfusion of blood.

Hematocrit, total plasma protein, and plasma kininogen were measured. The plasma kininogen concentration was determined according to the method of Diniz and Carvalho (2), modified by Greeff and collaborators (4), as follows: the plasma was heated with trichloracetic acid for 30 minutes, neutralized with Tris buffer, and incubated with trypsin at 37°C for 30 minutes. The incubate was then denatured in ethanol and vacuum-dried at 35°C. The residue was dissolved in isotonic saline and its biologic activity was tested on the rat uterus according to the method of Horton (7) and Konzett and Sturmer (9). Strength of uterine contraction was recorded on an x-y writer and compared to a standard dose of synthetic bradykinin (Sandoz). The preshock concentration of plasma kininogen was considered as the normal control value (100%); changes occurring during shock were expressed as percent of control. All rabbits were sacrificed at the end of the experiment because the repeated sampling of blood produced too severe an anemia for recovery to be expected.

RESULTS

As shown in Figure 2, hematocrit and plasma proteins decreased during shock by 40% and 30%, respectively; there was no significant difference between treated and untreated animals. The kininogen level decreased 45% in the control animals, but only 10% in the treated animals. This difference was significant ($P < 0.05$). After retransfusion and restoration of normovolemia, hematocrit and plasma protein values returned nearly to preshock levels. However, the plasma kininogen content of untreated animals remained approximately 25% lower than normal. We concluded from these data that the kininogen deficit in the untreated animals was not simply a function of the fall in plasma proteins, as had been suggested by Haberman (5). The percent decrease in plasma protein differed significantly from that observed in plasma kininogen level. On the other hand, a fall in plasma kininogen *per se* is no absolute proof for liberation of kinins, as will be discussed later.

Additional experiments were carried out in dogs to evaluate the possible role of vasoactive kinins in the pathophysiology of cardiogenic shock. Sicuteri and co-workers (19) have drawn attention to the possible involvement of the plasma kinin system in the development of the hypotensive state after coronary occlusion. Since kinins are known to decrease blood pressure, produce pain, and increase capillary permeability, this triad would fit well into the symptom complex of myocardial infarction. It was postulated that proteolytic enzymes may be released from the necrotic region within the myocardium. These enzymes, in turn, would liberate kinins from their inactive precursors present in

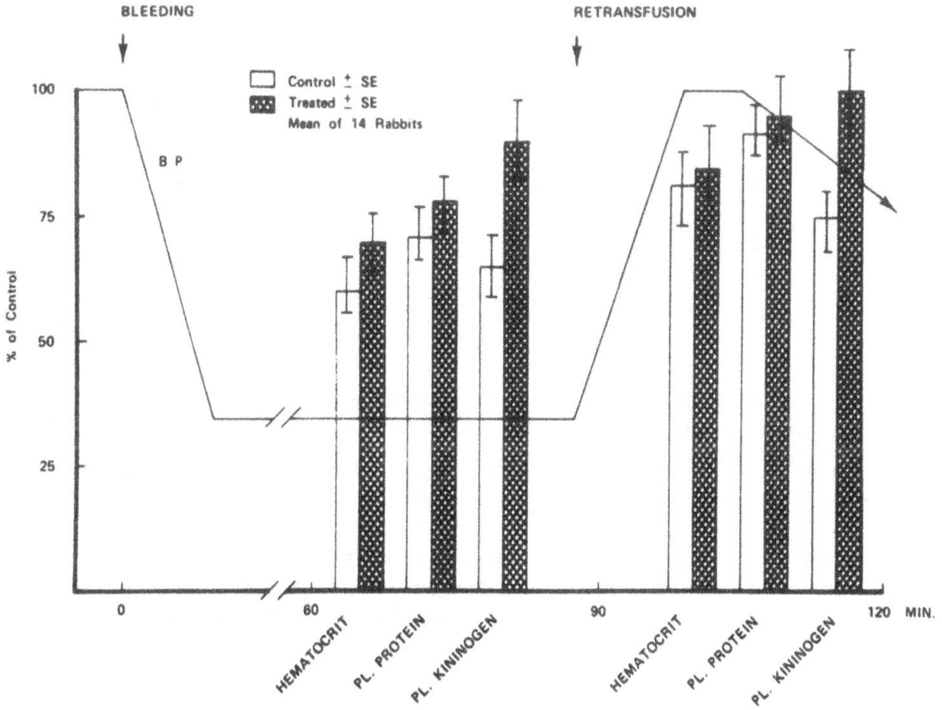

FIG. 2. Hematocrit, plasma protein, and plasma kininogen levels of 14 rabbits during hemorrhagic shock and after retransfusion. Seven animals were treated with 10,000 KIU of aprotinin per kilogram of body weight, while seven controls received an equal volume of saline. (Courtesy of Anesth. Analg. 50:970, 1971.)

---

the plasma. Measurements obtained on patients in the immediate postinfarction period demonstrated a marked decrease in kininogen level, which was interpreted as a sign of kinin liberation. These values returned to normal as the patients recovered from their infarction.

We decided, therefore, to measure plasma kininogen levels in dogs which were subjected to ligation of one coronary artery. The animals were anesthetized with sodium thiopental, the chest was opened, and the ramus descendens of the left coronary artery was ligated. Blood samples were obtained from the sinus coronarius immediately before and at frequent time intervals after ligation. As shown in Figure 3, a mean drop in kininogen level of 45% of the preocclusion measurement occurred between the first and third minute. After the third minute, the value returned to about 90% of normal but dropped again slightly within the next 20 minutes. The blood pressure, however, did not change markedly during this

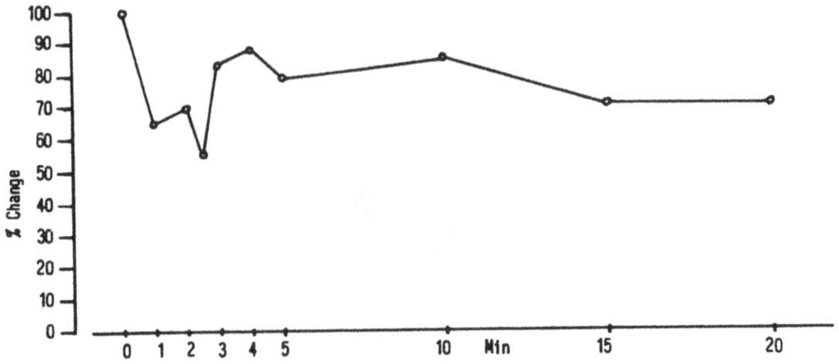

FIG. 3. Kininogen changes in blood sampled from the sinus coronarius. Data points represent mean values from five dogs (control = 100%; occlusion at time zero).

procedure. Of course, it is interesting to speculate whether the absence of pain during general anesthesia might have been a factor. While these experiments failed to establish a clear-cut correlation between kinin formation and cardiogenic shock, they confirmed earlier observations that kininogens are reduced after coronary occlusion.

These findings should be evaluated critically in the light of the following theoretical considerations. A change in plasma kininogen content can be due to: (a) liberation of kinins, (b) enzymatic destruction without formation of kinins, (c) a change in hematocrit, and (d) a change in plasma protein.

A change in hematocrit could mimic a change in kininogen by the following reasoning. If the relative volume of the cellular components of the blood decreases in hemodilution, plasma volume will increase. It follows that each milliliter of this more-dilute plasma contains less alpha-2-globulin fraction. By the same mechanism, a change in plasma protein content could give the mistaken impression of a kininogen change, since a loss in globulins would result in decreased kininogen levels, without kinin formation necessarily having taken place. Since both hematocrit and plasma protein values often change dramatically during shock, kininogen data must be interpreted with caution (17). Unfortunately, direct measurements of kinin formation *in vivo* are very difficult to obtain because of the minute quantities involved and their rapid breakdown by serum kininases. Pending development of better methods for the determination of kinin formation, we will have to rely on approximations such as the measurement of the kininogen deficit.

Proteolytic enzymes not only play a role in the activation of kinins, they are known to interfere with normal blood-clotting processes. The studies of Hardaway and others (6) have demonstrated that disseminated intravascular clotting is frequently present in shock and may be one of the causes of irreversibility. Small thrombi and sludging in the microcirculation are thought to interfere with metabolic processes in vital organs which cannot recover their normal function even after correction of the hypovolemia. Damage to the lysosome membrane and release of lysosomal enzymes into the circulation have been documented in both traumatic and endotoxic shock (8). Whether the bulk of these enzymes is released from tissue cells or from leukocytes remains undetermined, but they appear to exert a strong effect on the blood-clotting mechanism. With this in mind, we asked ourselves whether use of a proteolytic enzyme inhibitor might be beneficial in low-flow states by preventing hypercoagulability.

To answer this question, we carried out the following experiments. Eight cats were anesthetized with ether and bled in two stages: at zero time, 1/20 of their body weight in milliliters of blood was removed via the femoral artery, and 20 minutes later this was repeated. Blood samples were obtained immediately before bleeding, and after 15 minutes and 30 minutes in shock. Figure 4 shows two thromboelastograms from animals pretreated with aprotinin or saline before shock was induced. Clotting time was markedly reduced 15 and 30 minutes after bleeding in the animal given saline. The treated cat had less shortening of the clotting time after bleeding and a return to control values in late shock. This would indicate that inhibition of proteolytic enzymes can prevent hypercoagulability associated with massive hemorrhage. We have preliminary evidence that aprotinin treatment may still be effective, even if instituted 30 minutes or more after induction of shock (17).

We have attempted to correlate these findings with direct measurements of proteolytic enzyme activity in the blood, using the esterolytic method. This method employs a synthetic ester, benzoyl-L-arginin ethylester (BAEE), which splits up into benzoylarginin and ethanol in the presence of kallikrein and other proteolytic enzymes. The acid freed in this process was titrated against sodium hydroxide in an automatic titration unit. Figure 5 compares the clotting-time changes with esterolytic activity. While clotting time is reduced after induction of shock in the untreated animals, it remains constant in the animals receiving inhibitor. The esterolytic activity increases markedly during early shock, indicating liberation of proteolytic enzymes; it falls somewhat in late shock. Again, little or no change follows inhibitor treatment.

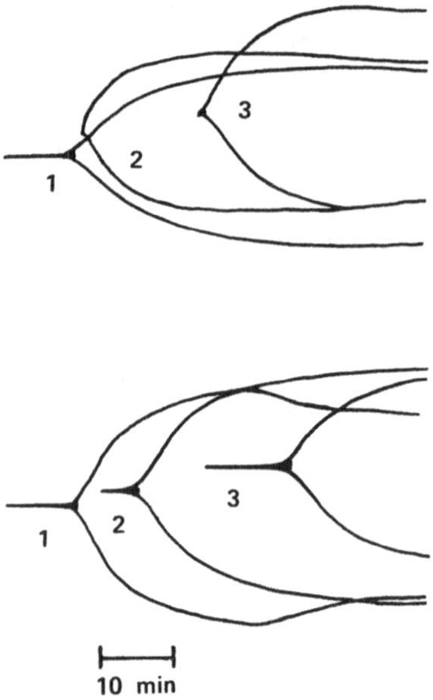

FIG. 4. Thromboelastogram of two cats before and after hemorrhagic shock. Upper tracings, control animal (receiving saline); lower tracings, animal receiving 10,000 KIU of aprotinin per kilogram of body weight before hemorrhage. Clotting time measurements: 1 = preshock control; 2 = 15 minutes after hemorrhage; 3 = 30 minutes after hemorrhage. (Courtesy of Anesth. Analg. 50:970, 1971.)

DISCUSSION

If we consider the results of our experiments along with those of Thal (20), Werle (22), Ludwig (14), and others (17,19), it becomes evident that the development of irreversibility in shock cannot be evaluated solely on the basis of hemodynamics. The well-known diagram of events causing perpetuation of shock consists of a circle beginning with blood loss and leading successively to reduced venous return, decreased cardiac output, and lowered blood pressure, followed by compensatory vasoconstriction, tissue hypoxia, and acidosis. It should be revised to include the activity of proteolytic enzymes and vasoactive polypeptides. We know that conventional shock therapy with blood transfusion, judicious use of peripheral vasodilators, and respiratory support often succeeds in breaking this cycle before manifestations of serious tissue ischemia appear. It must be assumed that in these cases normal defense mechanisms, such as the actions of naturally occurring proteolytic enzyme inhibitors and kinin-destroying enzymes, remain

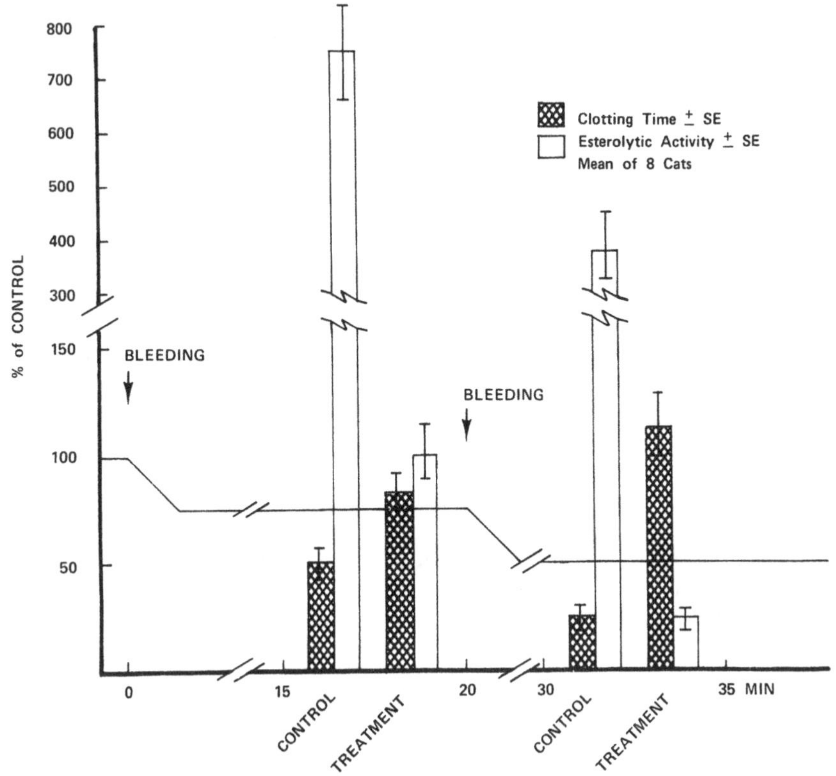

FIG. 5. Comparison between clotting time changes and esterolytic activity during a two-step hemorrhage. Four treated cats received 10,000 KIU of aprotinin per kilogram of body weight prior to bleeding; four controls received an equal volume of saline. (Courtesy of Anesth. Analg. 50:970, 1971.)

sufficiently operative to prevent intravascular clotting, perivascular edema, and myocardial depression. However, since it will always be difficult to predict whether a given patient in shock is threatened by serious microcirculatory disturbance, the early use of aprotinin might be considered as a possible adjunct in shock therapy. A significant reduction in mortality has been claimed in clinical trials with aprotinin by European investigators. The preparation is currently available in the United States only for investigational use.

SUMMARY

Proteolytic enzymes are present during hemorrhagic, cardiogenic, and endotoxin shock. They may contribute to the pathophysiology of low-flow states by at least three mechanisms: (a) the release of kinins, causing hypotension and capillary leakage; (b) the induction of hypercoagulability of the blood, followed by disseminated intravascular clotting; and (c) the activation or release of a myocardial depressant factor into the circulation. It appears that some of these processes can be mitigated by administration of a proteolytic enzyme inhibitor.

ACKNOWLEDGMENT

The aprotinin (Trasylol) used in this study was kindly supplied by Dr. Gerd Haberland, Farbenfabriken Bayer, Wuppertal-Elberfeld, Germany.

REFERENCES

1. Crowell, J.W., and A.C. Guyton. Evidence favoring a cardiac mechanism in irreversible hemorrhagic shock. Am. J. Physiol. 201:983-986, 1961.

2. Diniz, C.R., and I.F. Carvalho. A micro-method for determinations of bradykininogen under several conditions. Ann. N. Y. Acad. Sci. 104:77, 1963.

3. Erdös, E.G. Hypotensive peptides: Bradykinin, kallidin, and eledoisin. Advan. Pharmacol. 4:1-90, 1966.

4. Greeff, K., K. Scharnagel, R. Luhr, and H. Strobach. Die Abnahme des Kininogengehaltes des Plasmas beim toxischen, anaphylaktischen und anaphylaktoiden Schock. Arch. Exp. Path. u. Pharmak. 253:235-245, 1966.

5. Haberman, E. Probleme der Pathophysiologie des Kininsystems. In: *Neue Aspekte der Trasylol-Therapic.* Stuttgart: Schattauer, 1969, vol. III, p. 37.

6. Hardaway, R.M., and D.G. Johnson. A new theory of shock. Mil. Med. 128:198-208, 1963.

7. Horton, E.W. Human urinary kinin excretion. Brit. J. Pharmacol. 14:125, 1959.

8. Janoff, A., quoted from: Gazzaniga, A.B., and N.E. O'Connor. Effects of intravenous infusion of autologous kidney lysosomal enzymes in the dog. Ann. Surg. 172:804-812, 1970.

9. Konzett, H., and E. Sturmer. Biologic activity of synthetic polypeptides with bradykinin-like properties. Brit. J. Pharmacol. 15:444, 1960.

10. Lefer, A.M. Role of a myocardial depressant factor in the pathogenesis of circulatory shock. Fed. Proc. 29:1836-1847, 1970.

11. Lefer, A.M., and J.B. Martin. Relationship of plasma peptides to the myocardial depressant factor in hemorrhagic shock in cats. Circ. Res. 26:56-59, 1970.

12. Lewis, G.P. Active polypeptides derived from plasma proteins. Physiol. Rev. 40:647, 1960.

13. Lillehei, R.C., F. Simeone, J.C. Melby, and V.J. Collins. Shock: Current concepts of pathogenesis and treatment (Symposium). New Physician 13:415-434, 1964.

14. Ludwig, H., and P. Tauber. Proteinaseninhibition im experimentellen Schock. In: *Neue Aspekte der Trasylol-Therapie.* Stuttgart-New York: Schattauer, 1970, vol. IV, pp. 125-149.

15. Massion, W.H. Role of biologic energy transformation during shock in the development of "irreversibility". Anesth. Analg. 48:263-267, 1969.

16. Massion, W.H., and E.G. Erdös. The effects of ATP and a proteolytic enzyme inhibitor in irreversible shock. J. Oklahoma Med. Assoc. 59:467-471, 1966.

17. Massion, W.H., G. Blümel, L. Peschl, and H. Rettenbacher-Daubner. The role of the plasma kinin system in cardiogenic shock and related conditions. In: *Symposium on Proteases and Anti-Proteases in Cardioangiology,* Vietri sul Mare, May/June 1969 (in press).

18. Meyer, A., and E. Werle. In: *Pathogenese, Diagnostik, Klinik und Therapie der Erkrankungen des Exokrinen Pankreas,* edited by K. Heinkel and H. Schon. Stuttgart: Schattauer, 1964, p. 299.

19. Sicuteri, R., G. Franchi, P.L. Del Bianco, and E. Del Bene. A contribution to the interpretation of shock and pain in myocardial infarction. Malattie Cardiovascolari 8:3-19, 1967.

20. Thal, A.P., and V.M. Sardesay. Shock and the circulating polypeptides. Am. J. Surg. 110:308, 1965.

21. Vogel, R., I. Trautschold, and E. Werle. *Natural Proteinase Inhibitors*. New York and London: Academic Press, 1968.

22. Werle, E. Biochemische Betrachtungen zur Regelung der Gewebsdurchblutung. Arztl. Forsch. 18:281-292, 1964.

23. Wiggers, C.J. *Physiology of Shock*. New York: Commonwealth Fund, 1950.

PROLYLCARBOXYPEPTIDASE IN BIOLOGICAL FLUIDS[1]

K. Sorrells, Ph.D., and E. G. Erdös, M.D.

Department of Pharmacology, University of Oklahoma
School of Medicine, Oklahoma City, Oklahoma

Prolylcarboxypeptidase (PCP) was discovered in the kidney by Yang, Erdös, and associates (1-3). Because the enzyme cleaved the Pro^7-Phe^8 bond in angiotensin II, it was called angiotensinase C. PCP was soon found, however, to hydrolyze many other peptide substrates with a general structure of R_1-Pro-R_2-OH. Here R_1 can be either a blocking group, a dansyl group, another amino acid, or a peptide. R_2 is an aromatic or aliphatic amino acid with a free carboxyl group. Substrates in which proline is replaced by another amino acid are not cleaved. The enzyme is most active at an acid pH. It is inhibited by di*iso*propyl phosphorofluoridate (DFP), and it differs from catheptic enzymes. In the body (2,4), PCP occurs in lysosomal fractions of the kidney and of human leukocytes, and elsewhere.

Because it has been demonstrated that shock can lead to damage to cells and subcellular particles such as lysosomes, elevated levels of lysosomal enzymes in the circulation may be an important indicator of the severity of shock. Although numerous studies have been done on this subject, many suffer from one or more of the following shortcomings. First, the tests for the enzymes are not sensitive enough. Second, the enzymes are not specific enough; *i.e.*, they occur in most tissues and are abundant in fractions other than lysosomes. Finally, the enzymes may have specific functions which are unlikely to contribute to the shock syndrome.

---

[1]This work was supported in part by Grants HE-08764 and 5T01-HE-05859 from NIH, USPHS, and by the Office of Naval Research Contract N00014-68-A-0496 and N00014-69-A00385.

We believe that PCP can be suitably used as a lysosomal marker enzyme in shock, since it is normally either absent from plasma and red blood cells or present in only minute quantities (1,2). We have developed a highly sensitive and accurate assay for the enzyme (4,5) in which ^{14}C-1-dimethylamino-naphthalene-5-sulfonyl (DNS) Cl is allowed to react with prolylphenylalanine. The resulting substrate, ^{14}C-DNS-Pro-Phe, is both radioactive and fluorescent. The product of the enzymatic hydrolysis, ^{14}C-DNS-Pro, is separated by thin-layer chromatography and localized under ultraviolet light. The spots are cut out from the sheets, placed in a vial containing a liquid scintillator, and radioactivity is measured in a scintillation counter (4,5). The assay is sensitive enough to determine picomole quantities of the product of enzymatic hydrolysis.

This technique was used to detect lysosomal damage by assaying PCP in various biological fluids. Among the sources of the enzyme investigated were synovia, plasma, urine, and lymph. In the synovia obtained from the knee joints of patients suffering from arthritis, a linear relationship appeared to exist between the number of leukocytes present and PCP activity. In normal urine, the PCP level was very low. In 10 normal healthy males, it averaged 398 (±63SE) pmole/ml per hour. Values were not significantly different in nephrotic patients. In two patients who received a transplanted kidney, however, PCP activity was 127% higher than the normal values. An increase of 50-100% was also noted in the thoracic lymph of dogs collected during hemorrhagic or endotoxin shock.

Finally, PCP was assayed in the plasma of dogs in endotoxin shock. These animals received 0.3 mg/kg *Escherichia coli* endotoxin (Difco), representing an LD_{80}. Figure 1 summarizes the results. Twenty minutes after the injection of endotoxin, the PCP activity in canine plasma increased from 540(±159SE) to 1832 (±700SE) pmole/ml per hour. The difference in the enzyme levels before and after shock was highly significant ($P < 0.01$). In contrast, no significant change occurred in β-glucuronidase activity nor in the concentration of plasma proteins. (β-Glucuronidase is a lysosomal enzyme frequently used to assess damage to these subcellular particles.)

SUMMARY

We have developed a highly sensitive assay for the lysosomal enzyme prolylcarboxypeptidase (PCP) that occurs in neutrophil granulocytes and in the kidney. The enzyme is released into various biological fluids. PCP activity increases in dog plasma during shock, while the level of the other lysosomal enzyme measured (*i.e.*, β-glucuronidase) did not change significantly.

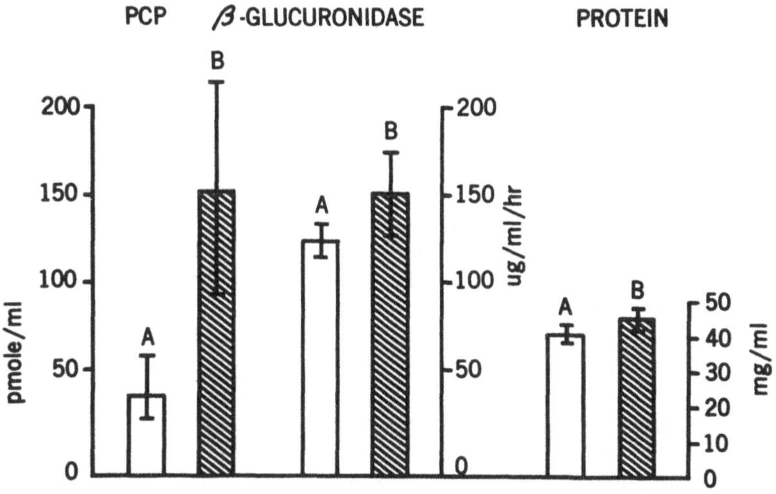

FIG. 1. Activity of prolylcarboxypeptidase (PCP) and β-glucuronidase in dog plasma before (A) and after (B) endotoxin shock. The activity of PCP was determined with ^{14}C-DNS-Pro-Phe substrate; β-glucuronidase activity was determined with phenolphthaleinglucuronide. Protein concentrations were determined by the biuret reaction. Vertical bars show the mean value ±1 SE. PCP assay, n = 6; in the other assays, n = 5. PCP activity = per ml/5 min.

REFERENCES

1. Yang, H.Y.T., E.G. Erdös, and T.S. Chiang. New enzymatic route for the inactivation of angiotensin. Nature (London) 218:1224, 1968.

2. Yang, H.Y.T., E.G. Erdös, T.S. Cniang, T.A. Jenssen, and J.G. Rodgers. Characterization of an enzyme that inactivates angiotensin II (angiotensinase C). Biochem. Pharmacol. 19: 1201, 1970.

3. Yang, H.Y.T., and E.G. Erdös. In: *Immunopathology of Inflammation*, edited by B.K. Forscher and J.C. Houck. Amsterdam: Excerpta Medica, 1971, p. 146.

4. Sorrells, K., and E.G. Erdös. Prolylcarboxypeptidase (angiotensinase C) in subcellular particles of leukocytes. Fed. Proc. 30:600, 1971.

5. Sorrells, K., E.G. Erdös, and W.H. Massion. Effect of prostaglandin E, in the shocked lung. Proc. Soc. Exptl. Biol. Med., in press.

DISCUSSION

DR. L. D. MACLEAN, *Panel Moderator (Montreal, Canada):* The papers we have heard must stimulate the clinicians to see whether we can't demonstrate these things and modify them into the clinical setting. Are there questions? Dr. Hardaway, would you like to comment on these activities?

DR. R. M. HARDAWAY, III *(El Paso, Texas):* It's very difficult for me to accept the idea that vasodilation is a mechanism for certain types of septic shock in that, if this is a mechanism, it's in the face of a high catecholamine level. And secondly, the high cardiac output and lowered resistance through the portal visceral capillaries ought to improve things rather than make them worse. So, it must be detoured through special beds or through arteriovenous shunts; but they don't seem to be going through the "real business" capillaries. It seems to be the worse types of shock that have the high cardiac output. The mortality rate in this type of shock is certainly very high.

Secondly, I'd like to comment on a mechanism in endotoxin. As you know, endotoxin causes a coagulation defect. If one desensitizes animals with increasing doses of endotoxin, the mortality rate is essentially zero for otherwise fatal doses. If this happens, there is no effect on the coagulation system. In other words, the mortality and the coagulation defect seem to go together.

Thirdly, I'd like to mention another toxic factor which we haven't talked about. If we had a hemorrhagic shock model which had a mortality of roughly 10%, and if we beat on a dog's hind legs with a rubber mallet under anesthesia prior to hemorrhage, the mortality was still about 10%. However, if one waits about 48 hours and then produces the hemorrhagic shock, the mortality rate goes up to about 90%. This seems to be correlated with an interesting finding, roughly peaking at 48 hours, where there is a large amount of pigment in the blood. It looks like hemolysis. I don't know what the pigment is. But if one then substitutes for the trauma a small amount of hemolysis, namely, about 20 cc of the dog's own blood which is hemolyzed by freezing and then given back to him, this will, in conjunction with the hemorrhage, produce the mortality of about 90%. So, something in either traumatized tissue or in hemolysis will tremendously increase the mortality rate. This, again, is correlated with the clotting defect.

DR. MACLEAN: Dr. Weil, do you measure catecholamines, serotonin, or hydrolytic enzymes from the cell in your shock unit?

DR. M. H. WEIL *(Los Angeles, Calif.):* No, I must admit that we do not. Of the indirect indices of cellular injury, the only parameters that we actually measure are the conventional enzymes: the transaminases, dehydrogenases, and, of course, amylase. I'm not sure, from the point of view of the complexity of the individual cases and the large assortment of measurements that are available, that we're inclined to rapidly saunter forth into this arena because of the difficulty of knowing what we start off with.

DOES ENDOTOXIN HAVE DIRECT OR INDIRECT EFFECTS ON THE HEART?[1]

Lerner B. Hinshaw, Ph.D.

University of Oklahoma Medical Center, Oklahoma City, Oklahoma

One of the perplexing questions about endotoxin shock is whether endotoxin acts directly or indirectly on the myocardium. In general, the role of the heart in shock is a knotty problem, since the heart is obviously susceptible to numerous influences—both direct and indirect. The contribution of the heart to the development of systemic hypotension and inadequate blood flow in the early, intermediate, and late phases of endotoxin shock needs to be clearly defined.

This manuscript summarizes recent research from our laboratory, as well as the work of others, on the role of the heart in shock. The answers to five basic questions are being sought: (a) Is the heart poisoned directly by endotoxin? (b) Is altered cardiac function an early contributing factor in irreversible endotoxin shock? (c) Do circulating adrenergic agents mask circulating myocardial depressant factors in endotoxin shock? (d) Do cardiodepressant substances circulate in the blood of animals shocked by endotoxin? (e) Does the heart ultimately fail in endotoxin shock, and, if so, what measurable parameters may be predictive of impending cardiac failure?

IS THE HEART POISONED DIRECTLY BY ENDOTOXIN?

The precise role of the heart in endotoxin shock has remained vague. Although the heart is thought to ultimately fail, its

[1]This research was supported by Veterans Administration Hospital and U.S. Navy THEMIS Project N00014-68-A-0496.

possible contribution to the genesis of the irreversible shock state is an unresolved question. Experiments on both the canine and primate species demonstrate that venous return drops dramatically very soon after endotoxin administration (20-22,53) due to intravascular pooling. Therefore, systemic hypotension is apparently precipitated largely by peripheral rather than direct cardiac mechanisms.

Weil and others (53) found no evidence for myocardial failure in the early phase of canine endotoxin shock: cardiac arrhythmias were absent, and no conduction defects were observed. Londe and others (32) found that large doses of endotoxin produced no perceptible effect on the myocardial extraction of oxygen and that the coronary vasculature was unaffected. Others have suggested that the heart is affected only indirectly by endotoxin because of unfavorable circulatory conditions (3). On the other hand, Solis and Downing (48) and Kadowitz and Yard (25) demonstrated cardiac depression early after endotoxin administration. In each instance, ventricular contractile force was diminished, and, in the studies by Solis and Downing (48), contractile force was depressed even when arterial pressure was maintained.

Studies of Cardiac Performance in Endotoxin Shock

Objectives and conditions of our experiments. To determine whether the heart contributes to the precipitation of irreversible endotoxin shock, we designed canine experiments in our laboratory in which cardiac function was assessed while hemodynamic and respiratory parameters were controlled. To better reveal possible direct toxic actions of endotoxin on the myocardium, aortic pressure, cardiac output, blood temperature, and respiratory rate and depth were kept constant for 2-3 hours after endotoxin administration. Blood was continously exchanged between an endotoxin-shocked animal and the isolated working heart-lung preparation (55).

Results. Our results failed to reveal a single instance of endotoxin toxicity on myocardial work performance or oxidative metabolism. Coronary flow increased markedly and coronary vascular resistance decreased, while myocardial oxygen uptake remained relatively unchanged during the shock period. Left ventricular contractile force and dP/dT (maximum change in ventricular pressure during isometric contractions) increased in all individual experiments after endotoxin administration, while stroke work and particularly cardiac power remained relatively constant during the 3-hour shock period. Left ventricular end-diastolic pressure (LVEDP) not only failed to increase in a single experiment after endotoxin injection, it ordinarily declined steadily. The presence of severe systemic hypotension and acidosis in the animal whose blood was exchanged with the isolated working heart failed to elicit detrimental cardiac responses.

Discussion. Our data offer no support for a direct toxic action of endotoxin on myocardial tissue. They are consistent with conclusions of some investigators (3,32,53), but not with others (29,48). Reports in the literature disagree about the precise role of the heart in hemorrhagic shock. Albert and others (2) defined primary heart failure as the initiating deleterious factor in hemorrhagic shock experiments. On the other hand, Siegel and Downing (47) reported that the heart is damaged only after prolonged hemorrhagic hypotension. Others have observed that cardiac function is only temporarily depressed in hemorrhagic shock, and that it ultimately recovers during the hypotensive state (6).

Lefer *et al.* (28-30) have identified a myocardial depressant factor (MDF) in the plasma of animals in late hemorrhagic shock. They have postulated that MDF may help initiate irreversibility in shock by depressing excitation-contraction coupling or by directly damaging the cardiac contractile machinery. Their work provides no evidence for the release of a myocardial depressant factor in the plasma of the endotoxin-poisoned animal. Conceivably, however, an inotropic adrenergic endogenous agent, released after the development of hypotension in endotoxin shock, could have masked the myocardial effects of a circulating myocardial depressant substance.

In a review published in 1960, Gilbert (15) commented that no evidence exists for a direct adverse effect of endotoxin on myocardial function. More recently, Siegel *et al.* (45) and Bell and Thal (4) have demonstrated myocardial failure in septic shock in patients, and a logical argument for a general "cardiac theory" of shock has been developed (11,12). Results from our study suggest that primary cardiac toxicity induced by endotoxin does not contribute significantly to the pathogenesis of septic shock. The data do not exclude the possibility that endotoxin may, by certain indirect effects, eventually compromise cardiac integrity.

IS ALTERED CARDIAC FUNCTION AN EARLY CONTRIBUTING FACTOR IN IRREVERSIBLE ENDOTOXIN SHOCK?

While agreement is general that the heart ultimately fails in shock, its contributory role in the development of irreversibility remains doubtful. Some have postulated that heart failure occurs only late in shock, after prolonged inadequate coronary perfusion (3). Others have developed a "cardiac theory", which assumes that irreversible shock is due to a sustained depressed output by a dysfunctioning heart, which fails as a relatively early event

(25,48). A cardiac-toxic theory has also been suggested in which a myocardial depressant factor is postulated to decrease cardiac performance (28,29,31).

Studies of Possible Direct Cardiac Damage by Endotoxin

Objectives and conditions of our experiments. We performed experiments on dogs to determine whether the heart is directly damaged by endotoxin or whether it fails as a result of hemodynamic or respiratory alterations set in motion by the shock state. In the first series of experiments, cardiac performance and metabolism were assayed in an isolated heart preparation after a 3-hour period of hypotension by requiring the heart to work at the precise preshock levels of cardiac output and aortic pressure. In the second series, the degree of hypotension and depressed cardiac output in the isolated heart preparation was mimicked by pump adjustment in the absence of endotoxin. In addition, cardiac function was evaluated at 180 minutes at the same cardiac output and aortic pressure observed at 60 minutes (23).

Results. Three hours of systemic hypotension and depressed cardiac output, followed by restoration of pressure and flow to control values by pump adjustment, revealed no statistically significant differences between the endotoxin-shocked and control animals. Myocardial contractility, cardiac power (work/second), dP/dT, O_2 uptake, and CO_2 production at 200 minutes after endotoxin administration were statistically unaltered from control pre-endotoxin values. These observations appear to preclude any significant direct toxic action of endotoxin on myocardial performance and metabolism. Although findings reveal a strong resistance of the myocardium to endotoxin, the effects of prolonged systemic hypotension may ultimately impair cardiac function. In one experiment in each of the endotoxin and control series, left ventricular end-diastolic pressure rose above control values at 200 min on restoration of aortic pressure and cardiac output.

Discussion. Our studies indicate that the hemodynamics of the endotoxin-shocked animal change markedly, apparently in an attempt to provide a high level of cardiac performance and metabolism. Coronary flow rises quickly when the heart is required to work at the preshock level, while the coronary venous oxygen content remains at a normally low value. Oxygen uptake is adequate even when the pH falls to significantly depressed values. Thus, increased blood flow (achieved by marked coronary vasodilatation coupled with an adequate oxygen extraction from capillary blood) and the ability of the heart to achieve normal oxidative metabolism in an acid medium meet essential requirements and thus permit the heart to operate at normal performance levels. Data from the study described above show that dP/dT, cardiac power, and aortic pressure are directly related to oxygen uptake of the myocardium. These results are consistent with the view that heart failure probably occurs only late in shock, after prolonged inadequate coronary perfusion (3). We obtained no evidence to support recent observations that, in hemorrhagic and endotoxin shock, a myocardial depressant factor is released which directly lowers cardiac performance (28,29,31). Our experiments failed to reveal a single instance of endotoxin toxicity on myocardial work performance or oxidative metabolism, thereby supporting the conclusions of some investigators (3,6,32,53) but disagreeing with others (4,25,45,47). The hypothesis that primary heart failure is an early event in shock (2,11-13), initiating the irreversible state, is not supported by any of our data.

The problem of the precise role of the heart in the development of irreversible endotoxin shock is complicated by events occurring in peripheral anatomic areas. These most assuredly depress cardiac output (15,21,22,42,53), on the basis of diminished venous return due to peripheral pooling of blood. In addition, the resultant prolonged systemic hypotension may set into motion a vicious circle, due to the adverse effects of diminished coronary perfusion pressure and flow on myocardial integrity. Our data suggest that careful future consideration be given to the indirect hemodynamic or respiratory effects on the myocardium, so that the role of the heart in septic shock may be elucidated (4,45).

DO ADRENERGIC AGENTS MASK MYOCARDIAL DEPRESSANT FACTORS IN ENDOTOXIN SHOCK?

A prevailing view is that the heart is one of the first organs to fail in shock (2,11,12,25). Solis and Downing (48) found that ventricular contractile force was diminished after endotoxin administration, even when arterial pressure was maintained. Lefer and others have identified a myocardial depressant factor (MDF) in the plasma of animals in hemorrhagic or endotoxin shock (28-31). They have postulated that MDF may be important in the pathogenesis of irreversibility by depressing excitation-contraction coupling or by directly impairing the cardiac machinery (31). Possibly MDF is a toxic substance gradually released by some ischemic organ. Or perhaps it represents a normally occurring metabolite which accumulates in the plasma and reaches toxic concentrations (28). On the other hand, Goodyer found that ventricular contractile capacity was enhanced in endotoxin shock as a result of increased sympathetic drive (18).

Studies of Cardiodepressant Action of Endotoxin *vs.* Myocardial Stimulation by Catecholamines

Objectives and conditions of our experiments. We performed experiments to determine whether a cardiodepressant action of endotoxin could be masked by a simultaneous myocardial-stimulating action of catecholamines released as a result of systemic hypotension. To evaluate these possibilities, adult mongrel dogs (intravenously anesthetized with sodium pentobarbital) were treated with heparin and their blood was exchanged with an isolated left ventricle. Propranolol, 0.5 mg/kg, was infused during a 15-minute period in a volume not exceeding 20 ml. Beta-adrenergic blocking activity was assayed by intracardiac injections of epinephrine or isoproterenol. Blockade was essentially complete for chronotropic, inotropic, and coronary vasodilatory responses to injected epinephrine. Blockade was evaluated periodically during the course of the experiments. At the end of the control period, an LD_{90} of *Escherichia coli* endotoxin, 1.2 mg/kg (Difco, Detroit), based on the weight of the dog providing the heart, was injected into the pulmonary arterial inflow of the isolated heart. An additional amount of endotoxin, based on body weight, was intravenously administered to the intact support animal (24).

Results. Results from this study indicate that endotoxin exerts no direct toxic effect on the myocardium. Even though all support animals were severely damaged from the effects of endotoxin (as manifested by extremely low arterial pressures and deaths occurring within 3 hours), isolated hearts performed normally, as shown by values of cardiac work and power, dP/dT, left ventricular end-diastolic pressure, and oxygen uptake.

Discussion. Goodyer (18) pointed out that ventricular contractility was enhanced in hemorrhagic and endotoxin shock due to increased sympathetic drive. Lefer and others, on the other hand, demonstrated the release of a cardiodepressant blood-borne factor in hemorrhagic and endotoxin shock (28-31). It seemed conceivable to us that both the excitatory and depressant influences could operate in endotoxin shock, each tending to cancel the effects of the other. One would expect the elimination of sympathetic influences on the heart by beta-adrenergic blockade (as done in the present study) to unmask a depressor effect. However, our results provide no evidence for the presence of a circulating cardiodepressant factor in the blood of animals dying in irreversible shock. Cardiac performance appeared to be well maintained, at least partly by increased coronary blood flow and decreased pH, which should increase oxygen delivery to myocardial tissue (19). The increase in coronary blood flow could not have been due to catecholamine release since this action was clearly blocked by propranolol.

Results from this study agree with the data of Weil and others (53), who found no electrocardiographic evidence for myocardial failure after endotoxin produced no perceptible effect on myocardial extraction of oxygen. They also agree with the report of Kutner and Cohen (27) that lethal doses of endotoxin did not affect myocardial contractility. Moreover, they are consistent with the findings of Alican *et al.* (3), who noted a resistance of the myocardium to endotoxin when arterial pressure was maintained.

Our findings do not disallow the adverse effects of prolonged systemic hypotension and progressive peripheral pooling on cardiac performance, which most assuredly occur. The data clearly suggest, however, that myocardial performance is not compromised by direct or secondary toxic effects of endotoxin or myocardial depressant substances circulating in the blood of irreversibly shocked animals.

DO CARDIODEPRESSANT SUBSTANCES CIRCULATE IN THE BLOOD AFTER ENDOTOXIN ADMINISTRATION?

Evidence for the presence of a circulating toxin or depressant substance has been previously described by Cannon (7), Shorr and colleagues (43,44), and more recently by others (29,31,37,50,52)—including Lefer, with the introduction of the "myocardial depressant factor" (29,31,50,52). The significance of such substances cannot be overestimated, particularly in regard to their possible adverse effects on myocardial performance in shock. Research from this laboratory and elsewhere (18,32) has strongly suggested that the myocardium performs normally in the early phase of endotoxin shock (from zero to 3 1/2 hours). However, no information is presently available to explain the mechanism of depressed cardiac output in the intermediate stage of shock.

Studies of the Possible Existence of a Circulating Myocardial Depressant Substance in Endotoxin Shock

Objectives and conditions of our experiments. We performed a study in our laboratory to extend the period of observation after endotoxin administration from 6 to 9 hours and to explore the possible existence of a circulating factor deleterious to myocardial performance. A donor heart from an animal not receiving endotoxin served as the test organ to receive blood from a previously shocked support dog. Experiments were designed to assay the myocardial effects of factors in the blood during the intermediate or terminal stages of shock. The dose of endotoxin was adjusted so that approximately 40% of all animals had died at the time of the heart donor transfer (5-6 hours). It seemed reasonable that this arrangement of both time and degree of lethality should be adequate in order to reveal the net effects of possible detrimental and/or beneficial blood-borne agents on myocardial performance (56).

Results. Experiments during the period 6-9 hours after endotoxin administration revealed no detrimental cardiac actions in the test organ. These included studies in which two endotoxin-treated support animals died during the assays of myocardial performance, metabolism, and hemodynamics. Changes in mean aortic pressure through the range of 75-150 mm Hg demonstrated that the responses of hearts receiving blood from animals in shock or from controls were, in general, indistinguishable. All individual hearts in both groups demonstrated notable increases in dP/dT, left ventricular systolic pressure, coronary blood flow, stroke work, power, oxygen uptake, and carbon dioxide production as functions of elevated afterload. In contrast, left ventricular end-diastolic pressure changed little during the initial increase in afterload, but it decreased within 30-60 seconds to a steady-state value little changed from the previous coronary pressure (homeometric autoregulation). Mean changes in dP/dT, stroke work, power (work/second), left ventricular end-diastolic pressure, O_2 uptake, CO_2 production, coronary blood flow, and coronary vascular resistance were similar or nearly identical in both groups. The differences between controls and experimental groups were statistically significant only at 150 and 100 mm Hg ($P < 0.05$); in the case of oxygen uptake, this was true only at 100 mm Hg ($P = 0.01$). Hearts receiving blood from endotoxin-injected animals appeared to have slightly higher rates of contraction with somewhat greater oxygen assimilation. Also, mean left ventricular end-diastolic pressures were slightly lower at all points in the endotoxin group, although the differences were statistically insignificant. These latter trends are consistent with the probability that the heart is driven by humoral adrenergic influences of a beneficial nature in the intermediate stage of shock, as suggested by Goodyer (18).

Discussion. Our findings offer no evidence of a circulating toxic or depressant substance damaging to the myocardium, as described or suggested by others (29,31,50,52). A number of years has passed since the classic descriptions of Cannon (7), Shorr, and others (43,44) of circulating toxic or vasodepressant factors, although Cannon (7) believed that the heart escaped injury from such substances even in the terminal stage of shock. Other findings strongly suggest that the myocardium is resistant to endotoxin (22,32,38,53) and is affected adversely only as a terminal event (26). Clearly, however, the present experiments examine only the *net* effects of "shocked blood" on the heart. Indeed, both stimulatory and depressant influences may impinge upon the myocardium simultaneously, each cancelling the other out.

The possible presence of circulating myocardial depressant agents is of utmost concern in the study of the pathogenesis of septic shock. The present study and an earlier report from this laboratory suggest that the endotoxin moiety itself possesses no direct myocardial toxic characteristics, and that if deleterious agents do circulate in the blood of an endotoxin-treated animal, they do not depress myocardial function, even in terminal shock. Myocardial damage or depression has been reported in animal experiments after endotoxin administration (29,48) and after hemorrhage (46,47,52), as well as in clinical septic shock (4,45). Observations from certain patient populations also suggest that left ventricular decompensation occurs in the later stages of septic shock (35). A possible explanation for the apparent differences between these previous reports and our study is that a constellation of factors may act to destroy cardiac integrity: (a) the combined cardiac effects of a hemodynamic insult depressing myocardial blood flow (1,3,40); (b) a neural dysfunction resulting from cerebral hypoxia (5); (c) interference with cellular metabolism due to a primary toxic defect (54) or coronary vascular obstruction (8); and (d) the circulation of abnormal products of metabolism (46-48,50).

DOES THE HEART ULTIMATELY FAIL IN ENDOTOXIN SHOCK?

The gravity of bacteremic shock has been emphasized in a recent report which estimates that 70,000 deaths each year result from bacteremia due to gram-negative organisms (34). Recent publications in the clinical literature (4,35,45) and results from experimental studies (8,29,48) have implicated heart failure or myocardial depression in septic or endotoxin shock. Some have suggested that the myocardium fails only terminally, while others point out that depression of cardiac function may occur during the intermediate stages of shock. Several investigators have provided data to suggest that the heart is relatively resistant to endotoxin or its released products during the early or intermediate stages of shock (3,18,23,24,32,38,53). The heart has also been reported to be relatively resistant to the effects of hemorrhage by some investigators (2,9,18,26,39) but susceptible to damage by others (2,11,29,47). A complication in determining whether the heart fails as a pump, or whether cardiac output falls because of peripheral pooling, is that venous return is reported to decrease in various animal species during early shock due to trapping of blood in peripheral tissues (22,53). At present, no experimental data are available which evaluate the relative contributions of peripheral and cardiac factors in the intermediate stage of shock and thus explain the decrease in cardiac output.

Evaluation of Myocardial Function in Late Shock

Objectives and conditions of our experiments. One of the most difficult problems in studying the pathogenesis of experimental septic shock is the evaluation of myocardial function during later phases of shock, when arterial pressure and cardiac output have been altered for extended periods. Therefore, we designed a study in which a canine model would be challenged with a dose of endotoxin large enough to seriously insult the animal but small enough to permit survival of at least half of the animals 5 hours after endotoxin administration. The hearts of the surviving animals were tested for performance characteristics during the period 6-9 hours after endotoxin administration (57).

Results. In contrast to previous studies carried out in this laboratory which demonstrated normal cardiac function up to 3 hours after endotoxin administration (23,24), the present work clearly demonstrated the ready susceptibility of the heart to failure when the duration of shock was extended to 6-9 hours. Heart failure, indicated by elevated left ventricular end-diastolic pressure (LVEDP) and relatively depressed dP/dT values, particularly at elevated afterloads, was observed in six of eight experiments. The failure was generally profound and irreversible. Epinephrine intervention was necessary in some instances to reverse elevated LVEDPs which had risen above 20 mm Hg, but cessation of infusion led to abrupt failure. The serious failure observed in most of the hearts was considered to be remarkable since, during the period of isolation and perfusion, mean coronary perfusion pressure and cardiac output of each heart were in the normal range and blood was continually exchanged with a large, control, nonshocked animal. One would expect these factors to have the net effect of assisting myocardial function. In nearly all instances, however, heart failure was profoundly irreversible, even after an extended period of perfusion and epinephrine infusion.

Discussion. An observation in the failing heart has been that the combined effects of increased mean aortic pressure (afterload) and LVEDP should increase myocardial contractility (36,51). Yet, our dP/dT values, on the average, increased less than expected in comparison to the control, nonshocked, heart preparations. Assuming that the inotropic state of the failing heart is constant, as mean aortic pressure (afterload) is increased, the preload (LVEDP) also rises. The resultant effect should be a rise in dP/dT greater than seen in the control hearts. Data from the present study are therefore consistent with the view that dP/dT decreases in the failing heart.

Our finding that oxygen uptake by the failing heart is no different from that of control hearts seems puzzling; however, studies of myocardial energy utilization in heart failure have yielded conflicting results. Oxygen consumption has been found to be unchanged from normal or slightly elevated (49). Since the failing hearts in our study apparently declined in contractility (as evidenced by a depressed dP/dT), one would think that oxygen uptake might fall. That such was not the case may be explained by the interaction of opposing factors: an increase in LVEDP suggests an augmentation of myocardial wall tension which should increase oxygen consumption, while the decrease in contractility should diminish oxygen uptake. The resulting assimilation of oxygen by myocardial tissue may therefore increase, decrease, or remain unchanged (10).

Another difficult finding to comprehend was that neither arterial pressure, heart rate, pH, nor hematocrit were observed to be predictive factors in assaying cardiac function of the dog prior to heart removal. Results from these studies suggest that procedures for evaluating left ventricular myocardial integrity in the septic shock patient should include measurement of LVEDP with altered afterloads.

Clearly, the factors which produce myocardial damage are extremely potent when enough time is permitted for their effects, although these factors remain unidentified at present. Adverse circulatory conditions may play a role, as suggested by reports of others (1,3,39,41,46,47). Defects in the autonomic regulation of the heart may intervene either as a result of sympathetic-vagal imbalance (8,16), a damaged central nervous system (5,14,17), or altered adrenergic circulating influences (16,18,33). Coronary vascular obstruction may occur, with coagulation products lodged in capillaries (8), both oxygen and pH may decrease (14), toxic or depressant substances may circulate in the blood (29,31,33,37, 43,44,50,52), or a primary cellular defect (25) may be unleashed to irreversibly damage the myocardium.

SUMMARY

Results from the previous five heart studies conducted in our laboratory suggest the following: Endotoxin exerts no direct cardiotoxic effect. No evidence exists for a circulating myocardial toxic factor. The heart is highly resistant to endotoxin and to defects in the hemodynamic and respiratory systems for up to 3 1/2 hours. After 4-6 hours, however, the heart ultimately fails. Cardiac failure cannot be uniformly predicted by prior changes of systemic blood pressure or pH after endotoxin administration. Moreover, it is severe and only temporarily reversible by adrenergic agents. The cause of the failure is unknown. The degree of failure is readily assayed by increasing afterload (mean arterial pressure) through a wide range (75-150 mm Hg) and monitoring changes in left ventricular end-diastolic pressure and myocardial contractility. The normal heart shows no signs of failure when perfused by blood from shocked or dying animals regardless of the time after endotoxin administration (6-18 hours).

These findings suggest that myocardial performance should be carefully assayed in patients in septic shock. Myocardial performance parameters should be carefully monitored after the mean systemic pressure has been elevated by therapeutic or test procedures. Some sort of myocardial performance curves are essential for the proper diagnosis of heart failure.

REFERENCES

1. Abel, R.M., and R.L. Reis. Effects of coronary blood flow and perfusion pressure on left ventricular contractility in dogs. Circ. Res. 27:961-971, 1970.

2. Albert, H.M., B.A. Glass, and R.L. Carter. The role of the heart in shock: Exsanguination studies. Ann. Surg. 34:48-52, 1968.

3. Alican, F., M.L. Dalton, and J.D. Hardy. Experimental endotoxin shock. Circulatory changes with emphasis upon cardiac function. Am. J. Surg. 103:702-708, 1962.

4. Bell, H., and A. Thal. The peculiar hemodynamics of septic shock. Postgrad. Med. 48:106-114, 1970.

5. Brown, R.S., P.A. Mohr, and W.C. Shoemaker. Effect of cerebral hypotension on the neural regulation of the cardiovascular system. Surg. Gynecol. Obstet. 131:436-440, 1970.

6. Bugg-Asperheim, B., and J. Kjekshus. Left ventricular pressure and maximum rate of pressure rise as determinants of myocardial oxygen consumption during hemorrhagic hypotension in dogs. Acta physiol. scand. 78:174-183, 1970.

7. Cannon, W.B. *Traumatic Shock*. New York: D. Appleton & Co., 1923, Chapter IV.

8. Cavanagh, D., R.S. Rau, D.M.C. Sutton, B.D. Bhagat, and F. Bachman. Pathophysiology of endotoxin shock in the primate. Am. J. Obstet. Gynecol. 108:705-722, 1970.

9. Chimoskey, J.E., and D.F. Bohr. Effects of hemorrhagic shock on contractility of papillary muscle. Proc. Soc. Exptl. Biol.

Med. 120:4-6, 1965.

10. Covell, J.W., E. Braunwald, and J. Ross, Jr. Studies on digitalis. XVI. Effects on myocardial oxygen consumption. J. Clin. Invest. 45:1535-1542, 1966.

11. Crowell, J.W., and A.C. Guyton. Evidence favoring a cardiac mechanism in hemorrhagic shock. Am. J. Physiol. 201:893-896, 1961.

12. Crowell, J.W., and A.C. Guyton. Further evidence favoring a cardiac mechanism in irreversible hemorrhagic shock. Am. J. Physiol. 203:248-252, 1962.

13. Crowell, J. Oxygen transport in the hypotensive state. Fed. Proc. 29:1848-1853, 1970.

14. Downing, S.E., N.S. Tolner, and T.H. Gardner. Influences of hypoxemia and acidemia on left ventricular function. Am. J. Physiol. 210:1327-1334, 1966.

15. Gilbert, R.P. Mechanisms of the hemodynamic effects of endotoxin. Physiol. Rev. 40:245-278, 1960.

16. Glaviano, V.V., and M.A. Klouda. Myocardial catecholamines and stimulation of the stellate ganglion in hemorrhagic shock. Am. J. Physiol. 209:751-756, 1965.

17. Golden, P.F., and J.A. Jane. Survival following profound hypovolemia: Role of heart, lung, and brain. J. Trauma 9:784-798, 1969.

18. Goodyer, A.V.N. Left ventricular function and tissue hypoxia in irreversible hemorrhagic and endotoxin shock. Am. J. Physiol. 212:444-450, 1967.

19. Haddy, F.J. Physiology and pharmacology of the coronary circulation and myocardium, particularly in relation to coronary artery disease. Am. J. Med. 47:274-286, 1969.

20. Hinshaw, L.B., R.P. Gilbert, H. Kuida, and M.B. Visscher. Peripheral resistance changes and blood pooling after endotoxin in eviscerated dogs. Am. J. Physiol. 195:631-634, 1958.

21. Hinshaw, L.B., T.E. Emerson, Jr., and D.A. Reins. Cardiovascular responses of the primate in endotoxin shock. Am. J. Physiol. 210:335-340, 1966.

22. Hinshaw, L.B., L.L. Shanbour, L.J. Greenfield, and J.J.

Coalson. Mechanism of decreased venous return in subhuman primate administered endotoxin. Arch. Surg. 100:600-606, 1970.

23. Hinshaw, L.B., L.T. Archer, L.J. Greenfield, and C.A. Guenter. Effects of endotoxin on myocardial hemodynamics, performance and metabolism. Am. J. Physiol. 221:504-510, 1971.

24. Hinshaw, L.B., L.J. Greenfield, L.T. Archer, and C.A. Guenter. Effects of endotoxin on myocardial hemodynamics, performance and metabolism during beta-adrenergic blockade. Proc. Soc. Exptl. Biol. Med. 137:1217-1224, 1971.

25. Kadowitz, P.J., and A.C. Yard. Circulatory effects of hydrocortisone and protection against endotoxin shock in cats. Eur. J. Pharmacol. 9:311-318, 1970.

26. Kim, S.I., and W.C. Shoemaker. Comparison of cardiorespiratory changes in surviving and non-surviving shock dogs. Arch. Surg. 100:275-279, 1970.

27. Kutner, F.R., and J.J. Cohen. Effect of endotoxin on isolated cat papillary muscle. J. Surg. Res. 6:83-86, 1966.

28. Lefer, A.M., R. Cowgill, F.F. Marshall, L.M. Hall, and E.D. Brand. Characterization of a myocardial depressant factor present in hemorrhagic shock. Am. J. Physiol. 213:492-498, 1967.

29. Lefer, A.M. Role of a myocardial depressant factor in the pathogenesis of circulatory shock. Fed. Proc. 29:1836-1847, 1970.

30. Lefer, A.M., and J. Martin. Relationship of plasma peptides to the myocardial depressant factor in hemorrhagic shock in cats. Circ. Res. 26:59-69, 1970.

31. Lefer, A.M., and M.J. Rovetto. Influence of a myocardial depressant factor on physiologic properties of cardiac muscle. Proc. Soc. Exptl. Biol. Med. 134:269-273, 1970.

32. Londe, S.P., H. Massie, W.W. Monafo, Jr., and H.R. Bernard. Resistance of the isolated canine heart to endotoxin. Surgery 61:466-470, 1967.

33. Lundsgaard-Hansen, P., C. Meyer, H. Riedwyl, and G. Zierrot. Cardiac metabolism in experimental hemorrhagic shock. Minn. Med. 52:23-28, 1962.

34. McCabe, W.R. Endotoxin and bacteremia due to gram-negative organisms. New Eng. J. Med. 283:1342-1343, 1970.

35. MacLean, L.D., W.G. Mulligan, A.P.H. McLean, and J.H. Duff. Patterns of septic shock in man: A detailed study of 56 patients. Ann. Surg. 166:543-562, 1967.

36. Mason, D.T. Usefulness and limitations of the rate of rise of intraventricular pressure (dP/dT) in the evaluation of myocardial contractility in man. Am. J. Cardiol. 23:516-527, 1969.

37. Moyo, C.T.B., J.B. Dossetor, and L.D. MacLean. Hemodialysis in the treatment of shock. J. Surg. Res. 4:380-384, 1964.

38. Priano, L.L., R.D. Wilson, and D.L. Traber. Cardiorespiratory alterations in unanesthetized dogs due to gram-negative bacterial endotoxin. Am. J. Physiol. 220:705-711, 1971.

39. Rothe, C.F., and E.E. Selkurt. Cardiac and peripheral failure in hemorrhagic shock in the dog. Am. J. Physiol. 207:203-214, 1964.

40. Sarnoff, S.J., R.B. Case, and P.E. Waithe. Insufficient coronary flow and myocardial failure as a complicating factor in late hemorrhagic shock. Am. J. Physiol. 176:439-444, 1954.

41. Sarnoff, S.J., E. Braunwald, G.H. Welch, Jr., R.B. Case, W.N. Stainsby, and R. Macruz. Hemodynamic determinants of oxygen consumption of the heart with special reference to the tension-time index. Am. J. Physiol. 192:148-156, 1958.

42. Selkurt, E.E. Status of investigative aspects of hemorrhagic shock. Fed. Proc. 29:1832-1835, 1970.

43. Shorr, E., B.W. Zweifach, and R.F. Furchgott. On the occurrence, sites and modes of origin and destruction, of principles affecting the compensatory vascular mechanism in experimental shock. Science 102:489-498, 1945.

44. Shorr, E., B.W. Zweifach, R.F. Furchgott, and S. Baez. Hepatorenal factors in circulatory hemeostasis. Circulation 3: 42-79, 1951.

45. Siegel, J.H., M. Greenspan, and L.R. Del Guercio. Abnormal vascular tone, defective oxygen transport and myocardial failure in human septic shock. Ann. Surg. 165:504-517, 1967.

46. Siegal, H.W., and S.E. Downing. Contributions of coronary

perfusion pressure, metabolic acidosis and adrenergic factors to the reduction of myocardial contractility during hemorrhagic shock in the cat. Circ. Res. 27:875-889, 1970.

47. Siegel, H.W., and S.E. Downing. Reduction of left ventricular contractility during acute hemorrhagic shock. Am. J. Physiol. 218:772-779, 1970.

48. Solis, R.T., and S.E. Downing. Effects of *E. coli* endotoxemia on ventricular performance. Am. J. Physiol. 211:307-313, 1966.

49. Sonnenblick, E.H., J. Ross, Jr., and E. Braunwald. Oxygen consumption of the heart: Newer concepts of its multifactoral determination. Am. J. Cardiol. 22:328-336, 1968.

50. Thalinger, A.R., and A.M. Lefer. Mechanism of the cardiac action of a myocardial depressant factor in shock. Proc. Soc. Exptl. Biol. Med. 136:354-358, 1971.

51. Wallace, A.G., N.S. Skinner, Jr., and J.H. Mitchell. Hemodynamic determinants of the maximal rate of rise of left ventricular pressure. Am. J. Physiol. 205:30-36, 1963.

52. Wangensteen, S.L., J.D. De Holl, S.F. Kiechel, J. Martin, and A.M. Lefer. Influence of hemodialysis on a myocardial depressant factor in hemorrhagic shock. Surgery 67:935-943, 1970.

53. Weil, M.H., L.D. MacLean, M.B. Visscher, and W.W. Spink. Studies on the circulatory changes in the dog produced by endotoxin from gram-negative microorganisms. J. Clin. Invest. 35: 1191-1198, 1956.

54. Wright, C.J., J.H. Duff, A.P.H. McLean, and L.D. MacLean. Regional capillary blood flow and oxygen uptake in severe sepsis. Surg. Gynecol. Obstet. 132:637-644, 1971.

55. Hinshaw, L.B., L.T. Archer, L.J. Greenfield, C.A. Guenter, and J.A. Miller. Effect of endotoxin on myocardial performance. J. Trauma, in press.

56. Hinshaw, L.B., L.J. Greenfield, S.E. Owen, L.T. Archer, and C.A. Guenter. Cardiac response to circulating factors in endotoxin shock. Am. J. Physiol., in press.

57. Hinshaw, L.B., L.J. Greenfield, S.E. Owen, M.R. Black, and C.A. Guenter. Precipitation of cardiac failure in endotoxin shock. Surg. Gynecol. Obstet., in press.

PULMONARY DYSFUNCTION AFTER SHOCK AND TRAUMA[1]

Brian D. Lowery, M.D., and Joseph H. Sugg, M.D.

Department of Physiology, McGill University, Montreal, Quebec; Departments of Surgery, The Johns Hopkins University, Baltimore, Maryland, and the University of Alabama, Birmingham, Alabama

In terms of patient survival, the immediate period of "shock," or low perfusion, from whatever cause, is not our real problem. We get patients through this phase quite well, although undoubtedly the stage is set for the progressive, multisystem organ dysfunction which becomes our therapeutic challenge. Survival is determined by the severity of vital organ damage during and immediately after the shock episode. This is true for the respiratory system as for the other vital organ systems. Such damage can obviously be ameliorated or worsened by therapeutic interventions.

Our real challenge, it seems, is to discover the nature of the first pathologic change, then to understand the progression of the pathophysiology until overt system failure is manifest. Only in this way is therapy likely to become rational and successful. Moreover, we must approach our investigations with a firm understanding of the basic system physiology. If not, we are likely to either err in our designs and waste time or repeat previous work, both good and bad.

In this presentation, we will discuss some basic defects in pulmonary function. We will use experimental work from our own laboratory as a springboard and discuss those areas of basic physiology which are pertinent to an understanding of the failure of the respiratory system.

---

[1]This work was supported by NIH Grants 5-TOIOGM-01541-04 and GMO-1924-04 and MRC of Canada Grant MA-3020.

BACKGROUND

Our interest in pulmonary dysfunction after severe hemorrhage and trauma was a direct result of caring for severely wounded young men in Vietnam. With our colleagues, Drs. Carey and Cloutier, we found (18), as did others (5,9), that most such patients developed systemic arterial hypoxemia associated with no central failure of respiratory drive. Some men also developed severe hypoxemia which was progressively refractory to increased O_2 concentrations in the inspired air. This is good evidence for an increasing fraction of cardiac output traversing the lungs without coming into contact with ventilated alveoli. We then turned to animal studies for a model which would predictably produce a functional respiratory failure similar to that seen in our patients.

Selection of Animal

We had specific reasons for choosing swine as an experimental animal. Swine lungs have a quite septate parenchymal architecture with heavy septae completely bounding the lobules. As shown by the classic work of Van Allen *et al.* (39), this anatomical arrangement permits little or no collateral respiration between adjacent pulmonary lobules. Several experiments from the respiratory group at McGill University, Montreal, are also pertinent. Brown and coworkers (6) demonstrated greater changes in certain measurements of lung mechanics in porcine lungs with artificially obstructed small airways than in canine lungs similarly obstructed. Hogg *et al.* (16), studying normal excised human lungs, found that the resistance to collateral air flow was much greater than the resistance through airways. The converse was true in emphysematous lungs in which the resistance to air flow through collateral channels was actually less than resistance through airways. The greater the degree of collateral respiration, the more likely that the gas-exchanging function of the lung will be preserved if airway obstruction occurs, particularly within a lobe. Dr. Macklem suggested to us that if the distribution of ventilation and the effects of airway closure were important in the pathogenesis of the pulmonary failure syndrome seen after shock and trauma, the pig might well be more like man and hence a more suitable animal to study than the dog.

Animal Groups and Experiments

Several aspects of pulmonary function were studied in the pig during conditions of severe hemorrhage, both with and without the return of shed blood. In brief, three groups were studied. Group I: control animals were prepared and studied exactly like their experimental counterparts but were not bled. Group II: after control measurements had been taken, pigs were bled approximately 50% of their calculated blood volume and then allowed to maintain pressure equilibrium between their arterial system and their shed blood in a reservoir positioned at a level equivalent to 35-40 mm Hg, relative to the midatrial position. These animals could thus shed or take up blood as their systemic blood pressure rose or fell; they stayed in this state for the duration of study. Group III: bled and reinfused animals were bled in the same manner as those in Group II, but transvenous return of the shed blood was performed 150-210 minutes after the onset of bleeding.

METHODS

Our methodology has been described in detail elsewhere (19,20, 30-33). Briefly, control animals were prepared just like their experimental counterparts. Male pigs, weighing 15-34 kg, were tranquilized, anesthetized, orotracheally intubated, and allowed to breathe spontaneously during all experiments. Their lungs were hyperinflated every 15-20 minutes. Monitoring catheters were placed in the thoracic aorta via a femoral artery and in the pulmonary artery and right atrium through an external jugular vein. A Teflon cannula was placed in the right common carotid artery for bleeding. This device had a side-port allowing for anticoagulant infusion (NIH formula A, acid-citrate-dextrose) simultaneously with the shedding of blood in animals which were bled. No systemic anticoagulant was given. Shed blood was collected through silicone rubber tubing into air-free polyvinyl chloride reservoirs, kept at room temperature and handled sparingly. Vascular pressures were measured through appropriate transducers with polygraphic recording. Blood and expired gas tensions were measured with standard electrodes. Platelet aggregation was assessed by the screen filtration pressure method of Swank (35). Other special techniques will be mentioned in the appropriate sections.

RESULTS

Development of Hypoxemia

In the first group of studies, 21 animals were randomly assigned to Group I, II, or III, after they were prepared as described. Figure 1 demonstrates the low systemic blood pressures attending hemorrhage in Groups II and III, with the subsequent return to control values in the Group III animals who were reinfused. The hemorrhage also resulted in great increases in minute ventilation (V_E) (Fig. 2) in the two bled groups with return to, but not

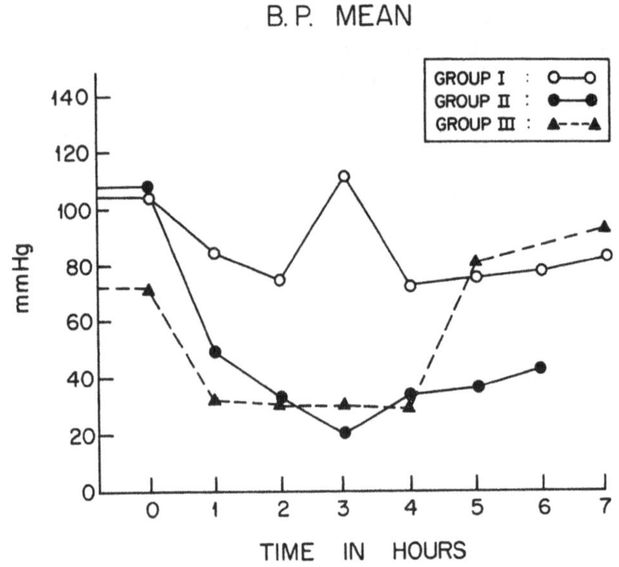

FIG. 1. Systemic mean blood pressure (mean ± 2SE). The control animals (Group I) are stable, while the two bled groups are profoundly hypotensive. Values in the Group III animals slightly exceed their control value after reinfusion.

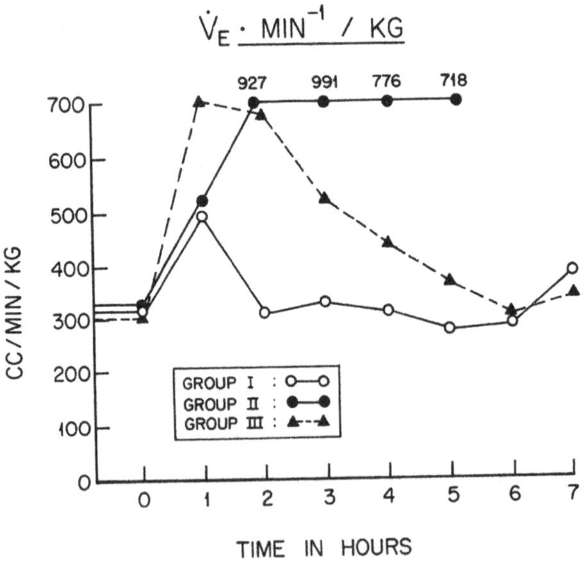

FIG. 2. Minute ventilation increases strikingly with severe blood loss and then returns to control values in Group III animals after return of shed blood ($\bar{X}$ ± 2SE).

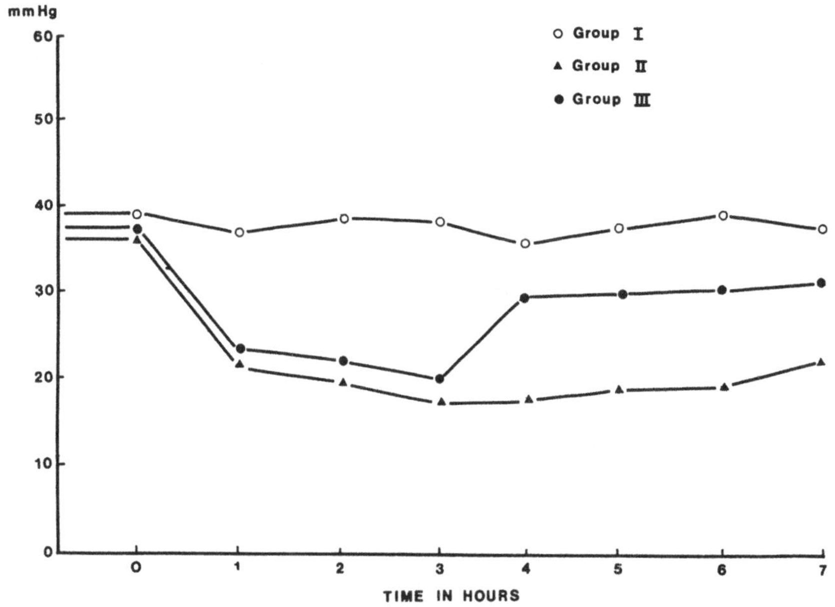

FIG. 3. Effects of hemorrhagic shock in the pig. Changes in arterial CO_2 tension (Pa_{CO_2}) follow the changes in ventilation in all groups ($\bar{X} \pm 2SE$).

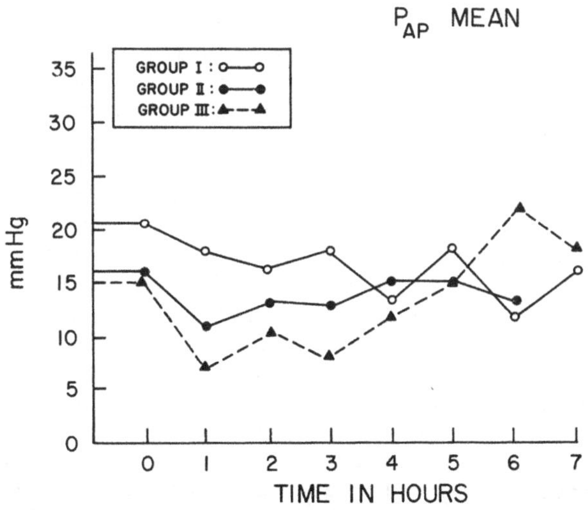

FIG. 4. Note that after reaching its low value, pulmonary artery mean pressure continues to rise in Group II over the day. Group III values rise slowly before reinfusion and then overshoot the control value after reinfusion ($\bar{X} \pm 2SE$).

below, control levels in Group III after retransfusion. The systemic arterial CO_2 tension (Fig. 3) varied, as could be predicted from the changes in ventilation. The pulmonary artery pressure (Fig. 4) fell in both Groups II and III, but began to creep back upward before reinfusion in Group III and continued to rise slowly in Group II. Finally, the systemic arterial O_2 tension remained quite stable in control animals but increased, as did the ventilation, in Groups II and III. However, in Group III animals, although ventilation was not below control levels, the arterial pO_2 fell significantly at the end of the day.

Platelet Studies

In the above groups, screen filtration pressures (SFP), using nickel screens with lines of 20 x 20 micron pores, 400 lines per inch, were measured *in vitro* on blood drawn simultaneously from the pulmonary artery and aorta. This test is a reliable measure of the *in vivo* formation of aggregates in the circulating blood, as shown by Swank (35). These measurements failed to change in control animals, but a very early rise was associated with hemorrhage (Fig. 5). The value from pulmonary arterial blood was always higher than that from blood from the thoracic aorta. This means that the platelet and/or leukocyte aggregates which promptly formed after the severe blood loss were either broken up by passage from the pulmonary artery to the aorta or lodged in the microcirculation of the lung.

We are quite aware of the normal regional differences in the distribution of perfusion ($\dot{Q}$) and ventilation ($\dot{V}$), which have been studied so extensively in intact dog and man as well as in excised lung preparations. Work in this area is well summarized by West (41). We have no reason to doubt that similar topographical gradients of ventilation and perfusion exist in the pig, with distribution of perfusion, particularly, being gravity-related. Because perfusion is normally greater in the gravity-dependent areas of lung, no matter what the body position of the animal or man, the "dose" of platelet aggregates delivered into and occluding the pulmonary microcirculation would necessarily be greater in the dependent lung. When pulmonary arterial pressure falls with severe blood loss, an even greater proportion of the right-sided heart output is directed to the dependent lung, while more of the "upper lung" (*i.e.*, the less dependent lung) fails to be perfused. During a period of hypodynamic circulatory function, the regional "dose" of any toxic material, particulate or humoral, will therefore be even more preferentially distributed to the dependent areas than during normodynamic function. Of course, if perfusion were evenly distributed throughout the lung, the factors in returning venous blood would necessarily be evenly distributed throughout the lungs.

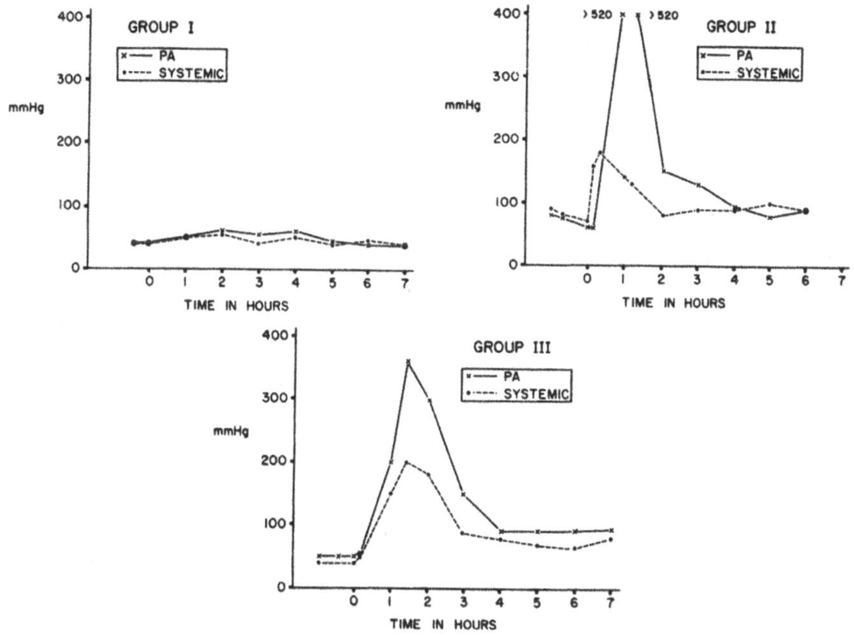

FIG. 5. Screen filtration pressures (SFP) from one representative animal from each group. Note that controls show no elevation and that the pulmonary artery blood SFP is always higher than that from the aorta. The rise in SFP is seen immediately after the severe blood loss.

Pathology

Our initial impressions of the altered morphology of these lungs have been described (19). We initially found Group I and II animals to be unaltered, both grossly and microscopically, with Group III animals showing moderate-to-severe congestion of focal small vessels, with interstitial and alveolar edema and hemorrhage, which was most marked in the dependent portions. A notable feature was the presence of polymorphonuclear leukocytes in the pulmonary capillary walls. As we studied more and more animals, however, we began encountering the same sorts of changes in Group II animals. It was, in fact, largely impossible to separate Groups II and III on the basis of microscopic appearance. The gross appearance of the lung always showed dependent congested consolidation and loss of crepitance. Control animals had similar but less severe damage.

Mechanical Properties of Lungs

A pump and valve system was devised whereby *in vivo* pressure-

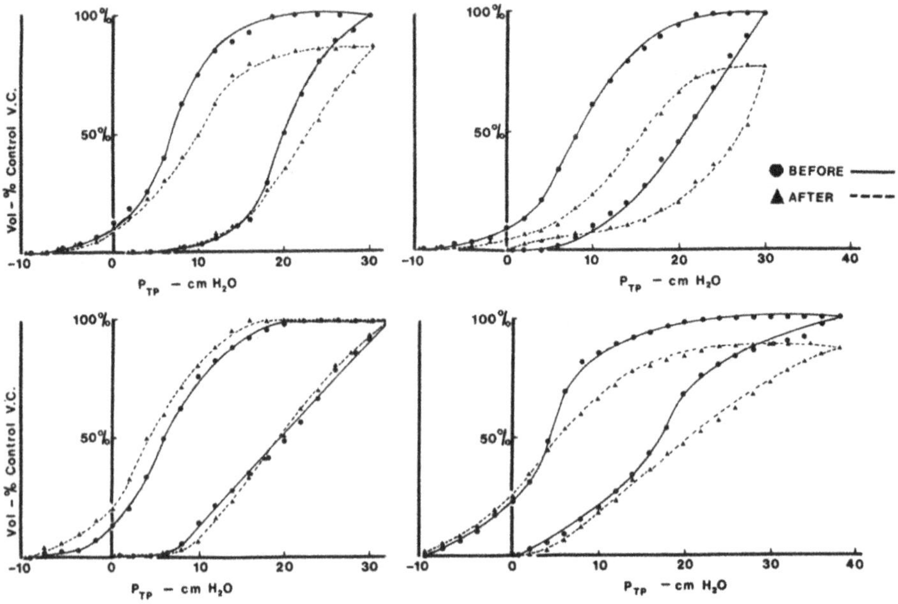

FIG. 6. *In vivo* pulmonary pressure-volume relationships during control period (solid line) and after bleeding (dashed line). Transpulmonary pressure, P_{TP}. (See discussion in text).

volume curves could be obtained sequentially. This work is described in detail elsewhere (31). In essence, whenever measurements of the pulmonary pressure-volume relationship were desired, the animal was temporarily paralyzed with succinylcholine. Room air was then slowly cycled in and out of the lungs, with the resultant transpulmonary pressure plotted directly against volume change on an X-Y recorder. Each curve required approximately 90 seconds, after which the animal was ventilated with a piston-driven respirator until spontaneous respiratory activity resumed. Residual volume of the lungs was measured by the helium-dilution technique and did not change significantly. In order to express changes which occurred in the pressure-volume relationship in time, all curves after control were replotted. The volume axis was expressed as a percentage of the volume (vital capacity) of the inflation and deflation limbs, respectively, obtained during the control period. The results from four bled animals shown in Figure 6 are representative of data obtained from 12 animals. After the severe blood loss, before the shed blood was returned, the pressure-volume curve shifted significantly down and to the right in 10 of 12 animals, with higher opening pressures frequently being demonstrated. These points are seen in three of the four animals whose results are shown in Figure 6. These curves resemble those obtained in the post-reinfusion period. Control animals showed no such shifts.

Distribution of Ventilation ($\dot{V}$) and Perfusion ($\dot{Q}$) Studied with Xenon-133

Animals were prepared as for all other studies. Four experimental (bled and reinfused) and two control animals had studies completed under this protocol. These are reported in more detail elsewhere (21), as are the methodologic details and calculations. In essence, these supine animals had sequential determinations of regional ventilation and perfusion over six regions of the left lung measured and compared to their control measurements. Figures 7 and 8 show the upper (least dependent) and lower (most dependent) areas from only one typical bled animal. We were not particularly surprised to see the decreased perfusion in the lower zone immediately after the hemorrhage, since we had previously postulated occlusion of the microcirculation in the dependent lung from formed cell aggregates, principally platelets. We were quite surprised to see the prompt diminution of ventilation to the lower lung, which persisted after the returned, shed blood had restored perfusion to control levels. Since these data were obtained from regions of finite volume, there may well have been focal areas within the counted region of zero ventilation which, with continued perfusion, would result in pure venoarterial shunts. Even areas with low ventilation-perfusion ratios will have increased alveolar-arterial O_2 differences and significant hypoxemia during room-air-breathing.

DISCUSSION

To begin to unravel this very complex problem, one must consider the principal functional defect together with the principal anatomic abnormality. Functionally, the respiratory failure syndrome we are discussing in man and animals is marked by an increasing venoarterial admixture, *i.e.*, "shunting" through the lungs. In the early stages, this may be due to low $\dot{V}/\dot{Q}$ ratios or a spread in the distribution of $\dot{V}/\dot{Q}$ ratios (42), in which there is a good response to pure O_2-breathing. In the later stages, this is manifest as ever-increasing $\dot{V}/\dot{Q}$ ratios of zero, *i.e.*, no ventilation but continued perfusion, or, pure right-to-left shunts. To adequately explain these findings we must delve much deeper into the fundamental changes in pulmonary function.

The most common anatomic abnormality is edema, first localized in the interstitium, and later, perhaps, becoming alveolar. The basic question to be answered is why fluid collects in the lung. Is it reasonable to assume that this is the factor which initiates the progressive cycle causing increased right-to-left shunts and failure of oxygenation? To answer this, we must consider the role of formed cell aggregates, of humoral substances which have endo-

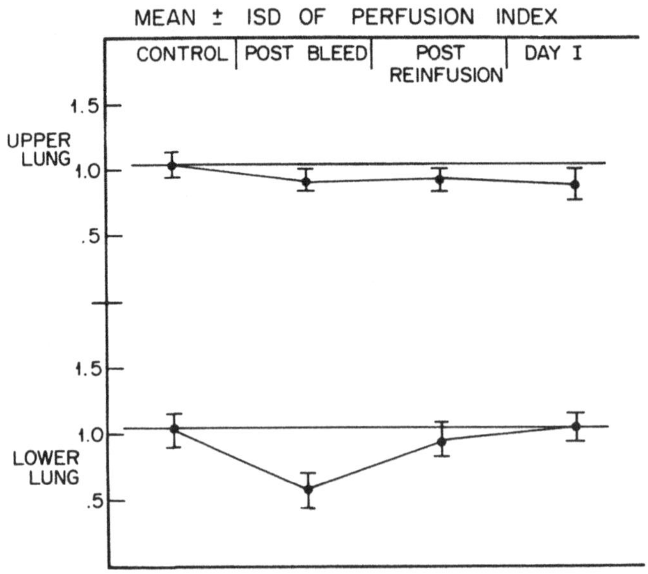

FIG. 7. Regional perfusion indices from the top and bottom (gravity-dependent) of lungs at the times indicated. Note the early decrease in perfusion to the dependent lung, with subsequent return to control.

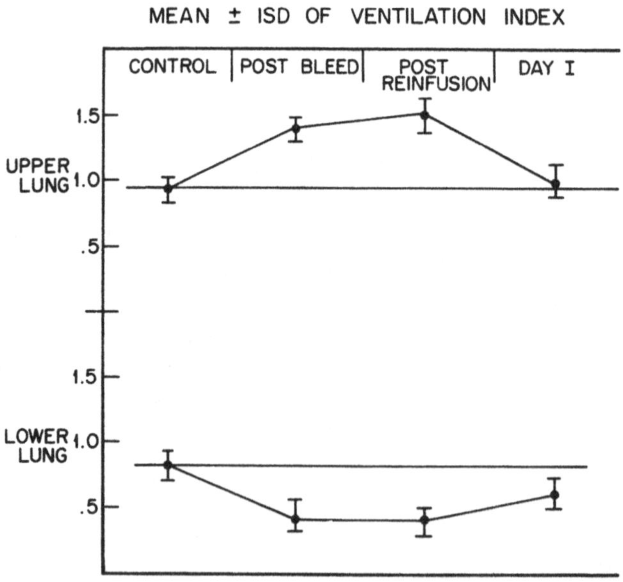

FIG. 8. Regional ventilation indices from the same lung regions as in Figure 7. The prompt and striking decrease in ventilation to the lower lung and its persistence is noted.

thelium-damaging effects as well as constrictor effects on vessels and bronchi. We must also consider neural influences, all of which can upset the balance of Starling forces in the lung capillaries and lead to interstitial edema, or even hemorrhage, and ultimate direct alveolar involvement if the "lesion" is severe.

Vascular Pressures

In modern times at least, Eaton (11) seems to have been the first to describe increases in pulmonary artery pressure after hemorrhage. He concluded that "an impounded pressure within the pulmonary artery following peripheral blood loss is evidence that an obstruction to normal circulation exists within the lung, the left heart, or both." His hemodynamic findings, in very careful work, were associated with an immediate increase in flow from the pulmonary lymphatic duct, increases in lung water content, and histology showing edema, capillary congestion, and hemorrhage. Both Henry *et al.* (13) and Veith *et al.* (40) have convincingly shown that left atrial pressure is not elevated after shock in dogs.

Why do vascular pressures in the lung rise? Veith's group feels that this occurs due to pulmonary arteriolar constriction, probably locally mediated; they believe that the initial pathologic changes are periarteriolar. One recognizes also that arteriolar constriction in itself would protect the capillary but might elevate capillary pressures in unconstricted areas of the lung. Sugg, Webb, and their colleagues feel that active constriction of small pulmonary veins causes the imbalance of Starling forces after hemorrhage (34). They also showed that total removal of a lung with immediate reimplantation protected that lung from morphologic lesions during subsequent systemic hemorrhage. Unfortunately, they did not measure blood flow through the two lungs. The reimplanted lung may well have been spared because little blood flowed through it, thus shielding it from any deleterious aggregates or substances in the circulation.

One recognizes that mechanical occlusion of an increasing percentage of the pulmonary vascular bed at any level of cardiac output should also elevate the vascular pressures in the unoccluded portion of the bed. Hence, aside from the effects of their chemical constituents, formed cell aggregates lodging in the microcirculation will cause elevated vascular pressures. The vasobronchoactive constituents of platelets are well known, and the release of serotonin, histamine, *etc.*, may result in local vascular constriction above and beyond that caused by the mechanical occlusion alone.

There is no work, of which we are aware, that isolates the role of central neural control in the pathogenesis of this lesion. The association of head injury and respiratory failure is recognized (10,28). With increased intracranial pressure, strong evidence exists that systemic hemodynamic alterations, mediated through the sympathetic nervous system, cause acute left-sided heart failure and resultant pulmonary damage (3,27,28). Moss (23, personal communication) has recently demonstrated the typical pathologic picture in the lungs of dogs whose arterially isolated heads are hypoxemically perfused (arterial pO_2 = 35 mm Hg). The lesion is prevented if a lung is removed and reimplanted, even if studied as long as 2 months after the reimplantation. Thus far, Moss has not measured perfusion through the reimplanted lung, but he feels that the defect is a hypothalamic function alteration, due to breakdown of glucose metabolism, and that this leads to pulmonary venular constriction.

Thus, three kinds of interrelated influences may alter vascular pressures within the lung: active neural stimulation, producing vasoconstriction (arteriolar and/or venular); local stimulation of vasoconstriction by circulating vasoactive elements; and mechanical obstruction of part of the vascular bed by platelet aggregates (leukocytes may be involved, as well), with subsequent release of their constituents. Currently, we support platelet aggregates as more important than neural influences in causing vasoconstriction, because the rise in pulmonary artery pressure after hemorrhage, in all the studies we know, is slow and progressive, as with the progressive filtration of aggregates leading to obstruction of increasing fractions of the vascular bed.

Formation of Edema

In addition to alterations in vascular pressures, decreases in serum albumin concentration occur after shock (7) which further favor the formation of interstitial lung edema. Moreover, there is increasing evidence (see Gaynor, this volume) of endothelial damage in shock. This was demonstrated convincingly in Dr. Gaynor's endotoxin infusion model. Gump *et al.* (12) have shown this in man after injury or major operation. Indeed, it seems inescapable, since the frequent concomitant of the edema is interstitial hemorrhage. Hemorrhage indicates a major alteration in vessels to allow such huge cells (relative to capillary structure and function) to pass out of them. One must recognize, additionally, that, once permeability is altered enough to allow large protein molecules into the interstitium, recovery of water becomes much more difficult, since the osmotic gradient favoring return into the capillary is lost. Certainly both platelet and leukocyte aggregates with high concentrations of proteolytic enzymes may play a role here, as well.

Platelet Aggregation

Influences are abundant in all forms of shock to induce platelet aggregation. These include elevated catecholamines, known to be elevated in man and in swine bled as we have described (L.C. Carey, personal communication). Acidosis, circulating or local ADP, serotonin, certain of the prostaglandins, and exposure of collagen are also active in this regard. We have discussed the possible role of platelet aggregates and their constituents in causing endothelial injury and/or vasoconstriction which subsequently leads to interstitial edema. The effects of platelet aggregation on lung perfusion have been well documented; the data indicate regional trapping and increased ventilatory dead space (1,24, 30,36). Furthermore, no doubt exists that such aggregates are capable of seriously damaging the lung and other organs (2,17,25).

One should remember that the agents causing vasoconstriction are also known to cause bronchoconstriction. They could well help induce decreased ventilation in the gravity-dependent areas of lung, in which the distribution of such aggregates should certainly be highest.

Space precludes a discussion of leukocyte aggregation in shock. For details of this subject, the reader may refer to the work of Wilson and his colleagues (43).

Changes in Mechanical Properties of Lungs

Much of the confusion regarding changes in lung compliance during shock is apparently due to methodologic differences between investigators. Suffice it to say that measurements of lung compliance using tidal volume and the pressure difference between points of zero flow are valueless without knowledge of the lung volume from which one makes these measurements. Frequency dependence of compliance must also always be considered, and respiratory rates should be reported.

Shifts in the pressure-volume relationship down and to the right, such as we have demonstrated, means that the work of breathing must increase to achieve the same volume change, since greater transpulmonary pressures must be generated. The curve shifts could have been due to a change in the irreversible elastic characteristics of the lung, atelectasis, qualitative or quantitative decreases in the surface-active alveolar lining layer, or a change in the dynamic relationships and/or geometric configuration of the small airways and alveoli in the lung. We have already stated that residual volume changes, which might have affected the curves, did not occur. Summarily, changes in the irreversible elastic properties of the lung did not occur, nor did gross atelectasis, although deep nonconfluent alveolar collapse could have taken place. The shifts are too rapid to be explained by quantitative decreases in the lung surfactant, although sufficient alveolar fluid will certainly alter its function. Henry (13) did find a definite decrease in the slopes of the deflation limbs of pressure-volume curves 18-36 hours after severe hemorrhage and reinfusion in dogs. He found no early changes. The late changes were associated with a decreased phosphorus uptake into lung phospholipids which, with other evidence, nicely demonstrated the decrease in surfactant production and activity.

Alterations in $\dot{V}/\dot{Q}$ Distribution

The same considerations which apply to alterations in lung mechanical properties also obviously pertain to shifts in ventilation seen early after hemorrhage. Certainly the stage is set very early for a broadening of the distribution of $\dot{V}/\dot{Q}$ ratios, which with worsening should lead to areas of true shunt. At this time, we are most intrigued by the possible alterations around small airways with minimal interstitial edema and by changes in the configuration of small airways which might be due to neural influences and/or bronchoconstrictor agents. These, as we have pointed out, exist in high concentrations in platelets. Milic-Emili, in studying patients with liver cirrhosis with no clinically or radiographically detectable edema, found significant increases in the lung volumes at which airways began to close in the bottom of the lung. This could not be explained by intrinsic bronchial disease (personal communication). Staub *et al.* (29) have shown, with some ingenious techniques, that pulmonary edema of various causes collects first around conducting vessels and extra-alveolar airways. His group has also shown that this may be associated with shifts in ventilation away from the dependent lung where the edema formation is greatest. Hughes and Rosenzweig (14,15) have also shown that small increases in lung water around very small airways may result in their closure at transpulmonary pressures greater than normal. Areas thus affected could, of course, have very low $\dot{V}/\dot{Q}$ ratios and would contribute significantly to hypoxemia.

We are aware of no studies of regional lung function after shock in man. We know of only two other animal studies of regional lung perfusion in this state, both using dogs. Tiefenbrun and Shoemaker (38), using radioactively labeled microspheres, found preferential perfusion of dependent lung early after severe hemorrhage. This was followed by local increases in vascular resistance in the dependent lung and a shift of blood flow upwards against the hydrostatic gradient. Naimark (24) made similar observations using the radioactive gas method.

SUMMARY

(a) Young domestic swine were studied during a control period, then at various times after hemorrhagic shock and reinfusion. Measurements included vascular pressures, blood gas tensions, screen filtration pressures, pulmonary pressure-volume relationships, and regional ventilation and perfusion indices.

(b) After hemorrhagic shock and reinfusion of shed blood, animals developed significant arterial hypoxemia which was not due to a failure of over-all ventilation.

(c) Screen filtration pressure increased more in the pulmonary artery than in the aorta after shock. This, together with a measured decrease in the number of circulating platelets, suggests that platelet aggregates were trapped in the pulmonary vascular bed after hemorrhagic shock.

(c) No change was noted in the slope of deflation limbs of pressure-volume curves after shock or reinfusion. Pressure-volume curves, however, shifted to the right. The combination of these findings indicates no change in the irreversible elastic characteristics of the lung, but suggests that ventilation to some areas of the lung requires greater transpulmonary pressure than required before shock.

(e) Regional blood flow and ventilation shifted away from the dependent lung after hemorrhagic shock. With reinfusion of shed blood, dependent regional blood flow returned to near control levels. Ventilation, however, did not return to dependent lung areas after reinfusion of shed blood.

(f) We conclude that hemorrhagic shock produces changes in the lung leading to arterial hypoxemia. Hypoxemia becomes apparent after reinfusion of shed blood and is associated with trapping of platelet aggregates in the vascular bed and increasing inequality of ventilation-to-perfusion ratios in different regions of the lung.

We have no doubt that a pulmonary dysfunction syndrome accompanies severe hemorrhage, trauma, sepsis, and other states well described in the literature. It may obviously be ameliorated or worsened by therapeutic measures. We have briefly reviewed factors in the pathogenesis of this syndrome which we feel are most important.

ACKNOWLEDGMENTS

All the studies reported herein were performed in the laboratories of the Department of Physiology and Joint Cardiorespiratory

Service, McGill University, Montreal, Canada. Additional collaborators were Dr. D. S. Mulder, Dr. Richard Martin, Dr. Mary Smith, Dr. N. S. Wang, Dr. W. M. Thurlbeck, Elisabeth Joyal, R.N., Gerald Fried, B.S., and Robin Davies, B.S. Drs. W. H. Palmer, D. V. Bates, J. Milic-Emili, P. T. Macklem, and N. R. Anthonisen provided important critiques and advice, as did Dr. Solbert Permutt and Baruch Bromberger-Barnea during the preparation of this manuscript.

REFERENCES

1. Allardyce, B., H.F. Hamit, T. Matsumoto, and R.V. Moseley. Pulmonary vascular changes in hypovolemic shock. J. Trauma 9:403-411, 1969.

2. Ashmore, P.G., V. Svitek, and P. Ambrose. The incidence and effects of particulate aggregation and microembolism in pump-oxygenator systems. J. Thorac. Cardiovasc. Surg. 55:691-697, 1968.

3. Bean, J.W., and D.L. Beckman. Centrogenic pulmonary pathology in mechanical head injury. J. Appl. Physiol. 27:807-812, 1969.

4. Blaisdell, F.W., R.C. Lim, Jr., and R.J. Stallone. The mechanism of pulmonary damage following traumatic shock. Surg. Gynecol. Obstet. 130:15-22, 1970.

5. Bredenberg, C.E., P.M. James, J. Collins, R.W. Anderson, A.M. Martin, Jr., and R.M. Hardaway. Respiratory failure in shock. Ann. Surg. 169:392-403, 1969.

6. Brown, R., A.J. Woolcock, N.J. Vincent, and P.T. Macklem. Physiological effects of experimental airway obstruction with beads. J. Appl. Physiol. 27:328-335, 1969.

7. Cloutier, C.T., B.D. Lowery, and L.C. Carey. Effect of hemodilutional resuscitation on serum protein levels in humans in hemorrhagic shock. J. Trauma 9:514-521, 1969.

8. Collins, J.A. The causes of progressive pulmonary insufficiency in surgical patients. J. Surg. Res. 9:685-704, 1969.

9. Collins, J.A., W.C. Gordon, Jr., T.L. Hudson, R.W. Irvin, T. Kelly, and R.M. Hardaway, III. Inapparent hypoxemia in casualties with wounded limbs: Pulmonary fat embolism? Ann. Surg. 167:511-520, 1968.

10. Ducker, T.B. Increased intracranial pressure and pulmonary edema. I. A clinical study of 11 patients. J. Neurosurg. 28:112-117, 1968.

11. Eaton, R.M. Pulmonary edema: Experimental observations on dogs following acute peripheral blood loss. J. Thorac. Surg. 16:688-694, 1947.

12. Gump, F.E., Y. Mashima, S. Jørgensen, and J.M. Kinney. Simultaneous use of three indicators to evaluate pulmonary capillary damage in man. Surgery 70:262-270, 1971.

13. Henry, J.N., A.H. McArdle, H.J. Scott, and F.N. Gurd. A study of the acute and chronic respiratory pathophysiology of hemorrhagie shock. J. Thorac. Cardiovasc. Surg. 54: 666-681, 1967.

14. Hughes, J.M.B., and D.Y. Rosenzweig. Factors affecting trapped gas volume in perfused dog lungs. J. Appl. Physiol. 29:332-339, 1970.

15. Hughes, J.M.B., D.Y. Rosenzweig, and P.B. Kivitz. Site of airway closure in excised dog lungs: Histologic demonstrations. J. Appl. Physiol. 29:340-344, 1970.

16. Hogg, J.C., P.T. Macklem, and W.M. Thurlbeck. The resistance of collateral channels in excised human lungs. J. Clin. Invest. 48:421-431, 1969.

17. Jørgensen, L., H.C. Rowsell, T. Hovig, M.F. Glynn, and J.F. Mustard. Adenosine diphosphate-induced platelet aggregation and myocardial infarction in swine. Lab. Invest. 17:616-644, 1967.

18. Lowery, B.D., C.T. Cloutier, and L.C. Carey. Blood gas determinations in the severely wounded in hemorrhagic shock. Arch. Surg. 99:330-338, 1969.

19. Lowery, B.D., D.S. Mulder, E.M. Joyal, and W.H. Palmer. Effect of hemorrhagic shock on the lung of the pig. Surg. Forum 21:21-22, 1970.

20. Lowery, B.D., J.H. Sugg, D.S. Mulder, and W.H. Palmer. A swine model developing respiratory failure after hemorrhagic shock. In preparation.

21. Martin, R.R., B.D. Lowery, J.H. Sugg, and N.R. Anthonisen. Regional ventilation and perfusion distribution in experimental "shock lung." Clin. Res. 19:803, 1971.

22. Moore, F.D., J.H. Lyons, Jr., E.C. Pierce, Jr., A.P. Morgan, Jr., P.A. Drinker, J.D. MacArthur, and G.J. Dammin. *Post-Traumatic Pulmonary Insufficiency*. Philadelphia: W.B. Saunders Co., 1969.

23. Moss, G., C. Staunton, and A.A. Stein. Cerebral hypoxia as the primary event in the pathogenesis of the "shock lung" syndrome. Surg. Forum 22:211-213, 1971.

24. Naimark, A., A. Dugard, and R.E. Rangno. Regional pulmonary blood flow and gas exchange in hemorrhagic shock. J. Appl. Physiol. 25:301-309, 1968.

25. Reeves, J.T., P. Jokl, J. Merida, and J.E. Leathers. Pulmonary vascular obstruction following administration of high-energy nucleotides. J. Appl. Physiol. 22:475-479, 1967.

26. Robb, H.J. The role of micro-embolism in the production of irreversible shock. Ann. Surg. 158:685-697, 1963.

27. Sarnoff, S.M., and L.C. Sarnoff. Neurohemodynamics of pulmonary edema: The role of sympathetic pathways in the elevation of pulmonary and systemic vascular pressures following the intracisternal injection of fibrin. Circulation 6: 51-62, 1952.

28. Simmons, R.L., T.B. Ducker, and R.W. Anderson. Pathogenesis of pulmonary edema following head trauma: An experimental study. J. Trauma 8:800-811, 1968.

29. Staub, N.C., H. Nagano, and M.L. Pearce. Pulmonary edema in dogs, especially the sequence of fluid accumulation in lungs. J. Appl. Physiol. 22:227-240, 1967.

30. Stein, M., and D.P. Thomas. Role of platelets in the acute pulmonary responses to endotoxin. J. Appl. Physiol. 23: 47-52, 1967.

31. Sugg, J.H., and B.D. Lowery. Pulmonary pressure-volume changes following hemorrhagic shock in swine. Submitted for publication.

32. Sugg, J.H., B.D. Lowery, M. Smith, R. Davies, and W.H. Palmer. Pulmonary platelet trapping associated with hypoxemia following hemorrhagic shock in swine. Submitted for publication.

33. Sugg, J.H., B.D. Lowery, and W.H. Palmer. Platelet changes and hypoxemia following hemorrhagic shock in swine. Fed. Proc. 30:217, 1971.

34. Sugg, W.L., W.D. Craver, W.R. Webb, and R.R. Ecker. Pressure changes in the dog lung secondary to hemorrhagic shock: Protective effect of pulmonary reimplantation. Ann. Surg. 169:592-598, 1969.

35. Swank, R.L. The screen filtration pressure method in platelet research: Significance and interpretation. Ser. Haematol. 1:146-167, 1968.

36. Swank, R.L., and M.J. Edwards. Microvascular occlusion by platelet emboli after transfusion and shock. Microvasc. Res. 1:15-22, 1968.

37. Thal, A.P., *et al. Shock: A Physiologic Basis for Treatment.* Chicago: Year Book Medical Publishers, 1971.

38. Tiefenbrun, J., and W.C. Shoemaker. Sequential changes in pulmonary blood flow distribution in hemorrhagic shock. Ann. Surg. 174:727-733, 1971.

39. Van Allen, C.M., G.E. Lindskog, and H.G. Richter. Collateral respiration: Transfer of air collaterally between pulmonary lobules. J. Clin. Invest. 10:559-590, 1931.

40. Veith, F.J., J.W.C. Hagstrom, A. Panossian, S.L. Nehlsen, and J.W. Wilson. Pulmonary microcirculatory response to shock, transfusion, and pump-oxygenator precedures: A unified mechanism underlying pulmonary damage. Surgery 64:95-109, 1968.

41. West, J.B. Regional differences in blood flow and ventilation in the lung. In: *Advances in Respiratory Physiology,* edited by C.G. Caro. London: Edward Arnold, Ltd., 1966, pp. 198-254.

42. West, J.B. Ventilation-perfusion inequality and over-all gas exchange in computer models of the lung. Resp. Physiol. 7: 88-110, 1969.

43. Wilson, J.W., N.B. Ratliff, E. Mikat, D.B. Hackel, W.G. Young, and T.C. Graham. Chest 59:36S-39S (Supplement), 1971.

DISCUSSION[1]

DR. L. J. GREENFIELD *(Oklahoma City, Okla.)*: From our experience, it's been very difficult to ascribe a primary role to surfactant. We have been able to demonstrate that the alveolar cells are injured. From what we know about the turnover rates, we would suspect that the usual sequence of replacement of surfactant would be affected adversely some 18 hours later, and this certainly does correlate with the late-stage pulmonary injury. But, again, I suspect this is not a primary role. It is much more attractive to incriminate the microvascular bed, where the changes of interstitial edema can permit the extravasation of fluid with albumin, both of which are known to denature surfactant and to permit or facilitate alveolar closure. Certainly, the alveolar cells have a strong capacity to recover. I think this is important to us clinically, so that, if we do provide ventilatory support for the patients over a period of 4-5 days, the turnover rate of these alveolar cells that are injured should permit them to restore normal levels of pulmonary surfactant. So, there is a time factor that is working in our favor.

DR. M. H. WEIL *(Los Angeles, Calif.)*: I have a number of questions because I'm left, as you may be, with the assortment of things that can go wrong, including interstitial edema and the possible deposition of substances within the capillary bed of the lung. I'm not sure, in your highly competent review, that I understand where some of your prejudice lies at the moment. You spoke about filtration pressures. Is this *in vitro* filtration pressure of the blood that was transfused into the animal?

DR. LOWERY: This was *in vitro* filtration pressures of blood from the animal, drawn simultaneously from the pulmonary artery and the aorta across the pulmonary capillary bed.

DR. WEIL: You also pointed to the potential effects of obstructing the terminal airway because of interstitial edema. Then, you also pointed to the differentials between both the airway or the alveolar pressures and the pulmonary venous pressure in terms of gradients of flow, also with regard to the hydrostatic height of the lung in various positions. Well, we're left, then, with three identifiable mechanisms for underventilation in perfused areas of lung or underperfusion of ventilated areas of lung. I wonder if you would care to order these for us in the light of your own experience—experimentally and, perhaps, clinically.

---

[1]This discussion also covers the presentation of Dr. Hinshaw (see preceding paper).

DR. LOWERY: I'm not sure that I can order them, and I think they may be operative with various percentage influences at different periods of time. Indeed, if one subscribes to the particulate matter theory, the first problem must be the occlusion of the perfused bed and whatever damage occurs to the capillary--whether this produces an abnormality of the Starling forces so that the capillary leaks without reason, or whether the endothelium is damaged directly. The idea of very small amounts of interstitial edema producing marked abnormalities in regional gas exchange in dependent areas of the lung evolves from Staub, West, and Emili; Staub demonstrated, by rapid freezing, that production of pulmonary edema was localized around small, terminal bronchioles. Emili, in studying patients with minimal pulmonary edema not detectable by any sort of clinical examination, demonstrated marked increases in the closing volume of the lung in the dependent portions. The full description of closing volume is not possible in these few seconds, but if there is reason for airways to close at the bottom of the lung, this is a gravity-related phenomenon. This may be studied using a xenon technique, in which a bolus of xenon is inspired, breathed out, and counted (at the mouth) for radioactivity. In patients who have cirrhosis and no clinically detectable edema, closing volumes may be as high as 50% or 60% of total lung capacity, which is considerably above the functional residual capacity or the resting and respiratory level.

DR. WEIL: May I make one very brief comment? I would recognize a tremendous advantage to putting in one other parameter, namely, colloid osmotic pressure. I can say, from a recent experience, that the colloid osmotic pressures in the type of patients that we have reference to are almost always significantly reduced. We can't account for the pulmonary edema because the reduction in colloid osmotic pressure is not sufficient to overcome the pulmonary capillary pressure. Now, if indeed the pulmonary capillary pressures that we measure with a random pulmonary artery catheter are not representative, and if now these measurements could be made on a regional basis and, in some context, could be integrated to look at the mean capillary pressure, it may very well be that the reductions in colloid osmotic pressure represent much more of the problem than would appear on the surface.

DR. LOWERY: I've heard of that and I think that must be explored. It remains a challenge to try to work out mean capillary pressures of any sort in this complex system. No matter how large a compartment model one goes to, it remains for the good people to do that.

BIOCHEMICAL-BIOPHYSICAL BASIS OF SHOCK

Linda L. Shanbour, Ph.D.

Program in Physiology, The University of Texas Medical School at Houston, Houston, Texas

Ultimately, lethal shock states overwhelm the total organism. The most dramatic and most easily measured events in shock occur in the cardiovascular system; these late events in shock constitute failure of the circulation to perfuse the various tissues of the body adequately with blood and its nutrients. Yet, at some earlier stage in the natural history of shock, the key pathophysiological events are adverse interactions between chemicals and susceptible portions of the cell. This constitutes cellular damage--interference with essential biochemical reactions within the cytoplasm.

Most explanations of the pathophysiology of shock, whether endotoxic, hemorrhagic, or traumatic, progress from cardiovascular to cellular changes. The many excellent papers presented at this symposium concerned primarily with biochemical alterations in shock, permit us to explain cardiovascular responses on the basis of changes at the cellular level. Although there are uncertainties about some of the biochemical events and about the importance of species variations, a scheme can be drawn to explain many responses which commonly occur in shock.

In this speculative scheme, the primary event is direct cellular damage. Each cell is defined spatially by its envelope, the cell membrane, a complex lipoprotein across which certain solutes and solutions readily pass and certain materials do not. The first contact between a shock-producing chemical, such as endotoxin or myocardial depressant factor, and the target cells takes place at that membrane. There is evidence that endotoxin or toxic factors act, at least partly, through impairment of the adrenergic nervous system. This would explain hypotension in the face of an increase or no change in the cardiac output. Dr. Gaynor presented excellent evidence that there is initial widespread damage to the shocked vascular endothelium in large and small vessels in the absence of fibrin formation. Endothelial desquamation occurred as soon as 5 minutes after onset of shock. Primary endothelial cell damage could subsequently induce platelet and fibrin emboli. As suggested by many, this would lead to arteriovenous shunting and hypoxia. Whether there is a real increase in oxygen consumption in shock states has not been resolved, as Gump noted, although Valeri presented opposite findings from Vietnam casualties.

Direct cell membrane alterations can be categorized as mild, moderate, and severe. Mild membrane alterations would affect membrane-bound enzyme systems, such as adenyl cyclase, which is responsible for the formation of cyclic AMP from ATP. Endotoxin was reported by Jacobson to activate adenyl cyclase. Changes in intracellular levels of cyclic AMP would influence many physiological processes, such as glycolysis and lipolysis. Horwitz showed an increase in free fatty acids with no change in total serum lipids, as well as hyperglycemia and hypoinsulinemia in shock. These changes could be mediated through cyclic AMP and would require an increased metabolic rate. Consequent needs for heat dissipation from cells could alter circulatory events, as suggested by Gump.

Moderate damage to the cellular membrane would disrupt membrane transport systems. This would result in an imbalance of electrolyte and other solute gradients, events that directly affect neuromuscular transmission and muscular contraction. In addition, electrolyte imbalance would alter intracellular enzyme activities. Smith has shown increased uncoupling of oxidative phosphorylation in shocked tissues. This again would lead to a need for heat transport with subsequent alterations in microcirculatory perfusion.

With more pronounced membrane damage, leakage of essential cytoplasmic ingredients would occur, along with augmented influx of ions and discharge of the electrical potential. The *milieu interieur* would be profoundly altered and its enzyme systems impeded. Disruption of lysosomal membranes would release proteolytic enzymes and induce widespread cellular damage. Mast cell degranulation would release histamine, thereby aggravating arterial hypotension. Subsequent release of epinephrine and norepinephrine would produce leukocytosis and increases in platelets which would further alter circulatory events.

Many assumptions are involved in this incomplete scheme, and the contributors to this symposium could offer pros and cons for each point. However, this scheme does explain many of the alterations which occur in profound shock states. The relative importance of the events outlined in this scheme depends upon the degree of shock and the species of animal being considered.

It is precisely at this level of biological function that we know the least about what shock does to the cellular apparatus, to its membrane, and to its enzymes. Future research will have to resolve the biophysical and biochemical abnormalities induced by shock.

AFTERWORD

Shock remains a therapeutic challenge in patients who fail to respond to volume repletion or drainage of septic foci. When patients are treated promptly after diagnosis, they usually respond satisfactorily, but, in some cases, complex disturbances alter responses in a variety of organ systems which defy generalization. The clinician must then resort to a mechanistic approach to therapy, based on his understanding of physiological processes, in an attempt to restore homeostasis. Here, the interests of the basic scientist and clinician converge, as an effort is made to translate the information obtained from experimental models into effective patient therapy. The proceedings of this symposium, recorded on the preceding pages, provide tangible evidence of this shared interest.

Departing from the concern in previous years with blood pressure and flow, this meeting has focused attention on events in the small blood vessels and at the cellular level during shock. Evidence of a vascular endothelial lesion has been presented by some workers, with alterations of functional significance demonstrated by other investigators in the microcirculation of the pancreas, liver, intestine, and lung. Experimental and clinical data indicate that these regional circulatory derangements are enhanced by microaggregation of platelets, presumably because of their demonstrated affinity for endotoxin. The net effects at the cellular level in terms of oxygen utilization, remain unclear despite a great deal of research effort. The demonstrated imbalances between oxygen delivery, oxyhemoglobin dissociation, and tissue utilization invite a variety of interpretations. Additional studies should clarify whether true arteriovenous shunting occurs or whether a toxic factor interferes with oxygen exchange.

The pendulum has also swung away from a primary concern with the kidney and splanchnic circulation. The heart and the lung now seem to share the investigative spotlight. Whether the heart plays a primary role in irreversible shock is still a subject of controversy, but workers agree on its ultimate failure along with other organ systems. The role of the lung is less clear, although pulmonary damage jeopardizes late survival as interstitial edema supervenes. Numerous abnormalities have been demonstrated at the cellular level, including a fundamental alteration in liver mitochondria with uncoupling of oxidative phosphorylation, the elaboration of the various lysosomal enzymes from injured tissues, and hypoinsulinism. The contribution of other vasoactive mediators remains unclear, although significant effects have been demonstrated from the elaboration of serotonin, histamine, catecholamines, vasopressin, angiotensin, and various kinins. In addition, some observations suggest that immunological factors may participate in the response to shock.

The investigations reported at this symposium have emphasized the value of a more accurate classification of clinical shock states and the need for a realistic approach to clinical staging, using both metabolic and hemodynamic parameters to permit accurate comparisons of therapeutic results. Moreover, directions for future research have emerged from both the formal and informal exchanges which took place at these meetings—perhaps representing the most significant contribution of the symposium.

Lazar J. Greenfield, M.D.

PARTICIPANTS AND SPECIAL GUESTS

Petar Alaupovic, Ph.D., *Cardiovascular Section, Oklahoma Medical Research Foundation, Oklahoma City, Oklahoma*

Irwin R. Berman, M.D., *Department of Surgery, New York University Medical Center, New York, New York*

Arthur B. Callahan, Ph.D., *Office of Naval Research, Department of the Navy, Washington, D.C.*

C. J. Carrico, M.D., *University of Texas Southwestern Medical School, Dallas, Texas*

Philip E. Cryer, M.D., *Barnes Medical Center, St. Louis, Missouri*

Louis R. M. Del Guercio, M.D., *Department of Surgery, Saint Barnabas Medical Center, Livingston, New Jersey*

John H. Duff, M.D., *Department of Surgery, Royal Victoria Hospital and McGill University, Montreal, Quebec, Canada*

Thomas E. Emerson, Jr., Ph.D., *Department of Physiology, Michigan State University, East Lansing, Michigan*

Ervin G. Erdös, M.D., *Department of Pharmacology, University of Oklahoma Medical Center, Oklahoma City, Oklahoma*

Geoffrey Evans, M.D., *Department of Surgery, McMaster University, Hamilton, Ontario, Canada*

Leo Fairchild, *The Upjohn Company, Kalamazoo, Michigan*

Ronald P. Fischer, LTC, MC, *Experimental Surgery Division, Walter Reed Army Institute of Research, Walter Reed Army Medical Center, Washington, D.C.*

Evelyn Gaynor, M.D., *Department of Hematology, Medical Division, Montefiore Hospital and Medical Center, Bronx, New York*

Thomas M. Glenn, Ph.D., *Department of Physiology, Medical College of Pennsylvania, Philadelphia, Pennsylvania*

Lazar J. Greenfield, M.D., *Department of Surgery, University of Oklahoma Medical Center, Oklahoma City, Oklahoma*

Clarence A. Guenter, M.D., *Department of Medicine, University of Oklahoma Medical Center, Oklahoma City, Oklahoma*

Chesterfield G. Gunn, M.D., *Department of Medicine, University of Oklahoma Medical Center, Oklahoma City, Oklahoma*

Frank E. Gump, M.D., *Department of Surgery, College of Physicians and Surgeons, Columbia University, New York, New York*

Marshall Guthrie, M.D., *Research and Development Division, Smith Kline & French Laboratories, Philadelphia, Pennsylvania*

Gert L. Haberland, M.D., *Farbenfabriken Bayer AG, Wuppertal-Elberfeld, Germany*

Robert M. Hardaway, III, M.D., *William Beaumont General Hospital, El Paso, Texas*

Clifford M. Herman, CDR, MC, USN, *Experimental Surgery Division, Naval Medical Research Institute, National Naval Medical Center, Bethesda, Maryland*

Lerner B. Hinshaw, Ph.D., *Department of Physiology and Biophysics, University of Oklahoma Medical Center, Oklahoma City, Oklahoma*

David L. Horwitz, M.D., Ph.D., *Department of Medicine, University of Chicago Hospital, Chicago, Illinois*

Eugene D. Jacobson, M.D., *Program in Physiology, The University of Texas Medical School at Houston, Houston, Texas*

Alice R. Johnson, Ph.D., *Department of Pharmacology, Emory University, Atlanta, Georgia*

John L. Kitzmiller, LCDR, MC, USN, *C.I.C. And Department of Obstetrics and Gynecology, U. S. Naval Hospital, San Diego, California*

Arisztid G. B. Kovách, M.D., *Experimental Research Department, Medical University of Budapest, Budapest, Hungary*

Tibor G. Kováts, M.D., *Institute of Experimental Surgery, Medical University, Szeged, Hungary*

Robert J. Laffan, Ph.D., *Cardiovascular and Pharmacology Section, The Squibb Institute for Medical Research, New Brunswick, New Jersey*

Allan M. Lefer, Ph.D., *Department of Biochemistry, The Hebrew University—Hadassah Medical School, Jerusalem, Israel*

Brian D. Lowery, M.D., *Department of Surgery, The Johns Hopkins Hospital and Mount Wilson State Hospital, Baltimore, Maryland*

Lloyd D. MacLean, M.D., Ph.D., *Department of Surgery, McGill University, Montreal, Quebec, Canada*

Walter H. Massion, M.D., *Department of Anesthesiology, University of Oklahoma Medical Center, Oklahoma City, Oklahoma*

J. Robert McNeill, Ph.D., *Department of Physiology and Biophysics, University of Oklahoma Medical Center, Oklahoma City, Oklahoma*

George Motsay, M.D., *Department of Surgery, University of Minnesota, Minneapolis, Minnesota*

O. R. Pavlovskis, Ph.D., *Department of Microbiology, Naval Medical Research Institute, National Naval Medical Center, Bethesda, Maryland*

Jack L. Ratliff, M.D., *Department of Surgery, The University of Mississippi Medical Center, Jackson, Mississippi*

David G. Reynolds, LTC, MSC, *Department of Gastroenterology, Division of Medicine, Walter Reed Army Institute of Research, Washington, D.C.*

Lawrence Rose, M.D., *National Institutes of Health, Bethesda, Maryland*

Benjamin F. Rush, Jr., M.D., *Department of Surgery, New Jersey College of Medicine and Dentistry, Newark, New Jersey*

John A. Schilling, M.D., *Department of Surgery, University of Oklahoma Medical Center, Oklahoma City, Oklahoma*

William Schumer, M.D., *Department of Surgery, College of Medicine, University of Illinois at the VA West Side Hospital, Chicago, Illinois*

Linda L. Shanbour, Ph.D., *Program in Physiology, The University of Texas Medical School at Houston, Houston, Texas*

William C. Shoemaker, M.D., *Department of Surgery, Mount Sinai School of Medicine, City University of New York, New York, New York*

Ian M. Smith, M.D., *Department of Internal Medicine, University of Iowa Hospitals, Iowa City, Iowa*

K. Sorrells, Ph.D., *Department of Pharmacology, University of Oklahoma Medical Center, Oklahoma City, Oklahoma*

John J. Spitzer, M.D., *Department of Physiology and Biophysics, Hahnemann Medical College, Philadelphia, Pennsylvania*

Kenneth G. Swan, LTC, MC, *Department of Gastroenterology, Division of Medicine, Walter Reed Army Institute of Research, Washington, D.C.*

Alan P. Thal, M.D., *Department of Surgery, University of Kansas Medical Center, Kansas City, Kansas*

C. Robert Valeri, CDR, MC, USNR, *Naval Blood Research Laboratory, Chelsea, Massachusetts*

Maurice B. Visscher, Ph.D., M.D., *Department of Physiology, University of Minnesota, Minneapolis, Minnesota*

Max H. Weil, M.D., *Shock Research Unit, School of Medicine, University of Southern California, Los Angeles, California*

Howard Whigham, Ph.D., *Shock Research Unit, School of Medicine, University of Southern California, Los Angeles, California*

Robert F. Wilson, M.D., *Department of Surgery, School of Medicine, Wayne State University, Detroit, Michigan*

GENERAL SUBJECT INDEX

Lightning Source UK Ltd.
Milton Keynes UK
UKOW07f2136190315

248150UK00016B/185/P